SAVE YOUR DIGNITY PUBLISHING

I0492335

It's Time for a Cure Too

My Relief From Your Pain
More Growth For Your Brain

By Roy Knight Jr
Damaged and Concerned Consumer
12/24/2017

ISBN-13:
978-1982031800
ISBN-10:1982031808
Imprint: Independently published

Industrial farming has changed the landscape of your dinner table. What has been sold as "healthy whole grains" have really been tainted grains, directly influencing today's pandemics of heart disease, cancer, dementia and every other disease of inflammation.

ACKNOWLEDGMENTS

This would not have been possible without the research and instruction given by Dr. David Perlmutter and Dr. William Davis and Dr. Daniel Amen, The British Medical Journal, the New England Journal of Medicine, NIH's PubMed and Wikipedia also were very important in the construction of this book an important part in the construction of this book. I tried to attribute every passage used from those sources.

Credit also goes to James, for without his comments," No one even knows or cares about this".

© Wolfberry | Dreamstime.com ©Ffatserifade|Dreamstime.com - Evolution

© Alain Lacroix | Dreamstime.com - Sugar consumption

Photos By:

© Nui7711 | Dreamstime.com - Stethoscope, medicine capsules and banknotes

© Jevtic | Dreamstime.com - Business partners on wheat field

© Walter Arce | Dreamstime.com - Yellow Crop Duster

© Wolfberry | Dreamstime.com - Health Risks of Obesity

© Pratin Charnnarong | Dreamstime.com - Pill

IMAGE COURTESY OF AREEYA AT FREEDIGITALPHOTOS.NET

© Wolfberry | Dreamstime.com

© Arrow | Dreamstime.com - Brain and solution

Foreword

This is the book that books two and three were supposed to be, had I known the whole truth prior to finishing the second one. I learned of the intentional poisoning toward and of the second book but had decided to put that in another book, due to the extent of the information.

This gave me an opportunity to research the evolution of our diet to get an idea of how this ketogenic diet can take us not just into space but it's the optimal diet to propel us into the future, as this diet is a cure for all of our major problems.

It kills the hunger cycle, so it will take care of starvation. It stops mosquito bites. That will stop malaria, dengue fever, Zika, Yellow fever or encephalitis. If the mosquitoes won't bite you, you can't contract the diseases. Since I've been on my ketogenic diet and eaten absolutely no carbs or sugars, I don't get bit by mosquitoes.

There the need to eat only one meal each day, to get the optimum results from this diet. That in itself will answer the food problem. If you eliminate hunger by eliminating the hunger cycle, you will automatically lower the total consumption of food, ensuring nobody starves. The trick is to be ghrelin resistant instead of loptin resistant

The key is to learn how to live and work on an empty stomach. Your work becomes so much easier when you're not locked into a hunger cycle controlling everything you do. Without getting hungry, you end the need for coffee breaks to chomp down that Danish or bagel. All you need is to sip on your coffee while you keep working. You don't have to stop in the middle of anything for a lunch break, you can keep working without getting hungry. When you feel the hunger pangs, you smile and wait for the release of Ghrelin, to get all the benefits of the growth hormones and anti-oxidants it creates.

When one can live with an attitude free of hunger, one can accomplish amazing things. The fact that this is my fifth book inside of 3 years attests to that. This all points to our next evolution in the human diet, to the ketogenic diet.

TABLE OF CONTENTS

FOREWARD Pg0

My Whole Wheat Story Pg2

PART 1 THE DEPENDENCE

1 Sugar-America's Deadliest Addiction Pg11

2 The Celebration of Our Addiction to Sugar and the

Price we Pay for It Pg15

PART 2 THE TAINTING OF YOUR FOOD

3 Calories, Do You Worry About Them? Pg33

4 New Dangers Of Grain Consumption Due To

Contamination By Glyphosate Herbicides Pg40

5 The Glyphosate Poisoning of America Pg46

6 The Grain Industry's Ruse To Feed You Disease Pg57

PART 3 THE INESCAPABLE DAMAGE

7 Diseases Created By Plaque Pg75

8 Glycation - The Real Poisoning of America Pg79

9 Can Your Cancer Be Cured of Just Treated? Pg108

10 Can Your Heart Disease Be Cured or Just Treated?.......................Pg119

11 Can Your Dementia, Osteoporosis, IBS/IBD, Asthma, or Other

Disease of Inflammation Be Cured or Just Treated Pg125

PART 4 REGULATION - WHOSE?

12 FDA's Take on Gluten Pg139

13 USDA Involvement Pg158

PART 5 NEW TOMORROW!!

14 Fasting and The Ketogenic Diet Pg178

15 Why I Stay in Ketosis Pg190

16 Understanding the Real Reason Why We Fight Pg187

17 God's Answer Pg208

18 The Evolution Of Our Diet Pg215

Afterthoughts Pg222

About the Author Pg226

Credits Pg233

My Whole Wheat Story

To easier understand my thoughts as you read through this dialogue, I thought you should have a little more background on the author, so I included this addendum to my story.

The first thing I remember is being given a bath in the kitchen sink. I remember a yellow dinette set in our kitchenette upstairs at my foster grandparent's house in Wayne. It was my father's foster parent's house in Wayne, one of two that they had along with a furniture store across the street. The house was basically on the opposite corner of the intersection where we ended up living in Wayne. I can remember sitting down on the top stair so I could scooch down the stairs to reach the bottom because I couldn't step down each step. My legs just weren't long enough. This is the only way a toddler can navigate a stairway until their legs are long enough to clear each step. I can vaguely remember the day I was able to walk down the stairs and how big I felt. I can, though, remember my mother scolding me for not walking down the stairs when I was able to but didn't (it was too easy to scooch). I guess she was tired of the butt in my pants wearing out so quickly.

My father was quite possibly the only foster child where he went to school in Wayne. He started school in West Millgrove, Ohio in a two-room school with a half dozen other students in grades 1-8, then transferred to Wayne school which was a 1-12 school when he reached the ninth grade. It was here where he met my mother, who grew up on a farm, two miles north of town. Even though he was born just outside of Toledo in Millbury, Ohio, the child placement agency who put my father in a foster home after he was abandoned by his mother and his father couldn't take care of him, decided to send him 25 miles south to West Millgrove, on the other side of the county. His siblings, two sisters and a brother were born in a different county in Toledo (Lucas County), so they were sent to a different foster home, separating my father from the rest of his family. If this never happened, I wouldn't be here as Dad would have never met Mom. They met in school in Wayne where Mom was in the same grade as Dad and even though they graduated approximately 4-5 years before I was born, the school had been transformed into an elementary school by the time I attended 1st and 2nd grades there.

I can remember standing by my grandfather in his red plaid robe, working on a jigsaw puzzle. Even though I can't remember his wife, my foster grandmother very well, I can remember a vision of her standing in her kitchen downstairs in that house we first lived in after Dad returned from his Air Force service at FE Warren AFB in Cheyenne, WY, where I and my oldest sister were born. My life in Wayne started 8 months after I was born in April 1954. It ended in Wayne when we moved to Tucson, Arizona in the fall of 1962. I had just started 2nd grade. I remember my teacher's name as Mrs. Stahl.

I finished 2nd grade, 3rd grade, 4th grade in Tucson, Arizona where we became resident tourists. I loved Arizona so much, I had to return there as soon as I graduated junior college. Although I started 5th grade in Tucson, we soon moved to Albuquerque, NM where I finished 5th and 6th grades. By the time I started 7th grade we had moved to Omaha, NE, where I completed 7th and started 8th grade. Halfway through 8th grade, we moved to Urbandale, IA, a suburb of Des Moines where I also finished 9th grade. From there, we moved to Fort Dodge, IA, where I graduated from high school and Jr College.

As soon as I graduated, I left for Arizona as I fell in love with the state when we lived there while I was in Elementary School. I moved to Phoenix where my sister was living as she had moved back two years earlier. I had planned to attend ASU to further my education in music since I'd taken piano lessons most of my life and was an OK - good pianist. Even in Wayne where I started piano lessons before I started School, there was someone better than I who was about the same age as I. I think this was the start of my self-image as being inferior. It seems for the rest of my life, I was always 2nd or 3rd best and never the best. It seems that this helped to develop an attitude in my mind of my inferiority and that I'd been destined to be a loser all my life. From the self-denigrating humor I engaged in all my life to the negativity I lived with most of the time, and how I felt about minorities and most people that weren't like me, it wasn't surprising I had set myself up for failure. Too bad I didn't know any better at that time.

I met my first wife in Ft Dodge, IA where I graduated from high school and college. It was a junior college in the town where my girlfriend/fiancée's mother worked as a teacher. Her father was a county psychologist. Having parents with that kind of education was a bit out of my league. I owe my life to them, for without their help I would have never survived my high school and college. As smart as I was, I had multiple learning disabilities that did more to hold me back than anything else. I think looking back on it now, I see that I had just enough ADD to make it difficult to learn anything in a classroom setting. I had the same problem then, that I have now, once I learn something, my attention is too easily distracted, to learn something new, instead of mastering the one already learned. That's because it's easier. I graduated with a GDP similar to that to Sen. John McCain, low, very low. Just like John (7th from the bottom of his class), my GDP was in that same neighborhood. I can only imagine what Irene thought when her daughter, Jane and I left for Arizona on our honeymoon the day after we got married. All I can only say, I'm sorry, Irene. I am truly grateful for everything you did for me throughout my school years in Ft Dodge and I failed to compensate you for your effort. If it's any consolation, I failed to repay my mother as well, before she passed. The biggest mistake in my life was when I let your daughter leave me. I didn't fight enough to keep her. She's still my soul mate, the love of my life. My greatest dismay is losing her.

I hear other people say "they'd never change anything they've done in their life." I can't say that. I've made far too many mistakes. If I could, I'd go back and change every one of them. But then, I would have to have had more foresight, which is something a 20-year-old has little of. Foresight can only be learned as it's the foundation of wisdom. I certainly could have used more of that, then.

When Jane and I landed in Phoenix, 3 days after our wedding in Iowa, we were excited and anxious to start work so we could establish residency to finish our schooling. I wanted to lower my tuition rates to the resident rates for ASU where I had planned to finish my degree in music since I'd been playing piano since the age of four, I thought my love of music could carry me through school. It possibly could have if I would have returned to school. But after working for a year, I failed to return to school. I lost sight of my goals. Worse yet, I didn't pay attention to my wife's goals. I'd like to blame it on not knowing her goals, but I have to take responsibility for that too, as I didn't ask her what her goals were. That was my bad. My decisions to keep working and not return to school laid out the pathway I would take from then on in my life and the life of my then-wife, Jane, and we both suffered because of it. I let us both down by not returning to school. I did more damage to Jane than I did to myself, as her odds of being successful were a lot greater than mine, simply because she was much smarter than I. Even though I knew it then, I was too proud to realize it consciously. That was probably why I didn't know what she wanted out of life, or what her goals were. A little foresight clearly would have prevented that regret.

Our decision to quit school came at the opportunity of low-cost housing, as we found a house for rent in north Phoenix for about the same price we were paying for our apartment in Tempe. Just 2 miles away from ASU where I wanted to continue my schooling. The house we moved to was 18-20 miles away, depending on the route we took to get back to Tempe. This move took us away from the school where we needed to be close to, to finish our education. This move virtually ended our prospects for further education. For all intents and purposes, we were dead in the water. This is where we started treading water and not getting ahead. This was also the start of the end of our relationship. From this point on, I became a loser.

I worked several jobs starting the best place I could, for an uneducated man, retail. Retail offered me an opportunity to learn how to get along with people, as retail sales is a people person's job. One thing my life had taught me was how to make friends. A life of moving from state to state transferring to different schools had taught me how to make friends and I made friends, well, very well. That would prove to be advantageous later on in my life after I lost everything as a result of injuries received in a car accident.

Making friends seemed always easy to me and that allowed me to dabble in several different areas of retail and sales, eventually leading me to a career as a life insurance agent. But since this was a career that came after the accident that's defined my life, it was more difficult to achieve. My life then has been a tale of two lives, pre-accident and post-accident.

BAD DREAM REALIZED

The last thing I remember before the accident was headlights coming at me fast enough to total the car I was riding in. The next thing I remember was that I had to get out of where I was. I was in the hospital and I didn't know why I was there. All I knew was that I didn't like hospitals or anything about them. I hated the way they smelled and the fact that's there's nothing to do in a hospital, especially if you're a patient. I didn't realize that I was a patient in the ICU. I'd learned later that they air evacuated me to St Joseph's in Phoenix, even though my fiancé had instructed the paramedics to send me to a closer hospital in Scottsdale.

They recognized that I had a head injury and sent me to St Joseph's hospital because of Barrows neurological clinic. My mother always said it was that clinic that saved my life. I don't know, I was in a coma. I have a faint memory of a formula that they fed me through my nose when I couldn't eat anything solid. I can also remember the tubes in my nose and when they pulled them out.

When I came out of the coma, I was paralyzed and didn't even know it. All I knew was that I had to get out of there, so I removed the straps around my wrists, crawled out of bed and fell flat on my ass. No one was prepared for that. I remember that I had defecated on the floor when I fell. I can remember an aide cussing about having to clean it up, along with me. My next memory was in the shower getting cleaned off. I learned the hard way about my paralysis. I thought I could walk when I couldn't even stand. I was bedridden and didn't even know it or why.

My first trip to therapy was on a gurney because I couldn't sit up in a wheelchair. I don't remember exactly when I graduated to the wheelchair, I just remember my first or second ride in it was with a tray on the arms of the chair, to support my upper body. I still couldn't sit up and needed to use the tray to lay my head on. I can remember going across a walkway from the hospital over to the rehab center every time we had to go to therapy. I can also remember yelling and swearing a lot at the therapists. Even though my mother was there all the time, she said little to nothing. All she could do was to tolerate my outbursts and scold me when it got too abusive.

This was the start of my new life. I was used to something completely different. I was used to a very active life. My biggest gripe was that I had to drive my truck to go bowling 3 times a week because I couldn't carry two or three bowling balls on either of my bikes. I rode my motorcycles a lot. Everyone thought the accident I was in, happened while I was on my bike, because of my head injury. (That's what I get for riding without a helmet all of the time.)

I was bowling so much because I thought I might be able to go professional. My average was 186 and bowled on two scratch teams. I needed to maintain an average of 205 to go pro and was practicing as much as I could to achieve that goal. Instead of saving my earnings, I invested them in my future, using the excuse of practicing, to do something I enjoyed immensely, like bowling.

My golf game was a different story. My best golf game was a 93 on a 7600 + yd course. I usually play the par 3's though because I always seemed to like to take the scenic route around the course, every time I golfed. If I was going to be good at golf, it would have taken way too long to be prosperous, so I stuck with the bowling.

That was until I decided to further my education by getting a degree or diploma in electronics. That was four months before the life-changing accident happened. My plans to change my life for the better had been put on hold...for how long was anyone's guess.

What I was about to find out was that the "how long" was going to be forever. My life still hasn't gotten any better. I've had to struggle more than most to achieve what I've had through life. Even though my life is yet to get better, my recovery has just started taking off, thanks to my change in diet.

Where I'm at now is a far cry from where I was when I came out of my coma. When you look at me now, you can't tell that I'm paralyzed. You can't even see it when I walk. You can only see it when I run or attempt to do anything athletic. And I used to be an athlete. I was a runner, a distance runner. I wish I knew then what I know now, how much better a diet of fat is to that of carbs. I could have saved myself a lot of grief just by following a different diet.

Now, since my disability is invisible, my biggest problem is that my disability is unrecognizable to the naked eye. I've perfected my appearance as much as I can, to make myself appear normal. The problem is, it takes a lot of effort just to maintain that illusion still, even with my improved health. But from laying around a doing little more than watch TV, this new ability I've gained to put my thought into print has given me a new life. If I could only instruct my fingers to stop fat-fingering" everything I type, my life would be able to move forward much easier. But that's part of my disability and I guess everyone with a disability has to work slower, but I don't appear like I should have to. I look completely normal and only those who know me closely know of my disabilities.

That has a tendency to create questions in people's minds about what kind of a person I really am since they see a completely normal person, but underneath has severe handicaps that keep me from functioning properly. I can only function haphazardly at best, because of the effort it takes just to appear normal. Fortunately, most people are more patient than I. But then, almost all others don't have the brain damage that I get to live with. Thus, the crux of my disability, the inability to see it, making my disability invisible if not completely invisible to the naked eye.

My days of selling life insurance came shortly after GMO seeds emerged from the laboratories at Monsanto. (Their success in patenting this new type of seed would later have deadly consequences on the public and their health and eventually take its toll on their minds.) My career selling life insurance didn't last more than 10 years because of the result of a second car accident that gave me a hernia. I was coming home from taking my wife to work across town when a car ran a red light to broadside my car while traveling somewhere around 40-45 MPH. The car was totaled and I suffered a hernia along with a knock on the noggin from the passenger side mirror after breaking through the passenger's window. I also suffered whiplash that still gives me pain today. This was the second severe accident I've been a victim of.

In the first accident on December 24, 1984, at 00:00 hrs, a drunk driver ran a red light and broadsided the car my fiancé was driving to put me in a come for a month, with a severe closed head injury. That head injury prompted two massive strokes which nearly took my life. Whether fortunate or unfortunate, I lived. When I came out of the coma I was completely paralyzed. I felt like a fly on flypaper except that I couldn't move at all. My first trip to therapy was on a gurney. Quite possibly my second trip was also. When I graduated to a wheelchair, they had to put a tray on the chair to support my upper body because I didn't have the strength to hold my upper body upright. Even though it's a vague memory I can remember my head laying down on the tray while in the wheelchair. I can also remember shouting and swearing at the therapists for what they were putting me through, but if they didn't put me through all that, I wouldn't be where I am today. I was literally a basket case, at best. The doctors told my family that I might have a 50-50 chance of survival, considering the injuries I sustained.

Because I was used to working all my life, my first goal was to get back to work, so I found the only work I could do, sitting and watching, as a security guard. Well, this job also involved walking around but I had relearned to walk by then, so I could handle at least that much. I just couldn't do much of anything else. (It's a good thing I didn't have to chase anyone.) All of my other skills were thrown out the window with my brain injury and subsequent strokes. Have you ever had a massive stroke? They're life changing, to say the least. I had two of them within a 30 minute period. This is what brought me to the brink of death on 12/24/1984.

They leave you with nothing but a shell of a body to work with and the shell you're left with can't function properly either, so you're stuck, like a fly on flypaper. There's not much you can do about it except years and years of therapy. By the time that's through, your life has been changed so much that you're in a whole new world that's never going to revert to your old normal one. The one you have now is so different (due to your lack of abilities that you're used to living with), all you can do is adapt and learn how to live again. This is very time-consuming. Regardless of what you had learned or been through prior to any injuries, your total focus is to return to your prior prowess.

Although this assumes that you had any prowess in the first place, it's safe to assume that I did have some, at least. At the age of 26, I owned my own home, had a successful career which I was in the process of changing, successfully at age 30. I was starting my own construction company, which I followed up on, later in my life,

I'm still trying to figure out why I'm still alive. For the most part of the past 30 years, I've languished in pain and loss of function, to the point that I still have problems with balance, coordination, reasoning, judgment and most of all residual weakness on my right side, the side that was paralyzed from the strokes. As much as I try to rid my body of those detriments, I can't. They're stuck with me for the rest of my life and there is nothing I can do about it except to accept it. That may be the hardest thing to live with and subsequently brought me to my search to regain some of my lost abilities. I had been told that I'd never regained them as brain cells don't grow back.

At least that's what I thought until I read Dr. Perlmutter's book *Grain Brain*. His book taught me that the brain damage I suffered wasn't at all permanent. He also taught me that a lot of the damage to my brain, I was doing myself, with my diet. I had always thought that brain cells couldn't grow back once they were lost. I was wrong; they can grow back in many parts of the brain. This gave me hope that what I have lost 32 years prior, might be brought back. I might be able to regain some of the intelligence that I had lost from the accident and ensuing coma and strokes. This is when I changed my diet and started to bring those lost cells back. I did it initially by stopping my bread intake. Subsequently, I've ended all carbohydrate consumption and I have no intentions of going back. The glucose just does too much damage to the body to be worth its little bit of energy.

Pre-accident I was smart but uneducated. This was because of my learning disabilities, ADHD. When I was a kid, ADHD was considered just a "rambunctious kid", a daydreaming kid who couldn't keep his mind on what he was doing because it became too boring. Today this is defined as ADHD, so what I live with now, is ADD. Actually, I like to call it AAADD, Age Attributive Attention Disorder. Mine's been magnified by my disability, brain damage from a severe closed head injury, that should have left me an invalid forever. My decline would be continuing if it weren't for Dr. Perlmutter's book *Grain Brain*. His book allows me to try his Keto diet recommendation after going carb free two years earlier.

The carb-free life did wonders for me but the keto diet is what's brought my mental abilities back along with some added, coordination returned to my right side, something I didn't expect. I explain how this has happened in my first book in the article on *Life without carbs*. Actually, I touch on it in several articles. It has to do with the effects that Ghrelin has on your body and the advantages of being Ghrelin resistant, instead of Leptin resistant, the condition of most carboholics. This is the sign of addiction. It was an addiction that I lived with for 59 years.

That's given me 59 years of damage that this food has done to my body. The plaque that I created in those 59 years still flows through my blood. It may until I die. That's a form of glycation that may not ever disappear. That means I made a wise decision to stop eating what was creating it. My health has only improved since I made that decision.

I mentioned earlier that I had lost everything from that car accident that put me in the coma, actually, I had thought I had lost everything, that was until I was in another accident 9 years later that left me with an inguinal hernia that has since left me with more problems since the repair surgery than prior. That's where my chronic severe pain comes from. The hernia repair left me with a damaged nerve trapped in scar tissue that's still creating pain today.

That drove me to a life on Oxycontin, Morphine, Oxycodone; the list goes for 23 different pain medications and anti-depressants which did little for me except to make me fat, lazy and stupid. Stupid I was for continuing that lifestyle. I didn't know what drove that lifestyle until I gave up bread. Breaking that addiction was the start of a whole new life for me. I was truly born again. No carboholic can ever know this. You have to give up the addiction to know it. But once you know it, you'll never go back to your old life of a glucose diet. (I've since learned that this is the best way to control that pain.)

That was post second accident. That's the one that has disabled me completely for 20+ years, mostly because of the drugs I was taking to manage the pain. These drugs did more to worsen my health, than my previous life of 40 years of carb ingestion had done to it. I can see now, the dependence I had in my addiction to glucose at that time. More than that, I can feel the effects of that dependence that I had on sugar (including bread). The effects of that dependence (addiction) are being felt now every time I get out of bed in the morning or whenever I nap. My back doesn't want me to move. It would rather that I stay in bed and not put any weight on it. I get to feel the pain every time I roll over in bed.

That's due to the IVD or degenerative disk disease I live with, in my lower back. That is directly due to the diet of bread that my mother raised me in my whole life. That was because that's what she was raised on. That's what my family, going back as far as I can track, was raised on. This addiction goes back to the dawn of history when man first started farming this grain. Because of that, this addiction has been with us forever and that's why it's so impossible to see when you're in it. But then nobody sees addictions they have, especially if that addiction was imposed upon them without their knowledge, which is exactly the problem of today's addiction. (Because they add sugar to baby food, anyone who's been fed baby food has been fed sugar. And if you've been fed sugar as a baby, you've had enough to be addicted. Try to remember the last day you didn't need to eat. That is a cycle you are addicted to. It's a dependence on a diet. What my new diet has taught me is a diet of sugar and carbs is a diet that needs to be re-fed every 2 or 3 hours. This is the nature of a carb diet, where the keto diet doesn't have any cycles. You're free from the glucose cycle of hunger and satiety. The problem is that I didn't learn this until three years ago.

So all this time, I was sabotaging my own life with my cycles of destruction, while I was on a carb diet. I never realized that until I changed my diet to a keto diet. Because of my emotional cycles, I went through several jobs. That gave me the varied experiences I needed, to see the picture that I'm putting together in this *Time for a Cure* series.

This carb diet that I led my life with, not only damaged my professional life, it damaged beyond repair, my body. It damaged my professional career by making me live my life within the cycle of hunger. You know what that cycle leads to. That's a cycle that leads to most other destructive cycles, as explained in Fighting Hunger Fights Terrorism Also, it's because it's caused by the hormonal action tied to your hunger cycle and it has a tendency to be destructive because it drives greed.

I can say this because I was in that world when I was on my carbohydrate diet when I was addicted to glucose. It's something you never see until you break the addiction and that why I didn't realize it for 60 years. Being raised on bread and pasta and cereal, I lived on bread and pasta and cereal all my life, up until 3 years ago. That was when the change started. It's continuing with these books.

That is a far cry from where I was 32 years ago, laying in a coma with a 50/50 chance of survival. What's remarkable is my recovery cycle. It was completely stagnant on a carb diet. It wasn't until I went low-carb diet and quit eating bread and pasta and cereal and everything that was breaded, that my health started to improve. The best part is it improved without medication and it automatically came with weight loss. I had quit all of the meds 9 years earlier when I started exercising.

I've always exercised all my life. Ever since I could walk, I've loved to run. So when I landed at St Joe's hospital by helicopter and they examined me for my injuries, 32 years ago, they saw by my brain scans that there were bruises on my brain that were creating swelling within my cranium. They had to put shunts in my skull to release the pressure. They told my parents that I would probably be a vegetable for the rest of my life and that they'd probably have to take care of me.

Fortunately for me, they encouraged me to stay in my home with my fiancée (we had just gotten engaged the night of the accident). We got married shortly after I was released from the hospital. The marriage lasted approximately 5 years. It was a marriage of love and hate, arguments, and lovemaking. It was a marriage of cycles tied to our glucose addictions. And we were addicted big time. That's why we argued as much as we did, and we loved to argue. That's because we loved our carbs, in spades. We were both skinny as bean poles, so we could eat this food without consequence, at least to our waistlines, while in our 20's. The weight comes usually in the 30's when your metabolism slows, but it's been coming earlier, lately. That's due to the GMO modifications done to the grains to make them Roundup® ready.

3 years ago, I decided to stop eating bread and everything else that the grain wheat was in. I didn't realize at that time, how this was going to manifest, but it turned out to be the best decision I have ever made. I have never been happier about making that decision. My health has improved steadily ever since I made that decision. What's most important, it continues to improve on a daily basis, and the best part is it's improving my brain's power. That's exactly the answer I've been searching for, for 30 years.

Thank you, Dr. Perlmutter!

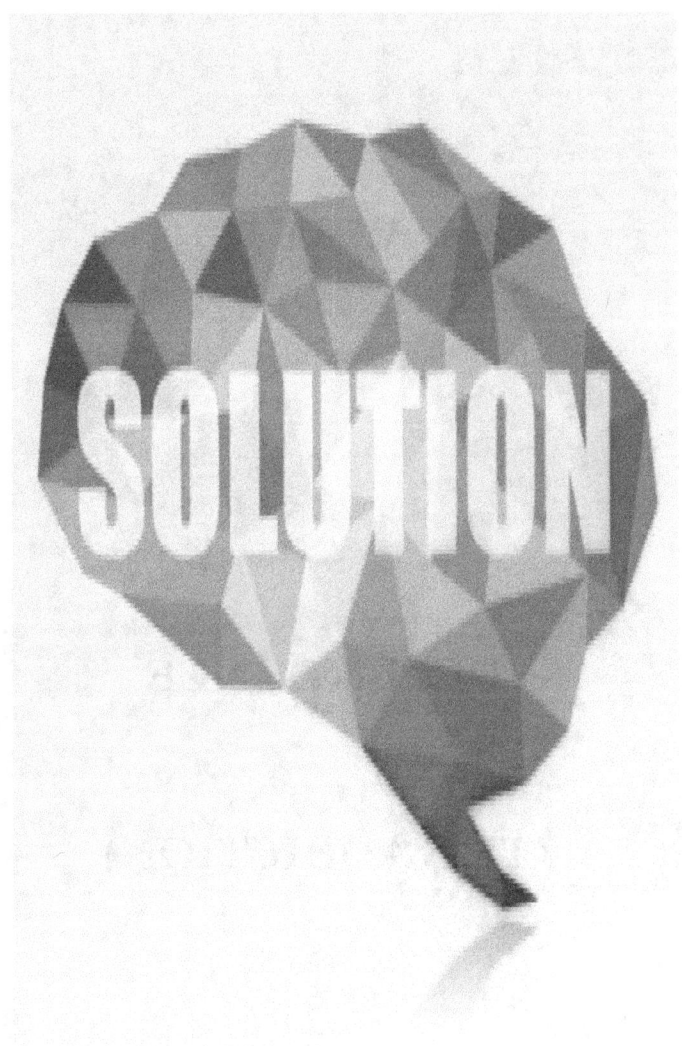

PART I

DEPENDENCE

(THE ADDICTION)

CHAPTER 1

Sugar! America's Deadliest Addiction.

Confessions of a Reformed Carboholic

Sugar, I love it. I grew up loving it. Because I grew up loving it, I'm now addicted to it. It's an **addiction** that was forced upon me by our food industry, telling my mother that she had to make refined and whole grains the most prevalent food in my diet. She fed me this food, supposedly, to keep me healthy. Aren't whole grains supposed to make you healthy? That was 60 years ago. I'm paying the price for that now, with my arthritis. I was paying the price for it just 30 months ago, by carrying 30 lbs more than what I carry right now and being borderline diabetic and in pain all the time. I'm about to debunk this myth that whole grains are healthy. There is a price to be paid for eating a (starchy) carbohydrate diet and you're paying it with every sandwich you eat, every corn chip you munch, and every noodle you eat.

My sisters are paying the price for it now, also. They are both obese and diabetic. My father has always exercised to keep his weight down. He's was always able to burn off the excess glucose, until he was about 35. Even though he's always jogged every day, since I was in 7th grade, he couldn't run away from this. After being borderline diabetic he couldn't change his downhill spiral. He's now taking an anti-diabetes drug  which has several side effects that are initially so small that they aren't noticed but after time, start to inflict other harm to the body, due to the effects of the chemical changes caused by the medication. His carb diet is starting to lead him down the same path as my mother, who passed away 4 months ago. My mother, in trying to be the best mother and wife she could be, went along with what the FDA, the USDA, and the ADA told her because she wanted to do what was right for her family. Guidelines from the ADA telling her that grains needed to be at the base of her all of her meals was what drove her to do this to our family. This is what doomed us to our current list of ailments, ailments like obesity and diabetes, arthritis, cancer, stomach ailments galore, and now, side effects from treatment for those ailments. It all comes along with a carbohydrate diet because all carbs break down into glucose. Even yet, *MyPlate.gov* suggests that whole grains be a part of a healthy diet. The evidence I'm going to show you is completely contrary to this notion.

Because sugar addiction is America's biggest **addiction**, that makes it, its worst addiction. It's an addiction that everybody grew up with and into. It's an addiction that's been with us for as long as we've been eating it. It's an addiction that's become far worse than it's ever been since we've been eating it over its 10,000-year history. It's an addiction that's built scores of empires, and then tore them all down. This addiction is far worse than any other addiction that plagues America. Whether it be today, yesterday or tomorrow, this addiction is the worst that Man has ever faced or may ever face. This is simply due to its propensity to expand its influence across the whole world. It's also driven by the greed of those condemned to this addiction. Their desire to feed their own addiction drives them to impose this addiction on the rest of the world, simply so they can make an extra buck. This addiction is at the root of almost every known form of dementia, heart disease, diabetes and everything that comes along with that, like cancers, cardiovascular diseases. The list is endless because sugar's worst instigator of inflammation, AGEs, or glycation is at the base of an arm-long list of disorders.

All of these disorders can be curbed simply by curbing carbohydrate consumption but addiction keeps this from happening. That's why fighting this addiction, in particular, is so important. It's life-saving at its simplest, just remove contaminating factors from the food source and the diseases cannot manifest themselves. The contaminating factor in this case? You guessed it, sugar. Sugar addiction is leading our society to the brink of destruction because of the nature of its addiction and what it does to the body. Its continued use only leads to discomfort and death. It's only redeeming factor is that it tastes good and satiates quickly. This is what makes it so deadly, though.

That's sad. I have to live with it too. I can't have what I love, what I've been addicted to. I have to say no, to stay healthy. So do you. I know that's exactly the opposite of what you've been told, but what you were told is wrong. For us, it's dead wrong. It should have never been pushed upon us to eat it in the quantities that it was. But pushed upon us it was. And we bought it. We bought into it big time and we're paying for it now. This is evidenced by the proliferation of Alzheimer's disease. How many lives does it have to take, before people wake up? How many families does it have to destroy, before people wake up?

Carbolism Should Be Treated Like Alcoholism

We need clinics for sugar addiction and they should be financed by the food industrial complex that imposed this diet on the people who now suffer the consequences of it. The administration of the clinic though should be done by trained medical professionals, because this is an addiction and should be treated as such.

Is this something that should be investigated? Should an industry be held accountable for the ruse that's been pulled on the American people, and now the world? The ruse is that this is healthy food when it's really not. Why are they still allowed to claim that it's healthy? Why are they still, allowed to advertise that it's healthy? It's clearly not, and it's clearly at the root of almost all of the deadliest diseases, that we're actively fighting right now. Diseases like Atherosclerosis, Endocarditis, and Hypertensive heart disease. That's just the CVD's. We haven't even covered the cancers or dementia. Those lists are much longer.

Can anyone tell me why this is still allowed to be advertised like it is today? It starts with what's put in baby food for starches and fillers and sweeteners. These fillers satiate babies quickly often putting them right to sleep after a short burst of energy. This is the first indication of sugar addiction and it starts at a young age. This is done for a purpose. That purpose is to addict you to its lure, so you'll buy into it when you're an adult.

It continues with your introduction to breakfast cereals and the load of sugars they carry when you see them advertised with the Saturday morning cartoons. I can remember for commercials for Sugar Pops, Sugar Frosted Flakes, and Captain Crunch. It starts young, real young and continues through your youth with candy and soda, and into your adult years with bread and baked goods (cakes, crackers, cookies).

It's been forced upon us. Nobody has had a choice in this addiction and that is what makes it so lethal. That also makes it profitable for the Pharmaceutical industry. This is what scares me. The Pharmaceutical industry used to be owned by the same industry the provided the crop seed for the farmers that grew the grain that provided the flour to bake all of those loaves of bread that causing so much disease.

The Perfect Ruse

It's almost the perfect scam. Sell crop seed to farmers that have been genetically modified, so that it feeds your customer base, food that will require them, in the future to purchase medications from your other companies. How convenient we've made it for this industry to take our money. We should be ashamed.

We would be ashamed if we knew that this was done intentionally, especially if it was done for nothing more than profit. That is why this is something that should be investigated. Regardless of how long it takes, we need to know who is responsible. This is a lesson that cannot be lost, like every other study done on these concerns, we cannot allow this to be swept under the rug. Even if they're no longer around, we need to hold their companies' accountable. This is the only way we can prevent this from happening in the future.

For 1,000s of years, we've been treating the symptoms of the diseases and disorders that carbohydrate digestion cause. Because of our addiction to it, we've never looked at the prospect of eliminating the cause completely. When a whole society is addicted to a staple that they've eaten their whole lives, how does one tell the truth about something that is so important to everyone on the planet? How does one tell everyone that what they're eating is killing them slowly, expensively, painfully, and worst of all, undignified because of all the lost memories of brain damage? How does one tell a whole society that a staple that they've lived on for close to 10,000 years has been, and continues to be, the one food that creates more disease and illness than any other one food in their diet? How does a world break their addiction, when the addicted are the majority of the world and only 5% of that population can recognize their addiction?

Dr. Perlmutter is trying to tell the people and continues to do so. I honestly feel that he thinks as I do, that if we don't dispel the consumption of these foods, our society is doomed. From what I've learned since I've broken the addiction, I see a collapse, due to out of control emotions, due to the wild glucose swings in the blood, making people under the control of a carbohydrate diet, under the control of those who impose this diet on the American public. It's in their interest to keep America addicted and the best way they can do this is to tell you that it's healthy and what you need to keep your body healthy. Only those who want to buy their pharmaceuticals, from them in the future, are ones who should buy their food products now, because, they eventually will.

By following what little advice I offer, to curb your carbs dramatically and as completely as possible, you can dramatically slow down if not eliminate many of the disorders and diseases within these pages. If it can't eliminate your disease, it will reduce the expression of your disorder. If it doesn't cure you, it will definitely extend your life. My goal is to extend it a minimum of 20 years. I would like to see everyone live to be 100 years old, or more. I know this diet lifestyle can do that (depending on your age and degree of addiction of course). To know this yourself, though, you have to change your diet.

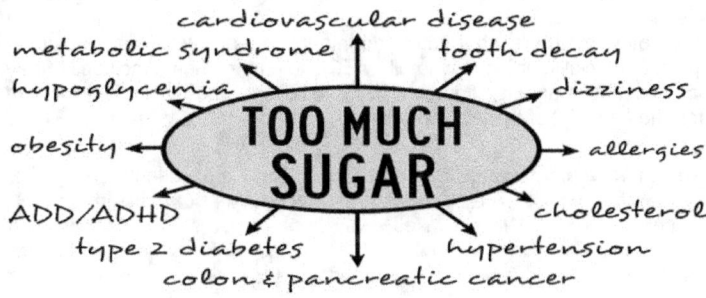

CHAPTER 2

Our Celebration of Our Addiction to Sugar and the Price We Pay For It.

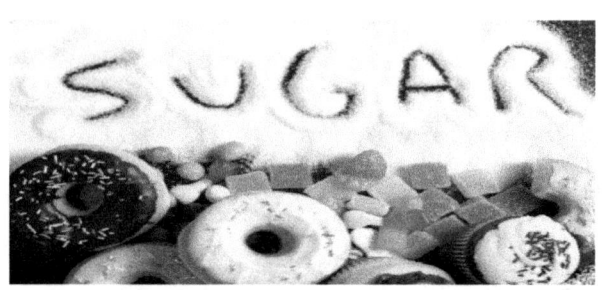

It's not hard to see how much you enjoy celebrating your addiction to carbs. It's displayed in everything that's said and done, in all aspects of the food industry. It's boldly advertised everywhere you go. Soon after following this celebration of addiction that you love to express, comes a parade of drugs that you'll be taking to treat all of the symptoms that come from succumbing to your addiction. This simple equation displays the need that we have to curb the influence of the grain and pharmaceutical industry on our health.

Failure to control this influence will not only lead to more disease and illness but more so, to greater health costs overall. How are we ever going to learn to live healthily and kick this habit, before it destroys our society? How are we ever going to put an end to diabetes? Or an end to Alzheimer's disease? Or cancer? Or heart disease? Or arthritis? Or hypertension? Hyperlipidemia? High Cholesterol? I would like to show just how our celebration of addiction to sugar is not only destroying our individual lives, it has the potential of destroying our entire civilization, if we don't curb is an influence.

I intend to show you how this industry hooks you in the first place, how they keep you hooked so in the future you're forced to buy into their drug habit. This drug habit involves NSAIDS (aspirin, Motrin, Advil, Aleve), anti-inflammatories, antacids, anti-gas and bloating, (Pepto Bismol, Gaviscon, Alka Seltzer) and we're just starting with the OCDs. For prescription medicine, we're looking at all opioids (Oxycontin, Oxycodone, Vicodin, Percocet), which again are addictive. More prescription NSAIDS like Celebrex, Relafen, Relifex, and Gambaran. We know that by the existing opioid abuse epidemic how dangerous these drugs are. Do you think this happened by chance?

Other prescription medicines that you're doomed to need if you continue your carbohydrate consumption (especially for those who allow ECC to control them), includes but are not limited to statins, vasoactive agents, fibrates, CETP Inhibitors, and niacin, just for starters. Statins are, by far, the far worst of these medications.

After spending 15 years giving care to and for seniors, I have seen the ravages statin drugs have taken on their bodies. They slowly rob their users from their mental faculties, then their muscles, then their lives. What it takes away from its users is in no way replaced by the treatment it offers. They are nothing more than invitations to a need to take more and more drugs. It seems that the drug industry has found ways to make you buy more of their wares.

Cholesterol, your body's fuel

This industry promotes that high cholesterol has something to do with heart disease, which couldn't be further from the truth and that high cholesterol is dangerous. This was first disputed close to 70 years ago. Cholesterol isn't the problem. Cholesterol is healthy. Your body has to use it to stay alive. Taking cholesterol away from your body only leads to more medication. I can see where this would benefit the drug industry.

High cholesterol isn't a heart problem. It's a diet problem. Your diet is responsible for your high cholesterol. Your major food source is your primary source of cholesterol and that is where the problem begins. Your high carbohydrate diet produces cholesterol in your body that is not clean cholesterol, meaning that it is dirty fuel, as cholesterol is your body's fuel. This is cholesterol you don't need. You need clean cholesterol that's been produced by fat. That is what powers our bodies.

Cholesterol is your body's fuel source. It's cholesterol that enters the cell to be used for fuel, so what's important is the kind of cholesterol that your body uses. Is it clean or dirty cholesterol? Cholesterol from carbohydrates is a dirty sticky fuel due to nature of which this cholesterol comes from. It comes from a sticky, icky, gooey, gluey substance, sugar or glucose and because of that, it has glycating effects on your body. This is what leads to plaque, the basis of almost all cancers, heart diseases and all dementias.

I've only talked about heart medications so far, I haven't even touched on cancer medication or cholesterol medication (many of which are related to heart medications like statins), nor have I covered other prescription medication for arthritis, high blood pressure, and memory loss. The list goes on and on. What a quagmire this has turned out to be. But I'm going to try to make some sense out of this quagmire, so that we're left with just a small puzzle leaving you wondering, like me, why?

I've already proven how the discontinuance of these foods leads only to better health and how continued consumption of these foods, only leads to a path of illness and disease. What I don't know, did this industry know what these foods do from the studies that have come out over the last 70+ years? Or did they remain electively ignorant of the reports? Or did they influence the cover-up of these reports? With as many reports that have come out, I seriously doubt it. There are just so many of them (701) that it's easy to miss most of them. Later I'll show you how this industry has had its problems in the courts. Some of it is not pretty.

I'll list just a few of the studies that have shown this damage going back over 70 years. The earliest study I found in 701 studies done over the years, was completed in 1939. I looked through page after page of studies that started in the 60's, 70's & the 80's. They seem to grow in number as time goes on. Studies have exploded since the turn of this century, as more and more people are starting to recognize the true dangers this food imposes on its consumers. Yet the majority of the addicted choose to remain ignorant to it dangers, as they're impotent in ignoring its lures. They are all controlled by their hormones which are controlling their emotions. This is a common trait of carbolism. The addicted have little to no choice in the matter. The need to feed the addiction is no less than that of any other addiction, which forces the addict to continue to feed the addiction. It's the way addiction works, it's the way carbolism works.

Celebration of sugar addiction

We're inundated with the commercialism of addiction on a daily basis. You see advertising for these foods and drinks everywhere. How many snack food companies are there? How many cereal companies are there? How many soft drink companies are there? Just how many beer and spirits companies are there? How many commercials do you see each day from these industries? All of those commercials are luring you into their web of addiction. The grain industry has found ways to infect our society, like seasonal flu or common cold affects all those who eat these grains. (And you thought your cold was just haphazard, something that you caught from someone else.)

We all know who profits from this today (Kraft, Nabisco, and Frito-Lay). But have you ever connected that with who is going to profit from it 10, 20, 30 years from now, the pharmaceutical industry? It seems that the grain industry's intent is to do nothing more than to fuel the drug industry. Whether it is their intent or not, it has been and is going to be, the end result. How long it continues to be, depends on how long you continue to allow your addictions to exist.

Drug companies, right now, are foaming at the mouth for all the business the food industry is sending them. Nobody is interested in breaking this addiction. What more could they ask for, a captive audience, all set up to need what they have an offer, to stop the pain, from the damage of their addiction at a cost that they set. You get to pay it or deal with your pain. Many times you have to pay it, just to stay alive. Do you wonder why medical costs keep going up or why insurance costs so much? The demand is so extensive, due to the addiction rate. Costs always rise when the demand for anything goes up.

If everyone would stop buying into this ruse, and find their cure by eliminating sugar and carbs (grains) from their diet, what would happen to the pharmaceutical industry? A huge drop in demand for their drugs would lower the price for the drugs. You could easily bring down the number of treatments, as well, just by stopping the bread. What would happen to the medical industry if nobody needed it except for emergency treatment for injuries, anymore? What if the need to treat disease diminished to nothing? It's not hard to see the impact that would have. What would be the cost of keeping people alive and healthier longer? What if you could allow more people to be more active longer? What if no-one needed medication anymore?

The underlying cause of sugar addiction

First off, let's define it. Dictionary.com defines addiction; *Noun, the state of being enslaved to a habit or practice or to something that is psychologically or physically habit-forming, as narcotics, to such an extent that its cessation causes severe trauma.-*

Wikipedia definition; *"Addiction is a medical condition characterized by compulsive engagement in rewarding stimuli, despite adverse consequences."*

I personally define addiction as a compulsion to consume a substance that the body craves but doesn't need because it actually harms the body. This definition rings true for heroin and opioids, sugar and alcohol, cigarettes and tobacco, the three most abused substances in the civilized algorithm, although not in that order. The worst of these addictions is that of sugar and alcohol, with sugar being by far, the meanest and vilest scourge ever committed upon the human race.

It starts with the placement of sugar and carbs in the baby food that's sold throughout the industry. It's obvious to me why they put it in baby food. That's because it's so palatable and goes down so easy making the food tastier so babies would be more likely to consume it. What baby doesn't love the taste of sugar? This taste for sugar soon turns into an addiction requiring it be fed to the body, every other hour or so. Whether or not this was the intended consequences of the marketing of this food, this consequence has become America's newest death sentence.

By showing how this addiction affects the body in *Carbs; The Newly Discovered Death Sentence,* I've shown how dangerous this food is to human physiology. Yet we continue to eat it and celebrate our addiction to it simply to enhance profits. Profits for the Grain industry are first to come, which includes all snack food companies, the beverage industry (they love the corn syrup), cereal companies, cracker industry as well as bread and pasta companies, then ultimately, profits for the pharmaceutical industry. All these are driven by our insatiable appetites for these foods, which is driven by the unending advertising that comes from this industry. It makes me ask is this the Devil incarnate, we've been afraid of all our lives? Is this the bane of civilization? Has this devil redirected our fears to the wrong cause, saying fat is bad and to eat carbs, or in the wrong way by telling us that we should fear something other than sugar? They've even blamed modern disease on meat and dairy which are perfectly healthy (dairy especially).

The major reason this addiction continues is due to the manner in which it is and has been promoted. The desire to create more and more ways and forms to entice everyone to eat and drink more of this deadly food is nothing short of astounding. It continues to amaze me how inventive we are at finding ways to kill ourselves with our own taste buds. Studies have been done, books have been written, the public has been warned, but it continues to happen. Every time I turn around I see another new way to kill ourselves in another appealing commercial. All this advertising encouraging us to consume more and more or their blood glucose raising, diabetes causing, HBP causing, dementia-causing foods is the driving force of this addiction and consequent expense. A carbohydrate diet requires that you feed it almost on an hourly basis. This is due to the fact that bread and sugar (glucose) create a hunger cycle.

A ketogenic diet, on the other hand, allows you to go all day without eating much of anything. Here's the secret, carboholics don't like to go hungry. They'll do almost anything they can to not go hungry. Those on a ketogenic diet don't mind going hungry. Actually, to us, it's not going hungry. It's simply going without eating. The hunger doesn't exist much, after the cycle of addiction has been broken. We feel the hunger pangs and many times, welcome them because we know that is where we build our better health. We do this by building Ghrelin throughout our systems because we know that Ghrelin works to build our immunity as well as making us a little smarter by increasing our brain power, through the addition of BDNF in our brains. Remember BDNF is that stuff that's the foundation of new brain cells. Remember the Nrf2, that ramps up the production of your anti-oxidants? Those are both benefits of Ghrelin in your system.

Your celebration of your addiction to this sugar is the industry's celebration of profits, both in the food, they sell us and the drugs we buy to relieve the pain. For them, it's a win-win situation. For the public who buys into this, it's a no-win situation. This is the prescription for future medications if you're in your teens and twenties. In your thirties, you'll start buying their headache and stomach ache medication. In your forties, it'll become insulin or anti-diabetes medication, then in your 50's and 60's and beyond, pick your poison, heart disease, cancer, Alzheimer's disease. Anyone or all of these are going to hit you when you least expect it. I know. I've experienced it. I pray that you heed my words and don't experience it yourselves.

Targeted Advertising

Almost everything I see advertised on channels marketing to younger viewers is encouraging everyone to buy more soda, energy drinks (most of which are laden with sugar), snack chips and cereals. Then when you're a few years older the ads are aimed at selling you crackers and pasta. Then into your 40's, 50's and 60's the ads are all aimed at selling you treatments and drugs for all the diseases and illnesses that your lifetime of consumption has brought you, drugs for diabetes, heart disease, cancer, arthritis, dementia, HBP, high cholesterol, etc, etc, etc. How long do I need to go on? Did I mention headaches or stomach aches?

When I watch programming on TV appealing to older viewers, like news broadcasts, I'm inundated with the commercials they show for drugs to treat heart disease (for there is no cure, only treatment), to treat cancer (again no cure), diabetes, high cholesterol, high blood pressure, arthritis, diabetes, and obesity. Drug companies are doing their best to sell their drugs to us to treat (not cure) us, for the illness and pain that they cause. And we buy it. We buy into it big time. We've bought into it our entire lives. The biggest problem here is most people are still buying into it. And they're buying into it in massive quantities, evidenced by pandemics of obesity, diabetes, Alzheimer's disease, heart disease, cancer, arthritis, HBP, etc, etc. What's being spent now, not just on snacks and beverages, but on staples like flour and sugar, pasta and cereal will be tripled, quadrupled, quintupled and even more, in payments to the pharmaceutical companies in the future, after your done paying the price for the damage all your years of consumption will cause. The only way to getting as close to a cure as you can is to give them up as completely as possible, otherwise, a continuance will only incur the need for drugs.

The drugs they'll be pushing on you, for heart disease or cancer, or even just for your headaches and stomach aches will be an array of *SIDE EFFECT* causing chemicals that will ultimately make it necessary for you to purchase more of their drugs to counteract the side effects of the drugs you've been taking for your treatment. You see proof of this everywhere. I experienced it myself when I was on 12 different medications just to treat an underlying chronic pain problem I had to take diuretics for my high blood pressure, anti-depressants because "they worked on the same receptors in the brain that the pain used", NSAIDS for the headaches I always used to get, opioids for the chronic pain I live with from the car accident. The diuretics were for my high blood pressure caused by my pain, or so I thought. After I quit the bread, the pain subsided. Maybe not completely, but it to encouraged me enough to quit all grains. When it subsided, even more, I decided to quit all carbs. My biggest benefits were the loss of my high blood pressure along with 30 lbs of weight and the disappearance of the worst of my pain.

When they advertise new drugs, the precautions and side effects of the drugs they want to sell you, take up more of the commercials, they show, than the explanations of their benefits. I have to wonder where the regulation is. Is it for the consumer (which it's supposed to be) or is this regulation for the benefit of the industry? How can drugs with that many precautions and side effects still be approved for sale? It appears to me that this industry has the FDA under their spell.

Which does it appear to be, to you? This industry is still allowed to market foods of disease and death while marketing treatments for those diseases and illnesses. Who knew that these industries are related? Before I started this, I didn't. I had to uncover this information, so I'll show you how all of this is connected and it's connected to take your money. Their manner of taking your money is clearly hazardous to your health. This is something you need to know because nothing is more important than your health.

The Industry that Feeds you Sugar and Grains, Force you into Buying Drugs from their Pharmaceutical Industry

The food industry which also includes the grain industry, which includes the crop seed industry that provides the farmers with the seed they need to grow the grains that they sell us to put on our tables for us to eat, is related to the pharmaceutical industry that makes all the drugs for all the diseases that these foods create. My question is how could we allow an industry responsible for our food, be also responsible to treat the diseases their food creates? (This is the worst kind of *catch 22* for the consumer.)

What we've allowed these related industries to do, in a nutshell, is drain our wallets at the grocery store by influencing us to buy their sodas, fruit drinks, snack foods, corn chips, pastas, breads, cereals and crackers, while draining our wallets again at the pharmacy to buy their drugs that treat the symptoms of the diseases their food is responsible for. We pay three times;

1. For the food, we're sold through their marketing....(and their advertising is pure magic to see and it's so easy to buy into). Their product tastes better than anything in the world. How much more could you ask for than a worldwide customer base that's addicted to your wares? Because it's addictive (like tobacco), you only have to make it more appealing than that of its competitors, of which it has plenty because the addiction is so strong. That makes it more deadly than heroin, simply because it's as prevalent as water. In some places, more prevalent.
2. We also get to pay their associates for the drugs we need to combat the diseases that their food has given us. And pay them we do. We'll pay them anything to get out of the pain that we've been inflicted with, from eating the food they so happily sold to us. We just don't connect that pain we feel with the food we've grown up with. But it is connected. It's connected in a big way. They first connected themselves toward the end of the 20th century with mergers and acquisitions bringing chemical, pharmaceutical, and crop seed companies under one roof.
3. The largest price we pay is detailed in the next section, *The Damage*. I cover it extensively in chapter 5 The *Real Poisoning of America – Glycation*.

The Perfect Sugar Ruse

This disturbs me and it disturbs me more and more every day. The company that produces the crop seed for the food I'm supposedly going to eat is the same pharmaceutical company that makes drugs for the illnesses and diseases this food is responsible for? Can this be legal? There's nothing illegal about it, it just happens and you buy into it.

This industry is so intent on keeping us addicted that sugar or corn syrup is quite often the #1 or #2 ingredient in baby food, meaning that if you're not one of the few that were raised on their mother's milk and had to grow up on baby food, you're condemned to an addiction that our grain and pharmaceutical industry has imposed upon you.

It's not surprising that we've ignored this addiction for as long as we've had it. We've ignored it because we grew up with it. Everyone has it, so as far as everyone is concerned, there is no addiction. After all, how can you be addicted to something that you need to survive? How can you live without something that you need to survive? That's where the question lies. Do you need it or not? If it's something you need to survive, why does it do so much damage? Do you really need this food or can you live without it? Allow me to be the first to tell you, you can live without it and you should live without it. To do this, you make your body not need it. Sounds simple, doesn't it? It is simple, it just isn't easy. This is one case where simply is not easy.

We've made it so easy for this industry to increase our addiction that we look forward to finding new ways to inflict more harm on our bodies. And this industry is more than happy to oblige us with their new creations to further our addiction. It's a win-win situation for them. They couldn't ask for anything more. Unfortunately for us, it's a no-win situation. We're paying the supply side for what we eat and the product side for drugs we take to treat what pain the food gives us. This is how Monsanto has engineered the state of your health for their pocketbook.

Monsanto's involvement

According to Wikipedia; *"Monsanto scientists were among the first to genetically modify a plant cell, publishing their results in 1983; five years later, the company conducted the first field tests of genetically engineered crops. Increasing involvement in agricultural biotechnology R&D in general dates from the installment of Richard Mahoney as Monsanto's CEO in 1983 This involvement increased under the leadership of Robert Shapiro, appointed CEO in 1995, leading ultimately to the divestment of product lines unrelated to agriculture."* This divestment of product lines is their disposal of their pharmaceuticals. Their venture into pharmaceuticals started in 1985 with their purchase of GD Searle, of NutraSweet fame. It was eight years after this that they filed for a patent for Celebrex. Did they know at this time, what their food was doing to their consumers? Had they seen any of the reports that started coming out in 1984 and continued until today? Are they aware of any of them now? It appears not, or they're choosing to be electively ignorant. I think it's the latter. Their history tells us it's the latter.

From Wikipedia; *"In 1985, Monsanto acquired G. D. Searle & Company, a life sciences company focusing on pharmaceuticals, agriculture, and animal health. In 1993, Monsanto's Searle division filed a patent application for Celebrex, which is 1998 became the first selectiveCOX-2 inhibitors to be approved by the U.S. Food and Drug Administration (FDA). Celebrex became a blockbuster drug and was often mentioned as a key reason for Pfizer's acquisition of Monsanto's pharmaceutical business in 2002."* Celebrex and arthritis, did they know the connection? What causes arthritis? Was this industry aware of the studies that started coming out in the 50's and 60's about the dangers of their product?

"In 1996, Monsanto purchased Agracetus, the biotechnology company that had generated the first transgenic varieties of cotton, soybeans, peanuts, and other crops, and from which Monsanto had already been licensing technology since 1991. Monsanto first entered the maize seed business when it purchased 40% of DEKALB in 1996; it purchased the remainder of the corporation in 1998. In 1998 Monsanto purchased Cargill's international seed business, which gave it access to sales and distribution facilities in 51 countries. In 2005, it finalized the purchase of Seminis Inc, a leading global vegetable and fruit seed company, for $1.4 billion. "This made it the world's largest conventional seed company at the time. Again, I have to wonder, had they seen the studies of what their products were doing to their consumers?

"1999: Monsanto sold off NutraSweet Co. In December, Monsanto merged with Pharmacia and Upjohn. The agricultural division became a wholly owned subsidiary of the "new" Pharmacia; Monsanto's medical research division, which included products such as Celebrex.

*"In 2007, Monsanto and **BASF** announced a long-term agreement to cooperate in the research, development, and marketing of new plant biotechnology products. "Through a series of transactions, the Monsanto that existed from 1901 to 2000 and the current Monsanto are legally two distinct corporations. Although they share the same name and corporate headquarters, many of the same executives and other employees, and responsibility for liabilities arising out of activities in the industrial chemical business, the agricultural chemicals business is the only segment carried forward from the pre-1997 Monsanto Company to the*

current Monsanto Company". This was accomplished beginning in the 1980s:

- *1985: Monsanto purchased G. D. Searle & Company for $2.7 billion in cash. In this merger, Searle's aspartame business became a separate Monsanto subsidiary, the NutraSweet Company. CEO of NutraSweet, Robert B. Shapiro, served as CEO of Monsanto from 1995 to 2001.*
- *1996: Monsanto acquired Agracetus, a majority interest in Calgene, creators of the Flavr Savr tomato, and 40% of **DeKalb Genetics Corporation**. It purchased the remainder of DeKalb in 1998.*
- *1997: Monsanto spun off its industrial chemical and fiber divisions into Solutia. In January, Monsanto announced the purchase of Holden's Foundations Seeds, a privately held seed business. By acquiring Holden's, Monsanto became the biggest American producer of foundation corn, the parent seed from which hybrids are made. The combined purchase price was $925 million. Also, in April, Monsanto purchased the remaining shares of Calgene.*
- *1999: Monsanto sold off NutraSweet Co. In December, Monsanto merged with **Pharmacia & Upjohn**, and the agricultural division became a wholly owned subsidiary of the "new" Pharmacia; the medical research divisions of Monsanto, which included products such as **Celebrex**, were rolled into Pharmacia.*
- *2000 (October): Pharmacia spun off its Monsanto subsidiary into a new company, the "new Monsanto". Monsanto agreed to indemnify Pharmacia against any liabilities that might be incurred from judgments against Solutia. As a result, the new Monsanto continues to be a party to numerous lawsuits that relate to operations of the old Monsanto. Pharmacia was bought by Pfizer in a deal announced in 2002 and completed in 2003.)*
- *2005: Monsanto acquired Emergent Genetics and its Stoneville and NexGen cotton brands. Emergent was the third largest U.S. cotton seed company, with about 12 percent of the U.S. market. Monsanto's goal was to obtain "a strategic cotton germplasm and traits platform." The vegetable seed producer **Seminis** was purchased for $1.4 billion.*
- *2007: In June, Monsanto purchased **Delta & Pine Land Company**, a major cotton seed breeder, for $1.5 billion. As a condition for approval from the **Department of Justice**, Monsanto was obligated to divest its Stoneville cotton business, which it sold to Bayer, and to divest its NexGen cotton business, which it sold to Americot. Monsanto also exited the pig breeding business by selling Monsanto Choice Genetics to Newsham Genetics LC in November, divesting itself of "any and all swine-related patents, patent applications, and all other intellectual property".*
- *2008: Monsanto purchased the Dutch seed company **De Ruiter** Seeds for €546 million, and sold its POSILAC bovine somatotropin brand and related business to Elanco Animal Health, a division of Eli Lilly in August for $300 million plus "additional contingent consideration".*
- *2012: Monsanto purchased for $210 million Precision Planting Inc., a company that produced computer hardware and software designed to enable farmers to increase yield and productivity through more accurate planting.*
- *2013: Monsanto purchased San Francisco-based **Climate Corp** for $930 million. Climate Corp. makes more accurate local weather forecasts for farmers based on data modeling and historical data; if the forecasts were wrong, the farmer was recompensed.*
- *2015 Monsanto tried to buy Syngenta for US$46.5 billion but failed.*
- *2016 Bayer offered to buy Monsanto for US$62 billion."*

Monsanto's involvement in the pharmaceutical industry and the AgroSciences has grown to monopolistic proportions. It not only controls what's grown to put on your table to eat, it's made that food so dangerous without you knowing, that it's forcing you to buy their drugs to treat your pain. This forces you into a cycle of their control. It started with the baby food you were given when you were young. It ends with the Ziploc bag full of drugs that your spouse will through away after your death.

It's not just crop seed that they manufacture; they also are responsible for the chemicals sprayed on the crops grown from their seed. Since it's been genetically modified to withstand the effects of their herbicide, Roundup, I've always wondered how much of those chemicals get into our food through this process. Roundup is a glyphosate herbicide, meaning that it's an enzyme inhibitor, that's not good for human health. For me, it's just not healthy enough for me to eat, especially for the problems I already live with. More chemicals in my body are not what I need to keep it healthy. You may want to chance it, but pesticides and herbicides in our diet have been linked to bladder cancer. Why would I want to chance that, just for the taste of something sweet or salty? You only think you're craving the salt when in all actuality, you're craving the carbs that come with the salt. The salt isn't addictive, the carbs are.

Below is just a little of Monsanto's bio-chemical industry. They're so good at manufacturing the chemicals for the herbicides and pesticides they manufacture GMO seed that is resistant to these chemicals. This may be good for the crops, but what about you? Though the plant may be resistant to the chemicals, does that mean that your body is? I don't think so.

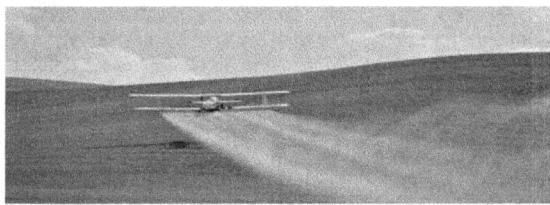

How glyphosate-based herbicides & GM seed combine to make consumption of grains dangerous.

Again according to Wikipedia; *"Monsanto chemist John E. Franz repurposed the chemical glyphosate as a systemic herbicide in 1970. Monsanto's last commercially relevant United States patent on glyphosate expired in 2000, and since then glyphosate has been marketed in the United States and worldwide by many agrochemical companies, in different solution strengths, and with various adjuvants, under dozens of trade names. As of 2009, sales of glyphosate represented about 10% of Monsanto's revenue due to competition from other producers of other glyphosate-based herbicides; their Roundup products (which include GM seeds) represented about half of Monsanto's gross margin."*

Glyphosate is an enzyme inhibitor, used not only in herbicides but also in many drugs. They allow the drug to be more specific to the treatment and incur fewer side effects, for the patient. Don't think that ingestion of Glyphosate now, through your grain intake, will prevent side effects of medications in the future. I can virtually guarantee that it won't.

What Wikipedia says about glyphosate; *"Glyphosate is absorbed through foliage, and minimally through roots, and transported to growing points. It inhibits a plant enzyme involved in the synthesis of three aromatic amino acids: tyrosine, tryptophan, and phenylalanine. Therefore, it is effective only on actively growing plants and is not effective as a pre-emergence herbicide. An increasing number of crops have been genetically engineered to be tolerant of glyphosate (e.g. Roundup Ready soybean, the first Roundup Ready crop, also created by Monsanto) which allows farmers to use glyphosate as a post-emergence herbicide against weeds. The development of glyphosate resistance in weed species is emerging as a costly problem. While glyphosate and formulations such as Roundup have been approved by regulatory bodies worldwide, concerns about their effects on humans and the environment persist."*

"Many regulatory and scholarly reviews have evaluated the relative toxicity of glyphosate as an herbicide. The German **Federal Institute for Risk Assessment** *toxicology review in 2013 found that "the available data is contradictory and far from being convincing" with regard to correlations between exposure to glyphosate formulations and risk of various cancers, including* **non-Hodgkin lymphoma** *(NHL)."*

A 2014 review article reported a significant association between **B-cell lymphoma** and glyphosate occupational exposure. In March 2015 the **World Health Organization's International Agency for Research on Cancer** classified glyphosate as *"probably carcinogenic in humans" (category 2A) based on epidemiological studies, animal studies, and in vitro studies. However in 2016 a joint meeting of the United Nations (FAO) Panel of Experts on Pesticide Residues in Food and the Environment and the World Health Organization (WHO) Core Assessment Group on Pesticide Residues (JMPR) concluded that based on the available evidence "glyphosate is unlikely to pose a carcinogenic risk to humans from exposure through the diet".* This last statement I wonder about. It also makes me wonder, "who influenced their decision to label this stuff as suitable to eat?" Apparently, they're not taking the rise in cancer rates into consideration.

Are you glyphosate-resistant? Can your body withstand the changes that glyphosate forces upon your body every time you have a corn chip or a sandwich? With Roundup being coated on most of the foods that you eat, how can you guarantee that none of it is in your body? How can you guarantee that it's not affecting your physiology? Can you guarantee that it's not affecting the actions of enzymes in your body that regulate your health? What guarantees do you have that this won't initiate more trips to your doctor?

What you think may not be of much importance, may be far more important that you believe. **Acetylcholine** is an important chemical in the body that's important for brain function and muscle function throughout the body as Acetylcholine is a neurotransmitter. For Acetylcholine to act as a neurotransmitter, it needs multiple enzymes that function in the central nervous system and the peripheral nervous system. Acetylcholine works as a neurotransmitter as well as a neuromodulator.

The body uses the enzyme **acetylcholinesterase** to help activate muscles by inhibiting the action of **acetylcholine**, and if glyphosate herbicides (Roundup weed killer) are enzyme inhibitors, how can the ingestion of grains laden with these herbicides, not affect the function of the enzymes in your body since you consume them every time you eat bread products of any sort? Corn chips and soy fall into this category also. (They may be worse.)

These Glyphosate herbicides are enzyme inhibitors that have the ability to alter or stop the cell signaling capabilities of enzymes. If they can do this to plants, where is the guarantee that it won't affect your body? Chances are, they're going to change how your body operates and in the long run be the precursor to many diseases. It's crucial for the body's proper function that the actions of certain enzymes are never altered. Where's the guarantee that these enzyme-inhibiting herbicides that your wheat has been sprayed with, won't affect your health? There is none except that if you eat this food, you will be affected.

According to Wikipedia; *"Acetylcholine receptor agonists and antagonists can either have an effect directly on the receptors or exert their effects indirectly, e.g., by affecting the enzyme acetylcholinesterase, which degrades the receptor ligand. Agonists increase the level of receptor activation, antagonists reduce it."* I would consider an enzyme inhibitor an antagonist as it inhibits enzyme function.

It's a little clearer to see now, how the altering of how enzymes work in our bodies, can have an effect on our health. I can see how this could come from a diet high in grains because of how much Roundup is sprayed on grain that's milled into flour. I can also see how this could present a huge gain for the pharmaceutical industry. Is this really the intent of Monsanto, the maker of Roundup, the widest used herbicide on the planet? Or is it just negligence? I have to wonder because of their previous ties with Pharmacia & Upjohn, makers of Celebrex. These are just a few of thousands of enzymes and cell signaling proteins that are affected by this enzyme inhibitor. How many corporate breakups don't include severance packages that include stock options? Is this what makes Monsanto want to continue their glyphosate spraying?

I for one, would not like to have this inhibitor flowing through my blood mucking up my system. Who knows what enzymes it's going to inhibit in your body? Fortunately for me, I don't have to worry about that anymore, as carbs aren't in my diet. They won't get a chance to muck up anything in my body ever again, I've gone keto and I'm not going back.

It looks to me like Monsanto is trying to lock up not only our digestive problems but the resolve of those digestive problems as well. They like to persuade you to buy their food products which you are more than happy to do, then they get your money again when you purchase your Celebrex to ease the pain of arthritis given you by their grains. The next step is to buy their drugs to counteract the side effects of the original drug you need to take for the pain. You don't want to know the step after that, my dad can tell you, it's not pretty and it involves, even more, drugs and more therapy and continued testing. It's a never-ending cycle that lasts until death.

Bayer's involvement

"It's not only Monsanto, Bayer has its own interest in the area of crop science, as explained by Wikipedia, " in 2002, Bayer AG acquired the Dutch seed company Nunhems, which at the time was one of the world's top five seed companies. In 2006, the U.S. Department of Agriculture announced that Bayer CropScience's Liberty Link genetically modified rice had contaminated the U.S. rice supply. Shortly after the public learned of the contamination, the E.U. banned imports of U.S. long-grain rice and the futures price plunged. In April 2010, a Lonoke County, Arkansas jury awarded a dozen farmers $48 million. The case is currently on appeal to the Arkansas Supreme Court. On 1 July 2011 Bayer CropScience agreed to a global settlement for up to $750 million. In September 2014, the firm announced plans to invest $1 billion in the **United States** *between 2013 and 2016. A Bayer spokesperson said that the largest investments will be made to expand the production of its herbicide Liberty. Liberty is used to kill weeds which have grown resistant to Monsanto's product* **Roundup.** *"*

Bayer's four divisions are related in their concerns to their contribution to our food industry as well as their contribution to the pharmaceutical industry. Bayer Pharmaceuticals, Bayer Crop Science, Bayer Animal Health, and Bayer Consumer Health are all related to our health. They too, like to charge us for the food they market to us, then charge us for medication to treat the symptoms of the diseases that their foods are responsible for. Their divested interests are Lanxess (Bayer Chemicals AG) Diagnostics Division, Diabetes Devices Division, Covestro (Bayer Material Science).

Astra Zenica / Syngenta's involvement

"Zeneca Agrochemicals was part of **AstraZeneca**, *and formerly of* **Imperial Chemical Industries**. *ICI was formed in the UK in 1926. Two years later, work began at the Agricultural Research Station at* **Jealotts Hill** *near* **Bracknell**." *"In 2004, Syngenta Seeds purchased* **Garst**, *the North American corn and soybean business of Advanta, as well as* **Golden Harvest Seeds**. *On 5 December 2004, the European Union ended a six-year moratorium when it approved imports of two varieties of* **genetically modified corn** *sold by Monsanto and its Swiss rival, Syngenta.*

AstraZeneca owned by Syngenta again is evidence of this industrial control over our lives. Syngenta is a Swiss biotechnology company that operates globally. According to Wikipedia; *"Syngenta AG is a global Swiss agribusiness that produces agrochemicals and seeds. As a biotechnology company, it conducts genomic research. It was formed in 2000 by the merger of Novartis Agribusiness and Zeneca Agrochemicals. As of 2014, Syngenta was the world's largest crop chemical producer, strongest in Europe. As of 2009, it ranked third in seeds and biotechnology sales. Sales in 2015 were approximately US$13.4 billion, over half of which were in emerging markets."*

The three agrichemical companies above are the largest in the world, controlling a majority of the foods we eat along with the medications we take. I've laid out the evidence of what their foods do to the human body, yet they continue to produce the seed for the crops to make the food they want us to put on our table to eat. They also produce the aspirin everybody takes for the headaches they get from eating their bread.

I've said before how convenient we've made it for this industry to take our money while slowly, painfully, and expensively, make us sick. But our money is not the only thing they rob us of. They rob us of our dignity as well, for their food does more than anything else to rob us of our memories. We allow them to do this because none of their foods require warning labels, like that of cigarettes. (The FDA doesn't seem to care about what it does to you, they only care that you know it's there, even though you don't know what it's doing to you.) Even the USDA's *myplate.gov* still recommends eating them.

We've put our health and lives in the hands of this industry by bending to their advertising and buying into their game. We allow them to addict us when we're infants by dumping sugar and corn syrup solids into the baby food we feed our kids. Then we allow them to continue their assault by buying into advertising schemes every Saturday morning with their cereal commercials. To fully hook us, they add sugar to this already sugar-laden food simply to make it more palatable.

When an industry does this, how are we supposed to fight the addiction? This makes every American who buys into this behavior a slave to this industry. Slaves make the best captive audience. They have no choice in what they do except to choose their device of demise. Will it be corn flakes or Wheaties?

What more do you need than a captive audience to sell your wares? This is why a Coke at a ballgame costs 3 times more than what you can get it for, at the grocery store. At the ballgame, you're a captive audience. It's the same when you're addicted. Every *'PUSHER'* knows this and they charge a premium price for it. This is exactly why everyone who remains in this trap makes themselves a slave, captive to the whims of these industries.

The Litigation Game

These industries are tied up with multiple lawsuits in other areas of their agrochemical businesses. For example, Monsanto has fought legal claims of false advertising, as explained again in Wikipedia;

1. *"In 1999, Monsanto was condemned by the UK **Advertising Standards Authority** (ASA) for making "confusing, misleading, unproven and wrong" claims about its products over the course of a £1 million advertising campaign. The ASA ruled that Monsanto had presented its opinions "as accepted fact" and had published "wrong" and "unproven" scientific claims. Monsanto responded with an apology and claimed it was not intending to deceive and instead "did not take sufficiently into account the difference in culture between the UK and the USA in the way some of this information was presented."*

2. *"In 2001, French environmental and consumer rights campaigners brought a case against Monsanto for misleading the public about the **environmental impact** of its **herbicide Roundup**, on the basis that **glyphosate**, Roundup's main ingredient, is classed as "dangerous for the environment" and "toxic for aquatic organisms" by the **European Union**. Monsanto's advertising for Roundup had presented it as biodegradable and as leaving the soil clean after use. In 2007, Monsanto was convicted of false advertising and was fined 15,000 Euros. Monsanto's French distributor Scotts France was also fined 15,000 Euros. Both defendants were ordered to pay damages of 5,000 Euros to the Brittany Water and Rivers Association and 3,000 Euros to the CLCV (Consommation Logement Cadre de vie), one of the two main general consumer associations in France. Monsanto appealed and the court upheld the verdict; Monsanto appealed again to the French Supreme Court, and in 2009 it also upheld the verdict.*

3. *"In August 2012, a Brazilian Regional Federal Court ordered Monsanto to pay a $250,000 fine for false advertising. In 2004, advertising that related to the use of GM soya seed, and the herbicide glyphosate used in its cultivation, claimed it was beneficial to the conservation of the environment. The federal prosecutor maintained that Monsanto misrepresented the amount of herbicide required and stated that "there is no scientific certainty that soybeans marketed by Monsanto use less herbicide." The presiding judge condemned Monsanto and called the advertisement "abusive and misleading propaganda." The prosecutor held that the goal of the advertising was to prepare the market for the purchase of genetically modified soybean seed (sale of which was then banned) and the herbicide used on it, at a time when the approval of a Brazilian Biosafety Law, enacted in 2005, was being discussed in the country."*

4. *"In March 2014 the **South African Advertising Standards Authority** (ASA) upheld a complaint, made by the African Centre for Biosafety, that Monsanto had made "unsubstantiated" claims about **genetically modified crops** in its radio advertisements, and ordered that these adverts be pulled. In March 2015 after considering further documentation from Monsanto, the ASA reversed its ruling."*

5. *"In 2009, Monsanto came under scrutiny from the U.S. Department of Justice, which began investigating whether the company's activities in the soybean markets were breaking **anti-trust** rules. In 2010, the Department of Justice created a website through which comments on "Agriculture and Antitrust Enforcement Issues in Our 21st Century Economy" could be submitted; over 15,000 comments were submitted including a letter by 14 State Attorneys General. The comments are publicly available. On November 16, 2012, Monsanto announced that it had received written notification from the U.S. Department of Justice that the Antitrust Division had concluded its inquiry and that the*

Department of Justice had closed the inquiry without taking any enforcement action. Opponents of Monsanto's seed patenting and licensing practices expressed frustration that the Department of Justice released no information about the results of the inquiry.

6. *"In 2009, Monsanto came under scrutiny from the U.S. Department of Justice, which began investigating whether the company's activities in the soybean markets were breaking* **anti-trust** *rules. In 2010, the Department of Justice created a website through which comments on* "Agriculture and Antitrust Enforcement Issues in Our 21st Century Economy" *could be submitted; over 15,000 comments were submitted including a letter by 14 State Attorneys General. The comments are publicly available. On November 16, 2012, Monsanto announced that it had received written notification from the U.S. Department of Justice that the Antitrust Division had concluded its inquiry and that the Department of Justice had closed the inquiry without taking any enforcement action. Opponents of Monsanto's seed patenting and licensing practices expressed frustration that the Department of Justice released no information about the results of the inquiry."*

This is a normal operating business for Monsanto, Syngenta, and Bayer. Too bad it isn't for you. All of these cases are a clear indication of the extent to which Monsanto is willing to push the limits. This is how corporate risk/loss assessment works. Sometimes the risk of paying a $15,000 find is worth the theft of a patent. My problem with this is they playing with my health. If I decide to eat their products, I get to play their game of disease and drugs. The problem is, what are their products? Who knows? Who knows who grow the crops for the corn flakes that you ate this morning for breakfast. Do you? I don't. But I now know it came from one of these companies. Monsanto's not the only one. Syngenta, as well, has been accused of making false claims about being involved in suits for false patent infringement;

"In 2001, the United States Patent and Trademark Office ruled in favor of Syngenta which had filed a suit against Bayer for patent infringement on a class of neonicotinoid insecticides. The following year Syngenta filed suits against Monsanto and other companies claiming infringement of its U.S. biotechnology patents covering genetically modified corn and cotton. In 2004, it again filed a suit against Monsanto, claiming antitrust violations related to the U.S. biotech corn seed market, and Monsanto countersued. Monsanto and Syngenta settled all litigation in 2008"

I mention this to point out the extent of their influence in the crop seed industry, where they have 15 of their own seed companies that all provide GMO crop seed for farmers to plant for their crops for food which ends up on our tables. Syngenta is the second largest corporation in the industry, Monsanto is even larger. (And we haven't considered Bayer CropScience, Dow AgroSciences or DuPont Pioneer.) Most of these cases involve patent rights to GMO seed with companies like Monsanto or DuPont Pioneer. It's not just patent problems that their litigation deals with; most of these companies like to make out that their chemical products are completely harmless to the environment when they've been proven otherwise.

"Syngenta was a defendant in a class action lawsuit by the city of **Greenville, Illinois** *concerning the adverse effects of* **atrazine** *in human water supplies. The suit was settled for $105 million in May 2012. A similar case involving six states has been in federal court since 2010." "In the US, Syngenta is facing lawsuits from farmers and shipping companies regarding Viptera* **genetically modified corn**. *The plaintiffs in nearly 30 states contend that Syngenta's introduction of Viptera drove down US grain market prices, leading to financial harm and that Syngenta acted irresponsibly by doing too little to enable shipping companies to export the grain to approved ports. Before Vipera's 2010 introduction Syngenta*

*secured all US and **NCGA**-recommended export approvals, but none from China. China had imported little to no US grain prior to 2010, and at the time was not considered a major partner, but it became a major partner in 2010 when it dramatically increased US grain imports. For three years, China imported U.S. Viptera grain without formal approval. In November 2013, Chinese officials destroyed a U.S. grain shipment containing Viptera grain, started rejecting all US shipments with the GM grain, but continued to accept it from all countries other than the US. That same year, US corn market prices dropped $4 per bushel, causing over $2.9B in losses, with just over half of that loss occurring prior to China's November rejection. China later approved the GM corn in 2014 but US corn grain market prices have not rebounded."*

I can only empathize with the farmers and the losses they've had to sustain. Their losses, fortunately, were only monetary. How many others have suffered losses of family members, like my family? Our losses were not only financial, they were family. It would be nice if money or the bottom line wasn't the most important thing in the industry. But it is. And we have to live with it. My choice is to not buy into it. I won't eat what they grow or take their drugs to fix the problems caused by what they grow. My choice is a choice of survival.

These are the kind of companies that are ultimately providing your food. Do you want them making your drugs, also? As you've seen, they already do. Do you wonder why the prevalence of these diseases is so rampant? It's in these industries' best interest that this cycle continues. Do you want this kind of industry to be responsible for your food or medicine? How about the medicine they make to treat the problems their foods create? We've allowed this to take place, right under our noses and we should be ashamed. Doesn't this sound a lot like a wicked witch luring small children with candy and sweets? Because of our addiction, we allow them to continue this behavior.

This addiction has and is costing America more money and lives than any other addiction that we've ever experienced. There are 24,000,000 deaths worldwide each year due to ECC, excessive carbohydrate consumption. There were 17.3 million deaths in 2013 alone due to cardiovascular disease. Cancer claims over 4 million each year and Alzheimer's take 5 million each year, yet I hear no outrage about it. All of these deaths and suffering can be curbed simply by curbing carbohydrate consumption. It's time to put an end to this addiction. It's time for a cure. But to stop the addiction, you first have to **DE-CELEBRATIZE** it. We have to stop celebrating its addictive qualities and exchange that celebration for the horror for what this addiction really does.

Everybody needs to think about what harm this food does before they put it in their mouth instead of thinking how good it tastes. Unfortunately for my generation and all those that have come along since, we're stuck in the quagmire of addiction that we have to carry for the rest of our lives. Even most natural causes of death happen in part, due to what this food has done to the body over the lifetime of the deceased. An autopsy will likely show some form of arthritis, as this is evidence of inflammation, oxidative stress and cell degradation that these foods cause. If the inflammation, oxidative stress and cell degradation exists in the joints, it has to exist elsewhere in the body and since it exists throughout the body, as inflammation exists in the blood, it has to affect everything it comes in contact with.

That means it affects your heart, your brain, and every internal organ. How can that not have an effect on your life? It has to, so I have to ask, why is this food still allowed to be sold without a warning about just how dangerous it is? Cigarettes are and require a warning. Alcohol is and it requires a warning also. Heroin is illegal and opioids require prescriptions. But not the one substance that minimizes all the damage caused by these other substances collectively, sugar from grains requires any warning for the damage it inflicts. Why is this not as important? Is this industry too big to fail? Is there a way they can change it? I for one, cannot wait, I can't afford to play their game.

Going back to the problems this industry has had in court, mostly protecting their own patents and falsely claiming that their products are nutritious when they're not. Most of the patent problems lie in the resistance their new crop seeds have to their pesticides and herbicides, which have proven to have adverse effects on the human body. Yet they are still allowed to spray their crops with these herbicides and pesticides. My question is, how much of these herbicides and pesticides trickle into our food supply? How confident are you that no chemicals are in what you eat? How confident are you that no enzyme controlling chemicals are not on your biscuits or crackers? How confident are you that your sugar addiction won't turn into diabetes? How confident are you that your addiction won't turn into heart disease or cancer? Whether you worry about it or not, you will experience brain loss. That's just in the science. You can't change it without saying goodbye to your addiction. This obviously isn't easy with a grain industry that feeds the pharmaceutical industry. It's even more obvious that they'll never let us know the damage their foods do to everyone who ingests them. That's up to you to know the dangers of sugar and grains, and now you do.

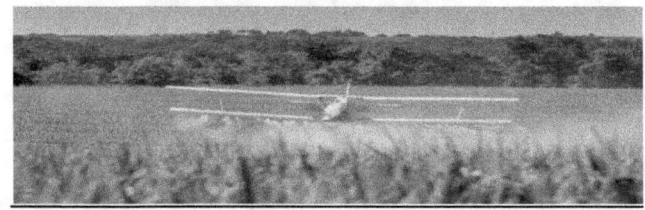

Do You Know Everything about What You're Eating?

Would you eat it if you did?

PART II

THE TAINTING OF YOUR FOOD

WHAT WERE ONCE "HEALTHY" CARBS

ARE NOW POLLUTED CARBS

THERE'S MORE DANGER

LURKING IN YOUR FOOD

THAN WHAT YOU

REALIZE

CHAPTER 3

CALORIES, DO YOU WORRY ABOUT THEM?

Calories, do you worry about how many you eat? If you do, you're not alone. A lot of people do the very same thing, they count their calories. If you're one of those who does, I have a suggestion for you. To help make your job easier and you healthier; you shouldn't worry about how many calories you eat, as much as you should worry about where the calories come from.

Calories are essential to survive, so they're absolutely necessary and yes if you eat more, you weigh more. If you eat less, of course, you weigh less. That does make eating fewer calories crucial yet eating less to control them can be very difficult at the least if you're on a carb diet. The simple reason to this is because carbs make you hungry. They create and maintain a hunger cycle that you have no control over, without removing them. That makes, where you get your calories from, more important than how many you eat.

Are the calories you get from the food you eat most, from carbohydrates or are the calories from protein and fat? If you're eating calories from carbohydrates, under the guise of **HEALTHY ENERGY**, you're allowing those carbs to make the fat that your body needs to use for that energy. If you're getting your calories from fat and protein, you're feeding your body exactly what it needs to survive and thrive. Eating fats and protein also allows your body to heal itself from virtually anything. It is very little our bodies cannot heal from, as long as they don't have the influence of the glycation that's the result of carbohydrates contaminating their systems. That means if your body needs glucose, let it make its own.

Whatever glucose you can get from carbs, your body can supply, on its own. When your brain (which is the only part of your body that needs glucose) needs glucose, it can supply the brain with all it needs through a process of gluconeogenesis. Your body reformulates the glycogen in your body to pull glucose out of it to use whenever the brain needs the glucose. (Remember, glucose used to be the name of glucose.)The interesting thing about this little-known fact is that your body makes this glucose, regardless of how much you already have in your body from the carbs you eat.

This all points to the fact that your body will make the nutrients it needs, provided you feed it the proper foods, to begin with, and carbs are not in that group. Carbs make your body make its own fat. It makes that fat out of the carbs you eat with the hormone insulin. (That's an enzyme you don't want to be inhibited.) A healthier way to live is to allow your body to make its own glucose instead of fat. This does wonder for the body. As long as you eat enough protein to compensate for the loss of muscle tissue from gluconeogenesis, you'll never lose vital muscle tissue.

This is why long fasts help you cure most diseases. After your body uses up its own fat to fuel your body, it resets your body to produce growth hormones that not only help keep you thinner; they keep you healthier by repairing your systems for you (usually without the need for medication).

It does this by changing your hormones. The way in which many hormones work is affected by eliminating carbs from the diet. Insulin is soon replaced by glucagon which regulates the gluconeogenesis that takes place in your body whenever it needs glucose. This hormone regulates how fat is burned in your body, whereas insulin controls how fat is stored in your body. As long as you're eating carbs you're creating insulin and it's instructing all the fat you're making to be stored, instead of to be used.

When you remove the carbs from your diet; your body changes, from increasing its production of insulin to increasing the production of glucagon which in turn ramps up the burning of your fat. This is why keto diets work so good. It's also why carb diets work so bad. In short, carb diets add fat to your body to be stored, keto diets take fat from your body to be burned. Which sounds healthier to you?

DIRTY FOOD GIVES YOU DIRTY FUEL

That means when you continue a diet of carbs, you're forcing your body to make its own fat out of those carbs and this is where your problem lies. The fat your body turns the glucose into is not a clean burning fat. It's a dirty fat at best. It leaves glycated residue wherever it's burned. That, in turn, gums up your cells…all of them, including your brain cells, your heart cells, your kidney cells, liver cells, every cell that blood flows through including the blood vessels they flow through. This is the true danger in carbohydrate consumption. This danger has been magnified by the glyphosate herbicide Roundup, with its enzyme inhibiting chemicals.

Some of the enzymes that get affected are enzymes that influence behavior. Some of these behavioral enzymes influence your appetite, as well as digestion, making this enzyme inhibitor responsible for more of your hunger and less of your nutrition. (It could actually detract from your nutrition.)

POLLUTED FUEL COSTS YOU, YOUR LIFE

Could that be why Monsanto is so adamant about their product being safe? They must know, if they reduce the use of their enzyme inhibitors on crops they're going to cut down on the need for their medications, to counteract the changes those enzyme inhibitors impose on the body and this could spell doom for their pharmaceutical industry.

If news like that were to leak out to the world, what would happen to the profits of the food producers that depend on the grain industry to provide them with their flour? What do you think that would to the profits of the pharmaceutical corporations Monsanto used to own? Don't you think that would have a major influence on them if everyone knew that it was actually all of the grain products that Monsanto is responsible for that is making them need the very medications that Monsanto's old pharmaceutical companies make?

I'm sure the pharmaceutical companies are still customers of Monsanto chemical division now, buying the same enzyme inhibitors to use in heart medication as well as many cancer medications. This practice leads only to more and more drug need by their consumers and this is how you get hooked. If you eat grains in any form you're one of their consumers.

This is what killed my mother and continues to kill over 20,000 mothers every day. This vicious cycle is courtesy of Monsanto's crop seed companies, Monsanto's herbicide companies through the production and spraying of Roundup, and what used to be Monsanto's corporate partner, Pharmacia. (Don't forget, they patented Celebrex 24 years ago.) Although I can understand if you did forget and why you forgot, it's in the food you eat. Now, can you see the danger?

Cutting down on the use of these herbicides will also cut down on the need to use these same chemicals to make the pharmaceuticals that help to counteract the damage done in the first place. This is the doom they've condemned our society to, an addiction that feeds itself into a pharmaceutical dependence. Their greed is more important to them than the health and safety of all America (and the world, for that fact). Their glyphosate ensures this for Monsanto even after their patent expired. It also ensures that America is not free, but still under the control of this industry and Monsanto.

ACCORDING TO WIKIPEDIA; *Glyphosate kills plants by interfering with the synthesis of the **aromatic** amino acids **phenylalanine, tyrosine**, and **tryptophan**. It does this by inhibiting the enzyme **5-enolpyruvylshikimate-3-phosphate synthase** (EPSPS), which **catalyzes** the reaction of **shikimate**-3-phosphate (S3P) and **phosphoenolpyruvate** to form 5-enolpyruvyl-shikimate-3-phosphate (EPSP). Glyphosate is absorbed through foliage and minimally through roots, meaning that it is only effective on actively growing plants and cannot prevent seeds from germinating. After application, glyphosate is readily transported around the plant to grow roots and leaves and this **systemic** activity is important for its effectiveness. Inhibiting the enzyme causes shikimate to accumulate in plant tissues and diverts energy and resources away from other processes. While growth stops within hours of application, it takes several days for the leaves to begin **turning yellow**.*

This is the damage it does to weeds but it can do the same kind of damage to your body by affecting the way your enzymes work. This makes your body waste a lot more energy, converting those glyphosated carbs into fat, so it can use them.

If you feed your body fat in the first place, you don't need to convert anything as the fat is "ready to use". This last little factor is what's important to know because it doesn't require your body to make fat out of the sugar. This is what drains your pancreas from its supply of insulin. It also glycates your blood and it's this glycation, that leads to more modern disease than any other one thing. If you can control glycation, you control all inflammation. Controlling all inflammation means that you're controlling all modern diseases created by inflammation.

This fact combined with the fact that Roundup affects the enzymes **phenylalanine**, **tyrosine**, and **tryptophan**, means that they're also affecting your hunger patterns, digestion, and sleep. That creates a double dipper for the food industry and pharmaceutical industry. And they do this legally, thanks to a patent law from 1954 and a ruling from an old Monsanto lawyer saying that modifying seeds for any purpose, is legal. I'm sure they didn't realize the consequences at the time their actions would have on humanity.

*One of the enzymes affected in your body is Phenylalanine, a precursor for **tyrosine**; the **monoamine neurotransmitters dopamine**, **norepinephrine** (noradrenaline), and **epinephrine** (adrenaline); and the skin **pigment melanin**.*

Affecting the phenylalanine is going to affect how your other hormones work that is influenced by these enzymes. Tryptophan is an enzyme that influences your hunger by influencing enzymes that affect hormones that are influenced by what you eat. This is why your hunger is greater now than it ever was in the past and this is why the obesity epidemic, diabetes epidemic, CVD epidemic, cancer epidemic and dementia epidemics have worsened alongside the increase of glyphosate sprayed on American crops.

That means you must get your calories from healthier sources like fats and protein. These are the foods your body prefers. It can live on carbs but carbs are only supposed to be used in times when we can't get the protein or fat and that's what makes cholesterol so important. Your LDL cholesterol is vital to your survival. If you accumulated this LDL from eating carbs, it's dirty LDL, which is going to leave a residue inside your cells and this is what turns carbs into poison. That residue is what leads to all the modern diseases known to man. If you can cut down on the residue, you can control all disease.

Protein and fat have been the basis of our diet as far back as our species dates. We're not going to change that overnight by converting to a diet of carbs. That's insanity in my opinion. Homo Sapiens went through well over 100,000 years evolving from eating protein and fat, supplementing it with carbs to gradually eating more complex carb such as root vegetables and truly whole grains, as they picked them directly off the stalk and ate them. (This is the only way to get whole grains from these grasses.)

Today, the basis of our diet is carbs and we supplement it with protein and fat. This practice urged on by a grain industry that's interested only in profits and not public health, has proven deadly for all Americans. Since the expansion of the use of Roundup, this practice has become the deadliest practice that anyone can take part in. (Not even the extensive exercise our ancestors had from running all the time could have saved them from the ravages of this weed killer.)

This weed killer has turned into a people killer, through its enzyme inhibiting functions and this is something Monsanto continues to deny. (They've made lying to the public legal, with their placements in the USDA, FDA, EPA and probably the CDC all to ensure their success in carrying out this grandiose ruse that grains are healthy to eat and that you need to eat more of them. Hold on to that thought because we're going to look into why they're pushing this on the public like they are.

Thousands of years ago in our Paleolithic state, we were primarily carnivores. Although we did eat some leafs and tubers, we primarily ate protein and fat in all the game we ate. Our species took close to 90,000 years to cultivate wheat, which we've been eating as a major part of our diet, instead of a minor part, as it had been for those 90,000 years.

This cultivation of wheat was the beginning of modern diseases showing up in our bones after our death. As our consumption grew, so grew the frequency of occurrence and severity of the disease. This is simply the nature of grain food which is ultimately glycating food. Its speed of glycation has grown over the years to the point it's at now, exponentially more than it was just 100 years ago.

This is an inherent problem with carbs, especially this starchy type of carb, grains. Eating carbohydrates have its bad side, and it's called glycation. Protein can't create glycation. Fat can't create glycation. They both need the glucose to do that. That makes glucose a natural toxin that we've been eating for over 10,000 years, only to be ramped up in the last 50 years or so to where the proliferation of its use is now sending hoards of people to their premature deaths. It's also making these same people very sick for extended periods of time before they die. It also makes people sick while they continue to eat, what now are really dirty carbs, due to the glyphosate herbicide sprayed on them as many as four times before they reach your table. Think about that for a minute.

The bread you make your sandwich with is toxic. It's been poisoned right under your nose without your consent, or knowledge, which forces you to need the pharmaceuticals that this same company produces. Who knew that this addiction that's been forced upon you would claim your health with every bite you take?

You should know what addiction this is by now and what you can do about it. What they're selling as safe has escalated death rates from diabetes to brain cancer, from Alzheimer's to atherosclerosis, all evidenced by the rise in cancer rates in the farmers that work with this weed killer.

It's also evidenced by the rise in autism since the start of spraying, 40 years ago. Autism rates climbed steadily for 15 – 20 years from the early 70's when they started using glyphosate, until they too, skyrocketed in the 90's when glyphosate usage multiplied. Now glyphosate is at an all-time high with every rate of modern disease at an all-time high as well.

Yet Monsanto and its industry refuse to acknowledge the true damage they're doing to our society. It's their greed that's driving every pandemic known to modern man. From destroying our health to destroying the environment, Monsanto is leaving quite possibly the largest footprint on our ecosystem, medical system, the pharmaceutical system as well as our agricultural systems and legal/political systems. They've mastered the industrial destruction of mankind and they've done it well from an investor's view. I just wish it could be that well from a consumer's viewpoint.

They have orchestrated legal covert terrorism on an unsuspecting public, by saturating our diets with toxic food, without telling us. What they should have shared with us, was that they were using us as guinea pigs, for their experiment on the impact glyphosate has, on human physiology.

Their experiment has been disastrous for the American people, as well as the world, as glyphosate is breaking records in sales every year, especially since the patent expired 16 years ago. But this isn't supposed to be about glyphosate. This is about the calories you eat and where you get them from. The glyphosate sprayed grains just tells you, not to get your calories from that source as that source is now tainted, severely.

Do you get your calories from a dirty source like carbs or do you get them from efficient foods like protein and fats? Remember where I said that a gram of sugar has 4 calories and that a gram of fat has 9 calories? That only points to the fact that fat is 225% more efficient as a food source. (This is something Monsanto has lied to you, for about 30 years.) With fat being that much more efficient than sugar, it's no wonder that it's that much healthier.

Eating the proper fats feeds your body exactly what it's been running on ever since we've been running as a species. A run we did in our Paleolithic years. We ran all day long, either hunting food, tracking down food, or just running down our food. The funny thing about this is, they were all running on empty stomachs, all day long, and not running out of energy. They could only do this by not eating many carbs. Their bodies had to run on ketones and fat, ramped up by adiponectin and other hormones in their bodies that set their brains to grow. (Many Paleolithic species had larger craniums and brains then we currently do. This is due to their low carb diet and its influence on their growth hormones. Fasting does this also.) The ketogenic diet they were on also does this.

It was this constant practice of exercising every day that made their bodies produce the hormones that allowed them to advance faster than the other species. It was our ability to sweat and cool our bodies that allowed our ancestors to run down their game to feed their families. It was this kind of diet that our bodies ate for 10's of 1,000's for years. Not until the last 60 years or so did we become sedentary and start eating more of what used to take us a half a day of gathering to eat. Most people now get their calories without the gathering or the hunting or the running so they never burn up those calories. They store them. This is the nature of a carbohydrate diet. The same hormone (insulin) instructs the fat it just made to store itself as visceral fat around your midsection until you need it. Your problem is, you seldom need it so it stays as fat.

The bad thing about that is that this fat you just made out of your carbs is going to demand more fat to join it. Fat in your body shuts down the action of leptin, the satiety hormone. When this hormone isn't working right to tell you when to put down your spoon, it's demanding that your body consume more carbs to satisfy it. This leptin resistance leads directly to you needing to eat more and more, just to produce enough leptin to satisfy your addiction. And this is precisely why you should get your calories from protein and a much more efficient fat, rather than carbs. This is a metabolic syndrome, a precursor to diabetes. This is why the keto diet is taking off so much. It's not only a fat burning diet, it's a brain growing, muscle growing diet that truly gives you the best body and brain you can have.

You're probably asking, what kind of fat is good to eat? I've always been told that fat is bad. Until I learned that it isn't at all. It's healthy. Actually, it's very healthy. The industry that told you it was bad had an interest in selling you that idea so you would eat more carbs. They even recommended for you to eat them over the fat. That's because the grain industry is behind the recommendations for what you eat and their interest is in supplying more grains for you to consume.

The healthiest fats to partake of are MCT fats, Medium Chain Triglycerides. They'll balance your cholesterol which is much healthier than just lowering it. Balancing is will actually lower your LDL by increasing your HDL. It's the HDL that cleans out your cells of the spent LDL that's been fed into them. If your body can't clean out the burned LDL out of your cells, the LDL backs up in your blood increasing your overall cholesterol. What could be worse?

Later they found out that a diet of fat won't lead you to any drug use. That's reserved for the carb diet and that may have been why this industry dissuaded everyone from consuming a diet of fat. Just like the sugar industry the grain industry has been lying to the public for greater than 60 years about the safety of their food. Now, they've amplified its danger by dousing it with more and more glyphosate right up until three days before harvest. How safe do you really think that makes the food you eat?

Remember the thought I asked you to hold on to earlier in this article, why Monsanto has been pushing the idea that grains are healthy to eat? The answer to that question is because this is a crop that can be marketed to farmers as making them more money by producing more crop. Yet they need to spread more Roundup, to do this, according to Monsanto. (This is something many farmers don't agree with and are actively trying to resist. Monsanto's push to own every farmer on North American soil has taken many of these farmers to court where Monsanto has tied them up for years at a time, often, to get them to use their own GMO seed.)

This includes Canada where a majority of canola comes from, which happens to come from another Monsanto glyphosated crop. This is another one that they like to spray with Roundup right before harvesting to save the lower oil pods that drop off the crop and shatter losing much of the valuable canola oil. For the farmer, it's Roundup to the rescue. For the consumer, it's Roundup to the dinner table where it can continue its enzyme inhibiting actions in the bodies of your family.

Right after Monsanto patented their first seed in 1980, they purchased GD Searle chemicals, makes NutraSweet in 1985. This was about 14 years after they patented Roundup. Their Roundup has done a bang-up job of bringing the senescence of glyphosate to humans. Roundup is advertised as working through senescence, on how it kills weeds. That senescence is rubbing off on our population. It was 7 years after they patented seeds that they patented Celebrex setting themselves up to be a provider of foods that require an early departure to drugs and a never-ending cycle that never lets up until a premature death. (This makes me think, they'd patent the glycation of America if they could.) This current cycle of disease, disorder, and death goes back to 1954 and the plant act. That's when they made it legal to patent seeds, later leading to genetic modifying of crop seed, later leading to genetically modifying crop seed to survive multiple uses of an enzyme inhibiting herbicide that induces senescence in humans. This is the genetic modifying of humans by modifying their food. This food that gets modified just happens to be an addictive food that's been made more addictive by its modifying. If this isn't criminal, I don't know what is.

To prevent your premature death, look to make fat and protein the core of your diet. You don't have to eat nearly as much, or as often, as it's that dreaded hunger cycle that never appears in the keto diet. That's because of the arguably worst manifestation of a carbohydrate diet is the hunger cycle that's tied to it. I don't know anyone who would agree to that kind of forced behavior. Especially when that hunger gets magnified by what's been sprayed on it multiple times. It's clear to me that the more glyphosate that Monsanto sells, the more disease the public is going to fight. From autism to Alzheimer's, all modern diseases have increased right alongside the increase of glyphosate usage.

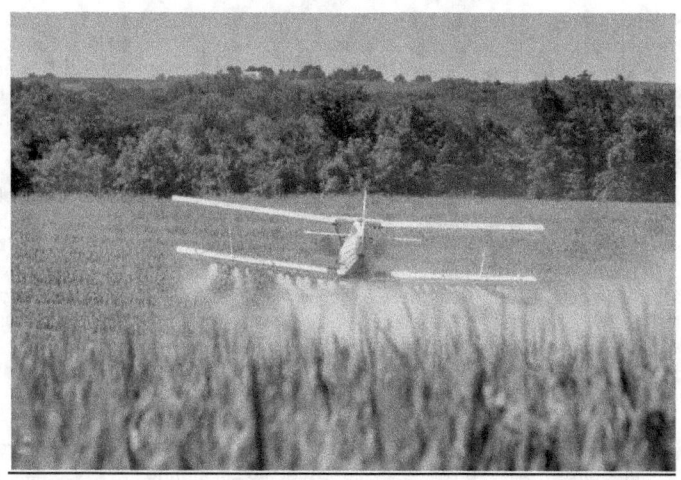

CHAPTER 4

NEW DANGERS OF GRAIN CONSUMPTION DUE TO CONTINUED CONTAMINATION BY GLYPHOSATE HERBICIDES

You know what Roundup is don't you? Would you drink it if you could? Probably not, I least, I wouldn't. Would you eat something that it's been drowned in it? If you knew what it was, you probably wouldn't touch that either.

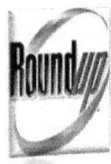 Do you realize that every bite of bread you take, you're eating Roundup, a glyphosate, enzyme inhibiting herbicide? Every corn chip you eat, you're eating glyphosate with it, also. It's in the nature of how this herbicide is used on all the grains it's sprayed on, and how it affects your body when you eat those grains. And you eat those grains every day in massive amounts. That should concern you more than anything else. Everything hinges on your health, if it's not the best, you're not your best.

This is something the food industry doesn't want you to know because it's the warning about genetically modified crop seed that's ready to accept the Roundup herbicide that kills all the weeds that rob the crops of their room to grow. This Roundup is a glyphosate herbicide responsible for inhibiting how enzymes work. That's how it kills weeds. That's also how it makes you sick. That means that the pharmaceutical industry doesn't want you to know either. Their survival depends on your pain, which is dependent on your consumption of these grains. (Monsanto found a way to ramp up that need 30 years ago when they formulated Roundup.) They inhibit enzymes that create senescence in plants. This also creates senescence in your body by inhibiting the same enzymes in your bodies. This has created a far greater need in pharmaceuticals leading to their record profits.

How sick it makes you, depends on how much of it you eat and how fast you eat it. If you eat any of the grains that this herbicide is sprayed on, you will experience future illness. The enzyme inhibiting glyphosate will see to that. The amount you ingest with each bite is so minute that you'll never notice the damage until it's too late. By that time, you'll be a slave to the pharmaceutical industry. Good luck then. Their only goal is to treat you, not cure you. Cures don't guarantee return customers, only treatment can do that.

Glucose, which used to be called glycose, is the sugar form of glycerin or glycerol. (Glycerol is a sweet lipid used for sweetening.) It's healthier than the sugar, because it's slower in satiating, and not as sweet as glucose or fructose, but that's beside the point. The point here is that fat (lipids) is healthier than carbs to eat. This points to why it's better for your body to make its own glucose instead of cholesterol, which is what it does when you feed it carbs and sugar. That's why eating only protein and fat is healthier for the body, as it allows the body to create its own glucose instead of feeding it that dirty glucose you get from carbs. Every time you eat carbs, you're getting dirty glucose at best. It's not only dirty, it's polluted with a carcinogenic glyphosate herbicide, called Roundup.

Farmers spray the Roundup on their crops to kill them, about two weeks before harvest, so they'll dry out quicker. This practice is called desiccating and it's a common practice in northern climates where the environment is a little damper like it is in North Dakota, the nation's largest wheat producer, where this is practiced on a regular basis. This is news that is not good. This news means that a good majority of bread and pasta that you eat has had Roundup sprayed on it within two weeks of harvesting, simply so the harvesting will go quicker. This puts more money in the pockets of farmers due to quicker turnover, but it puts most of the extra cash in Monsanto's pockets by selling more Roundup. It's easy to see now, how 2.6 billion pounds of it were sprayed in the US alone, in the last 20 years. What you need to do is consider how this may affect your health and if there is anything you can do about it.

Roundup, the very same Monsanto-made product which contains the recently-declared carcinogenic chemical glyphosate (along with inert ingredients that are also extremely dangerous), is sprayed on your food just weeks to months before you eat it.

According to Natural Society's website; *Most heavily Glyphosate sprayed grains;*

Which Crops Exactly? Monsanto **recommends spraying for***:*

Wheat, Oats, Non-GMO Canola, Flax, Peas, Lentils, Non-GMO Soybeans,

Dry Beans, Sugar Cane.

*That amounts to just about every grocery store food you can think of – after all, what **DOESN'T** contain wheat, oats, soy, or sugar cane just for starters?*

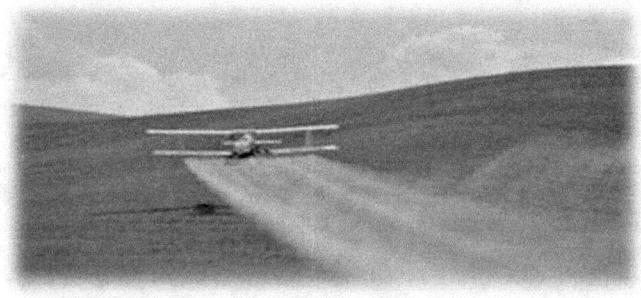

What grains do you eat, cereal grains or legume grains? (Do you like beans like I did. I was raised on them.) It really doesn't matter. They've all doused over and over again with the glyphosate herbicide, Roundup. Do you eat sugar? You should already know how bad sugar is for you. I guess Monsanto didn't think it was bad enough. They want to make it more dangerous. Even cane sugar gets desiccated before harvest. Why?

They claim it's to help farmers. It's really to sell more Roundup. My guess is it has something to do with their involvement in the pharmaceutical industry. Having owned Searle pharmaceuticals and being merged with Pharmacia less than twenty years ago, it leaves little doubt in my mind why they're motivated to continue this deadly ruse. I know where their investments were, so I have a good idea of where they are.

The only unfortunate thing about this ruse is, you're the victim of it by buying into it. That means every time you buy your corn chips, you're buying into this ruse. It's a ruse to control your appetite by controlling your hunger. It's basically pretty simple. Whenever you eat any kind of grain it breaks down to its simplest form in your body, and that's glucose. Glucose regulates your hunger. Glucose does this by controlling your hormones, which in turn, control your emotions, with hunger just being one of them.

What most people don't realize is that hunger is just as much an emotion as fear or anger. Incidentally, fear and anger are both controlled by hunger. So are composure and sobriety. Those emotions are much higher on the tone scale than fear and anger, though. This only shows the danger of the hunger cycle and the emotions it controls.

That all points to the fact that if you can control hunger you can control everything it controls. So how do you control hunger? To control hunger you must control that which creates hunger. There's one thing in your diet that influences hunger more than anything else. That one thing is sugar.

Sugar influences your hunger by playing with your hormones, Leptin and Ghrelin first and foremost. Leptin is your satiety hormone. It tells you when you're full and to stop eating. Ghrelin, on the other hand, is your hunger hormone. It makes your stomach growl when your sugar levels get low. This is the secret to controlling hunger. Control your sugar levels and you can control your hunger. Sounds simple, doesn't it?

It is simple. It's just not that easy. But it's vital to accomplishing this step if you want to control your hunger. That means that you should eliminate as many grain foods as possible for this task to be accomplished. This will have multiple benefits for your health.

1. It will cut down on most all glycation that takes place in your body.
2. It will reduce the number of glyphosate herbicides that you ingest with every bite you take of your bagel, croissant or sandwich. (all sandwiches are contaminated)
3. It will reduce the extra glycation that the glyphosate creates
4. It will keep you off of future drug needs
5. That will save you tons of dollars in medical costs meaning no more;
6. Treatments
7. Therapy
8. Surgery
9. Time wasted in doctors' offices reading magazines that you'd never read in the first place

Don't you have enough things to do? Can you really afford to spend that much time in a doctor's office waiting for treatment or a prescription for your pain? I used to spend half of my day dealing with doctors. Going to the appointment, waiting to see the doctor or therapist at the appointment, then waiting for more at the pharmacy for the prescription I was given to treat my pain. Notice that I mentioned, treat. That's all doctors do anymore. They're there to treat your pain not cure it. Curing it would mean that you wouldn't need their services too much anymore. That's why it's far more lucrative to treat you and not cure you.

This is what I've learned in my 30+ years of treatment for my disabilities and pain. My disabilities were created by a car accident when a drunk driver ran a red light into the car I was riding in. My pain was created by my diet. It was this diet that I had been consuming for most of my life that was at the root of almost all of my pain. That's because I followed what the USDA recommended for our diet. The USDA recommends a diet based on what farmers can provide and not what is healthy to eat and this where the problem with America's pandemics of diabetes, heart disease, cancer and Alzheimer's disease come from.

What initially started out as a problem with glycation has turned into extreme glycation due to

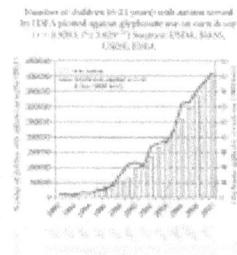

the amounts of glyphosate herbicide sprayed multiple times as ~~ordered~~ recommended by Monsanto for their farmers. As you just read above, they told to spray it just days before harvesting. This ensures that it gets into your food supply, regardless of what you eat, unless you're not eating the grains (cereal or legume). It's these foods that create a lions portion of the glycation, to begin with. Now, Monsanto wants to help that glycation along by forcing the enzyme inhibiting weed killer down your throats.

It's no wonder cancer, diabetes, dementia and all disease involved with inflammation have run rampant for the last 30 years. This also includes Parkinson's as displayed by this graph. This is a graph of the rise in Parkinson's deaths since the use of Roundup started over 40 years ago. Most of the increase has come in the last 20 years since the use of it has spread worldwide.

I hope it's easier to see now, how this industry does not have your best health in mind while growing the food you put on your table, for your family to eat. Now that you know what's at the root of all modern disease that has been plaguing the world ever since we've been eating grains, you also know that it's been amplified exponentially over the last 40 years. Grains which have always thought to be a healthy staple are inherently bad for us. Although they're able to sustain us, they're just as able to shorten our lives by the glycation that they create in the body. Now you know the missing link in this puzzle of why mankind has been plagued by these modern diseases ever since the start of civilization and why those diseases have been ramped up over the last 40 years, and really intensified in the last 20 years.

Monsanto denies this. They have to. Their business plan relies on the public not knowing this information. If the public knew that they were eating poisonous glyphosate herbicide every time they had a corn chip or bagel, or even just their oatmeal in the morning, how long do you think Monsanto's business would continue to thrive?

Here's your first clue to what this food does to you; my health since I quit eating it has improved so much that I experience very little pain now. I never take medication. I never get sick. I always have energy. From the time I get up in the morning (which is a little after sunup) until the time I go to bed (which is always 12 AM – 2 AM). I take very few breaks, if any, once I start working and I don't stop to eat. I pause to make a cup of Hot Chocolate around 8 or 8:30 PM, one of two or three that I'll drink before I go to bed, and then go right back to work, sipping my Hot Chocolate while I work.

Since I started my keto diet 3 years ago, I've lost my hunger cycle along with an expanded stomach that I had to keep full of carbs, just to keep my appetite under control. What I didn't know at that time was that my appetite was never under my control. It was always under the control of the industry that fed me. That's because I followed their advice. That the largest part advice that I followed was to make grains you're doing. But of my diet. So I ate grains every day, just like because I've you still get sick, I don't. I won't get sick broken the habit, the addiction that keeps you from kicking your habit.

This is a habit that's been imposed upon you and not by your choice, consciously. You were inflicted with this addiction when you were an infant and had no control over the food you ate. Too bad your mother didn't know then what she was doing to you, to guarantee your addiction. The food industry knew. That's why there's so much sugar in baby food, formula, and medicine. It's because it satiates so quickly it immediately calms a baby down. Whenever you can quiet a crying baby, it's assumed you're being a good mother. How many "good mothers" have addicted their kids by not knowing?

1. The dangers of sugar
2. The addictive nature of sugar
3. The glycative effects of sugar
4. The addition of Roundup to all sugar

Is this the kind of food you want your baby to eat? It's the kind of food you're eating. This is the kind of food that's giving you headaches and stomach aches. I know. I lived it for close to 60 years. It was imposed on me by my mother. She thought she was feeding me clean healthy food to grow on. It may have been food to grow on, but it wasn't healthy or clean. The clean food factor didn't come around until Monsanto invented their glyphosate herbicide, Roundup. After the emergence of Roundup on the market, modern diseases skyrocketed and have not slowed down since. The rate of these diseases will continue to increase until Roundup is no longer used. (What will happen to the millions of dollars invested in Monsanto when their products are deemed carcinogenic?)

This is why Monsanto can't afford this profitable, yet deadly behavior to discontinue. Their bottom line depends on this ruse continuing and continuing for as long as they can make money off of it. It depends on it, from two angles, from the crop seed side as well as the pharmaceutical side (even though they've supposedly divested themselves of their pharmaceutical holdings). I'm sure they all still have multiple stock options in both industries and if you think that won't influence their decisions, I think, you need to think again.

The use of Roundup is not going to wane as long as Monsanto is making millions of dollars on the sale of it. Over the last 20 years over 2.6 billion lbs of Roundup have been sprayed on U.S. farmland, according to ECOWatch.com With all that herbicide sprayed on your food, how much of do you think you could stay away from? If you eat food from a grocery store or a restaurant, you're eating Roundup with the food you eat. Monsanto makes certain of that. They have for the last 40 years. Are you starting to see the correlation of the addition of the herbicide and the condition of your health?

Whatever glycation these grains create in the first place is magnified by the Roundup that's been sprayed on the crops these foods come from. Your addiction to these crops and their subsequent foods is what's behind the pandemics of cancer, diabetes, heart disease, hypertension, dementia (including Alzheimer's and Parkinson's diseases) and ALL other diseases involved with inflammation. Basically, that means that if you're eating these grains, both cereal and legume, you're subjecting your body to poisons that are not only carcinogenic, they're atherosclerotic and inflammatory, to say the least. If they are even close to being responsible for cancer, I'm not going to chance to eat them ever again. Now I'm really happy I quit and it explains why I've felt so good since I quit. It's easier to understand now why so many people are going ketogenic.

Remember when I mentioned that glyphosate is an enzyme inhibiting chemical that's an active ingredient in Roundup that it's also used as a component in many medicines to make the medicine more effective? This is the legal corporate engineering Monsanto has formulated over the last 30+ years, to take more and more of your money. And it's all for the sake of profits. Health? Well, that's just collateral damage.

Enzyme inhibitors are commonly used in medicine as well. The same enzyme inhibitors that are used in the roundup are also used in some heart medications. (I'll bet if the person knew that the food that this industry gave them to eat for the last 30 years, gave them that food to get them to buy their medicine years later, they would have made better choices when they had the option to.) I've got to hand it to Monsanto, though, in terms of business savvy. This is the ultimate ruse. It's a gargantuan ruse perpetrated on the public without anyone finding out until now.

Now I also know why so much drug use leads to more and more drug use. It's a true

dependence inflicted upon you by Monsanto. First, they addict you to sugar. Then they addict you to the drugs you'll need to fight the pain created by the sugar. Then they'll addict you to a cycle of prescription medication that will continuously create a need for more medication until the cycle ends in premature death. The saddest part of this story is you'll probably never believe it…until you break your addiction. The next saddest part is that you were never told, until now.

The industry has formed its own "*Industry Task Force on Glyphosate*" to disseminate information on how healthy glyphosate is and how much benefit it is to the environment, yet more and more consumers are becoming aware of its inherent dangers. More and more people are waking up to the true poisoning that this enzyme inhibiting herbicide inflicts on the uneducated public.

Isn't it bad enough that the grains they grow glycate proteins and cholesterol? Do they really need to make it more poisonous? It's already at the heart of all major modern disease, isn't that enough? Are they really that greedy that they're willing to poison the whole world to increase their profits, even more? Wouldn't you consider this criminal?

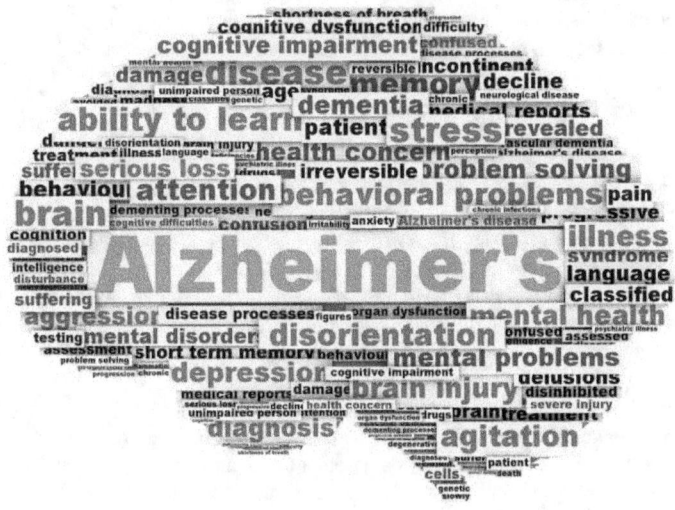

CHAPTER 5

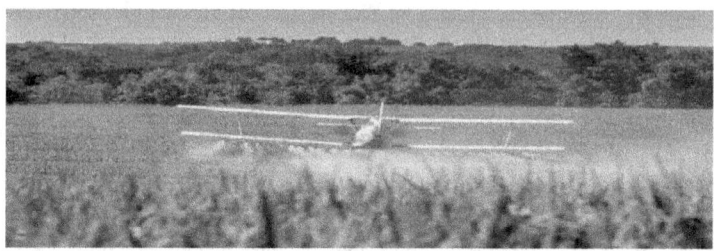

THE GLYPHOSATE POISONING OF AMERICA

Monsanto's Clandestine Chemical Terrorism

Who knew that our greatest terrorist threat would be a clandestine threat from inside our country and it doesn't carry a gun or bomb, or any kind of explosives, for that fact. This threat is a completely hidden threat, making it the worst threat we've ever faced. This threat comes from your diet. It's been forced upon you since you were a baby. This threat comes right from the core of the glucose ruse. This threat **is** the glucose ruse.

It's in something you eat multiple times a day. In all actuality, your hunger cycle is the instrument of your destruction, with this threat. It's your hunger cycle that locks you into the cycle of destruction that glycation is responsible for, as its the glucose that's responsible for all inflammation, which in turn, is responsible for all modern disease. Since it's glucose that's at the heart of all glycation, that puts it at the heart of all inflammation, as well. Being at the heart of inflammation means it's at the heart of all modern disease.

This glycation gets compounded exponentially by an herbicide that gets sprayed on it as a crop, multiple times, as late as two weeks before it's harvested. The herbicide that's widest used in the industry, is glyphosate, patented in 1970 by Monsanto. They lost their patent in 2000, so the *Roundup* brand weed killer can now be sold under any name, making it the widest used herbicide ever. (2.6 billion lbs of glyphosate have been sprayed over the last 20 years.) All of that glyphosate was sprayed on what you eat, meaning if you bought your groceries at a grocery store or ate at a restaurant, you ingested a good portion of what was sprayed.

Glyphosate is an enzyme inhibitor. That's how it works. It works through senescence. Senescence is the science of aging, and that's how these enzyme inhibitors work. They age the weed so fast that it dies within three days. This may be great for the farmer and his crop, but it's having a disastrous effect on your health. This is due to all the glyphosate that's sprayed on these crops over their lifetime. The last time is to desiccate the crop two weeks before harvest. This is done so there's less green seed in the crop, for a better harvest. Green seed isn't good for grinding, as it's too wet.

No crop that I know of gets washed off before it goes to the mill for grinding. That means that you're eating what's just been sprayed on these crops every time you eat any grains that it's been sprayed on. (And it's sprayed on almost all grains. Monsanto is doing as much as they can to own every farmer in the country to distribute these GMO crop seeds too.) Monsanto seems to want to spread as much glyphosate around the world as they possibly can and it's not doing anybody's health any good. Increased rates of heart disease, cancer, and Alzheimer's disease prove this. An increase of autism follows the same line on the same graph for the same amount of years. There is a correlation. Enzyme inhibiting is not conducive to good health. The two don't go together.

All this damage from the enzyme inhibitors in the glyphosate that's done to your hormones, when you eat this food, is no small matter. These hormones are important hormones affecting digestion, hunger, and sleep. (Those are the very same things affected by your diet. also.) Where's the similarity? It's explained in the way it affects its targeted enzymes, like tyrosine, tryptophan, and phenylalanine. These are all enzymes that influence your hunger, digestion and sleep hormones. If you have problems in any of these areas, this is your answer why.

It involves your consumption of glyphosate. (I'll bet you didn't know that, did you?) Would you eat it in the first place, if you knew? You probably would because you've been addicted to what they spray this substance on, without even knowing it. This was literally done right under your nose, when you were fed, as a baby. The industry makes certain that this substance gets into most all baby food. This ensures that you have no choice in this addiction. It ensures your lifetime of compliance in feeding the addiction. It also guarantees your compliance in the second half of the glucose ruse, the need for pharmaceuticals for the greatest portion of your life.

This is displayed in all these graphs below, as the increase of glyphosate usage mirrors the increase in disease. Are you one of these statistics? If you eat bread, I'm afraid you will be, if you're not now.

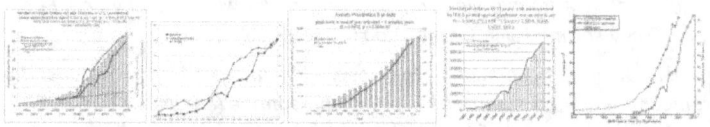

Targeted enzymes that influence the senescence of plants also influence the senescence of your body. They are important enzymes your body uses for digestion, sleep and controlling hunger;

Glyphosate is absorbed through foliage, and minimally through roots, and transported to growing points. It inhibits a plant enzyme involved in the synthesis of three aromatic amino acids: tyrosine, tryptophan, and phenylalanine. Therefore, it is effective only on actively growing plants and is not effective as a pre-emergence herbicide. An increasing number of crops have been genetically engineered to be tolerant of glyphosate (e.g. Roundup Ready soybean, the first Roundup Ready crop, also created by Monsanto) which allows farmers to use glyphosate as a post-emergence herbicide against weeds. The development of glyphosate resistance in weed species is emerging as a costly problem. While glyphosate and formulations such as Roundup have been approved by regulatory bodies worldwide, concerns about their effects on humans and the environment persist. Many regulatory and scholarly reviews have evaluated the relative toxicity of glyphosate as an herbicide. The German Federal Institute for Risk Assessment toxicology review in 2013 found that "the available data is contradictory and far from being convincing" with regard to correlations between exposure to glyphosate formulations and risk of various cancers, including non-Hodgkin lymphoma (NHL). A meta-analysis published in 2014 identified an increased risk of NHL in workers exposed to glyphosate formulations. In March 2015 the World Health Organization's International Agency for Research on Cancer classified glyphosate as "probably carcinogenic in humans" (category 2A) based on epidemiological studies, animal studies, and in vitro

*In November 2015, the **European Food Safety Authority** published an updated assessment report on glyphosate, concluding that "the substance is unlikely to be **genotoxic** (i.e. damaging to **DNA**) or to pose a **carcinogenic** threat to humans." Furthermore, the final report clarified that while other, probably carcinogenic, glyphosate-containing formulations may exist, studies "that look solely at the active substance glyphosate do not show this effect. In May 2016, the Joint FAO/WHO Meeting on Pesticide Residues concluded that "glyphosate is unlikely to pose a carcinogenic risk to humans from exposure through the diet", even at doses as high as 2,000 mg/kg body weight orally.*

These targeted enzymes are important for digestion and hunger

1Tyrosine *influences hunger by controlling enzymes that control how receptors react to stimuli that control your hunger. Tyrosine is a precursor to Dopamine, your primary hormone influencing hunger. This is the hormone triggered by leptin, your satiety hormone. If it takes more leptin to trigger the dopamine, it's going to take more food to trigger the leptin. Was this engineered intentionally?*

2Tryptophan *is also a precursor to serotonin and melatonin. Serotonin is another feel-good hormone that's affected by glyphosate. Melatonin is the hormone that allows you to sleep, without it, you're going to have trouble sleeping. Is it no wonder why so many people suffer from insomnia now? (They sell medicine for that, don't they?)*

3Phenylalanine *Phenylalanine is a precursor to **tyrosine**; the **monoamine neurotransmitters dopamine, norepinephrine** (noradrenaline), and **epinephrine** (adrenaline); and the skin **pigment melanin**. That was according to Wikipedia. All of those enzymes influence your hunger.*

The WHO has finally recognized glyphosate as a **GROUP 2 CARCINOGEN**, meaning that it probably causes cancer. We know that it affects your sleep, hunger, and digestion, let's see if these chemicals can be responsible for cancer. The evidence for this lies in the multiple graphs showing the increase of glyphosate increasing right alongside the increase of multiple disorders and disease, including autism.

Monsanto's Roundup Ruse

In Monsanto's desire to spread as much of this on the earth as possible, they're poisoning every bit of food you eat, unless you grow your own and raise and butcher your own. All forage for feed is sprayed multiple times, maybe even more than the grain used for your bread. Cattle slaughtered for beef, never live long enough to get cancer, yet it goes into their food supply. 1,8 billion lbs in 20 years have been dumped on your food supplies. Ultimately, it goes into your body in multiple avenues, increasing the amount you consume, thereby increasing the number of enzyme inhibitors affecting your health. This has brought the pharmaceutical industry record profits, not to mention what it's brought Monsanto and their crop seed companies, pharmaceutical companies, and chemical wing of their manufacturing. Monsanto has engineered clandestine distemper on our health without us even knowing or approving of it.

It's not been good for the unsuspecting public who are still condemned to eating this food to feed their addiction as evidenced by these studies from PMC;

Glyphosate, pathways to modern diseases III: Manganese, neurological diseases, and associated pathologies

Glyphosate is a likely cause of the recent epidemic of celiac disease. Glyphosate residues are found in wheat due to the increasingly widespread practice of staging and desiccation of wheat right before harvest. Many of the pathologies associated with celiac disease can be explained by disruption of CYP enzymes. Celiac patients have a shortened life span, mainly due to an increased risk to cancer, most especially non-Hodgkin's lymphoma, which has also been linked to glyphosate. Celiac disease trends over time match well with the increase in glyphosate usage on wheat crops.

Glyphosate is also neurotoxic. Its mammalian metabolism yields two products: Aminomethylphosphonic acid (AMPA) and glyoxylate, with AMPA being at least as toxic as glyphosate. Glyoxylate is a highly reactive glycating agent, which will disrupt the function of multiple proteins in cells that are exposed. Glycation has been directly implicated in Parkinson's disease (PD). Glyphosate has been detected in the brains of malformed piglets. In a report produced by the Environmental Protection Agency (EPA), over 36% of 271 incidences involving acute glyphosate poisoning involved neurological symptoms, indicative of glyphosate toxicity in the brain and nervous system.

In the remainder of this paper, we first introduce the link between glyphosate and manganese (Mn) dysbiosis and briefly describe the main biological roles of Mn. We then describe how glyphosate's disruption of gut bacteria may be a major player in the recent epidemic of antibiotic resistance. We then explain how glyphosate can influence the uptake of arsenic and aluminum, and propose similar mechanisms at work with Mn. In the next section, we describe how Mn deficiency can lead to a reduction in Lactobacillus in the gut, and we link this to anxiety disorder. We follow with a discussion on mitochondrial dysfunction associated with suppressed Mn superoxide dismutase (Mn-SOD), and then a section on implications of Mn deficiency for oxalate metabolism. The following section explains how Mn deficiency can lead to the overexpression of ammonia and glutamate in many neurological diseases. The next two sections show how Mn accumulation in the liver is linked to cholestasis and high serum low-density lipoprotein (LDL), and how this can also induce increased susceptibility to Salmonella poisoning. We then identify a role for Mn in chondroitin sulfate synthesis and the implications for osteomalacia. The next two sections explain how glyphosate exposure can lead to Mn toxicity in the brain, and discuss two neurological diseases that are associated with excess Mn, PD and prion diseases. After a section on the link between male infertility and Mn deficiency in the testes, we discuss evidence of exposure to glyphosate and end with a short summary of our findings.

The report goes on to detail how this herbicide is involved in suppressing dopamine which leads to an overactive thyroid. It's also involved in ;

1. MICROBIAL ANTIBIOTIC INTOLERANCE

Manganese (Mn) is an often overlooked but important nutrient, required in small amounts for multiple essential functions in the body. A recent study on cows fed genetically modified Roundup®-Ready feed revealed a severe depletion of serum Mn. Glyphosate, the active ingredient in Roundup®, has also been shown to severely deplete Mn levels in plants. Here, we investigate the impact of Mn on physiology, and its association with gut dysbiosis as well as neuropathologies such as autism, Alzheimer's disease (AD), depression, anxiety syndrome, Parkinson's disease (PD), and prion diseases. Glutamate overexpression in the brain in association with autism, AD, and other neurological diseases can be explained by Mn deficiency. Mn superoxide dismutase protects mitochondria from oxidative damage, and mitochondrial dysfunction is a key feature of autism and Alzheimer's. Chondroitin sulfate synthesis depends on Mn, and its deficiency leads to osteoporosis and osteomalacia. Lactobacillus, depleted in autism, depend critically on Mn for antioxidant protection. Lactobacillus probiotics can treat anxiety, which is a comorbidity of autism and chronic fatigue syndrome. Reduced gut Lactobacillus leads to overgrowth of the pathogen, Salmonella, which is resistant to glyphosate toxicity, and Mn plays a role here as well. Sperm motility depends on Mn, and this may partially explain increased rates of infertility and birth defects. We further reason that, under conditions of adequate Mn in the diet, glyphosate, through its disruption of bile acid homeostasis, ironically promotes toxic accumulation of Mn in the brainstem, leading to conditions such as PD and prion diseases.

2. MANGANESE DYSBIOSIS DUE TO GLYPHOSATE

Remarkably, Mn deficiency can explain many of the pathologies associated with autism and Alzheimer's disease (AD). The incidence of both of these conditions has been increasing at an alarming rate in the past two decades, in step with the increased usage of glyphosate on corn and soy crops in the United States, as shown in Figures

3. ANALOGY WITH ARSENIC AND ALUMINUM

Chronic kidney disease is clearly associated with multiple environmental toxicants. There has been an epidemic in recent years in kidney failure among young agricultural workers in Central America, India, and Sri Lanka, particularly those working in the sugar cane fields. A recent paper reached the unmistakable conclusion that glyphosate plays a critical role in this epidemic. A growing practice of spraying sugar cane with glyphosate as a ripener and desiccant right before the harvest has led to much greater exposure to the workers in the fields. The authors, who focused their studies on affected workers in rice paddies in Sri Lanka, identified a synergistic effect of arsenic, which contaminated the soil in the affected regions. This paper is highly significant because it proposes a mechanism whereby glyphosate greatly increases the toxicity of arsenic through chelation, which promotes uptake by the gut. Glyphosate also depletes glutathione (GSH) and glutathione S transferase (GST) is a critical enzyme for liver detoxification of arsenic. As a consequence, excess arsenic in the kidney causes acute kidney failure, without evidence of other symptoms such as diabetes usually preceding kidney failure.

4. ANALOGY WITH ARSENIC AND ALUMINUM
5. MN-SUPEROXIDE DISMUTASE AND MITOCHONDRIAL DYSFUNCTION

6. *GUT BACTERIA DYSBIOSIS AND ANXIETY*
7. *AMMONIA, GLUTAMATE, AND NEUROTOXICITY*

In this section, we will show that both glutamate and ammonia are implicated as neurotoxins in connection with autism and other neurological diseases, and we will offer the simple explanation that Mn deficiency leads to impaired activity of glutamine synthase and arginase, both of which utilize Mn as a cofactor. Mn deficiency can also explain the increased risk of epilepsy found in autism, due to the fact that Mn decreases T2 relaxation time. Mn-deprived rats are more susceptible to convulsions.

Many diseases and conditions are currently on the rise in step with glyphosate usage in agriculture, particularly on GM crops of corn and soy. These include autism, AD, PD, anxiety disorder, osteoporosis, inflammatory bowel disease, renal lithiasis, osteomalacia, cholestasis, thyroid dysfunction, and infertility. All of these conditions can be substantially explained by the dysregulation of Mn utilization in the body due to glyphosate.

It may seem implausible that glyphosate could be toxic to humans, given the fact that government regulators appear nonchalant about steadily increasing residue limits, and that the levels in food and water are rarely monitored by government agencies, presumably due to lack of concern. However, a paper by Antoniou ET AL. provided a scathing indictment of the European regulatory process regarding glyphosate's toxicity, focusing on potential teratogenic effects. They identified several key factors leading to a tendency to overlook potential toxic effects. These include using animal studies that are too short or have too few animals to achieve statistical significance, disregarding IN VITRO studies or studies with exposures that are higher than what is expected to be realistically present in food, and discarding studies that examine the effects of glyphosate formulations rather than pure glyphosate, even though formulations are a more realistic model of the natural setting and are often orders of magnitude more toxic than the active ingredient in pesticides. Regulators also seemed unaware that chemicals that act as endocrine disruptors (such as glyphosate often have an inverted dose-response relationship, wherein very low doses can have more acute effects than higher doses. Teratogenic effects have been demonstrated in human cell lines. An IN VITRO study showed that glyphosate in parts per trillion can induce human breast cancer cell proliferation.

8. PARKINSON'S DISEASE

9. PRION DISEASES

10. OSTEOMALACIA AND ARTHRITIS

This is only a partial list of what this herbicide is responsible for. Visit the link at the head of this section for the full story. You should visit it, if only for your health's concern. This just points out the fact that what you eat has more impact on your health than anything else. It would be nice if you could get away from it, but you can't. The pollution is everywhere you go for food. You have to produce your own food to be completely free from this curse.

It's cursing you not only through the grains you eat but through the damage done to feed crops, contaminating beef, pork, chicken, turkey and even dairy cows, poisoning even the cheese, milk and butter you buy. The only way you can get around this ruse is to grow your own food and raise and butcher your own meat. Monsanto has every other path sewn up, tighter than a drum. To eat grains is to court death. It's become that simple. These reports from PubMed give you an idea of what over 150 other reports say;

Celiac disease, and, more generally, gluten intolerance, is a growing problem worldwide, but especially in North America and Europe, where an estimated 5% of the population now suffers from it. Symptoms include nausea, diarrhea, skin rashes, macrocytic anemia, and depression. It is a multifactorial disease associated with numerous nutritional deficiencies as well as reproductive issues and increased risk to thyroid disease, kidney failure, and cancer. Here, we propose that glyphosate, the active ingredient in the herbicide, Roundup®, is the most important causal factor in this epidemic. Fish exposed to glyphosate develop digestive problems that are reminiscent of celiac disease. Celiac disease is associated with imbalances in gut bacteria that can be fully explained by the known effects of glyphosate on gut bacteria. Characteristics of celiac disease point to impairment in many cytochrome P450 enzymes, which are involved with detoxifying environmental toxins, activating vitamin D3, catabolizing vitamin A, and maintaining bile acid production and sulfate supplies to the gut. Glyphosate is known to inhibit cytochrome P450 enzymes. Deficiencies in iron, cobalt, molybdenum, copper and other rare metals associated with celiac disease can be attributed to glyphosate's strong ability to chelate these elements. Deficiencies in tryptophan, tyrosine, methionine, and selenomethionine associated with celiac disease match glyphosate's known depletion of these amino acids. Celiac disease patients have an increased risk of non-Hodgkin's lymphoma, which has also been implicated in glyphosate exposure. Reproductive issues associated with celiac diseases, such as infertility, miscarriages, and birth defects, can also be explained by glyphosate. Glyphosate residues in wheat and other crops are likely increasing recently due to the growing practice of crop desiccation just prior to the harvest. We argue that the practice of "ripening" sugar cane with glyphosate may explain the recent surge in kidney failure among agricultural workers in Central America. We conclude with a plea to governments to reconsider policies regarding the safety of glyphosate residues in foods.

GUT BACTERIA

We then show that glyphosate is associated with an overgrowth of pathogens along with an inflammatory bowel disease in animal models. A parallel exists with celiac disease where the bacteria that are positively and negatively affected by glyphosate are overgrown or underrepresented respectively in association with celiac disease in humans.

CYP ENZYME IMPAIRMENT AND SULFATE DEPLETION

RETINOIC ACID, CELIAC DISEASE, AND REPRODUCTIVE ISSUES

ANEMIA AND IRON

Glyphosate's chelating action can have profound effects on iron in plants. Glyphosate interferes with iron assimilation in both glyphosate-resistant and glyphosate-sensitive soybean crops. It is therefore conceivable that glyphosate's chelation of iron is responsible for the refractory iron deficiency present in celiac disease.

MOLYBDENUM DEFICIENCY

SELENIUM AND THYROID DISORDERS

INDOLE AND KIDNEY DISEASE

NUTRITIONAL DEFICIENCIES

Glyphosate disrupts the synthesis of tryptophan and tyrosine in plants and in gut bacteria, due to its interference with the shikimate pathway, which is its main source of toxicity to plants. Glyphosate also depletes methionine in plants and microbes. A study on serum tryptophan levels in children with celiac disease revealed that untreated children had significantly lower ratios of tryptophan to large neutral amino acids in the blood, and treated children also had lower levels, but the imbalance was less severe.

Cancer

Chronic inflammation, such as occurs in celiac disease, is a major source of oxidative stress and is estimated to account for 1/3 of all cancer cases worldwide. Oxidative stress leads to DNA damage and increased risk of a genetic mutation. Several population-based studies have confirmed that patients with celiac disease suffer from increased mortality, mainly due to malignancy. These include increased the risk to non-Hodgkin's lymphoma, adenocarcinoma of the small intestine, and squamous cell carcinomas of the esophagus, mouth, and pharynx, as well as melanoma. The non-Hodgkin's lymphoma was not restricted to gastrointestinal sites, and the increased risk remained following a gluten-free diet.

Proposed transglutaminase-glyphosate interactions

Evidence of glyphosate exposure in humans and animals

Kidney disease in agricultural workers

In another study in the PMC database of over 164 studies done on this subject;

Republished study: long-term toxicity of a Roundup herbicide and a Roundup-tolerant genetically modified maize

Biochemical analyses confirmed very significant chronic kidney deficiencies, for all treatments and both sexes; 76% of the altered parameters were kidney-related. In treated males, liver congestions and necrosis were 2.5 to 5.5 times higher. Marked and severe nephropathies were also generally 1.3 to 2.3 times greater. In females, all treatment groups showed a two- to threefold increase in mortality, and deaths were earlier. This difference was also evident in three male groups fed with GM maize. All results were hormone- and sex-dependent, and the pathological profiles were comparable. Females developed large mammary tumors more frequently and before controls; the pituitary was the second most disabled organ; the sex hormonal balance was modified by consumption of GM maize and Roundup treatments. Males presented up to four times more large palpable tumors starting 600 days earlier than in the control group, in which only one tumor was noted. These results may be explained by not only the non-linear endocrine-disrupting effects of Roundup but also by the overexpression of the EPSPS transgene or other mutational effects in the GM maize and their metabolic consequences.

Our findings show that the differences in multiple organ functional parameters seen from the consumption of NK603 GM maize for 90 days escalated over 2 years into severe organ damage in all types of test diets. This included the lowest dose of R administered (0.1 ppb, 50 ng/L G equivalent) of R formulation administered, which is well below permitted MRLs in both the USA (0.7 mg/L) and European Union (100 ng/L). Surprisingly, there was also a clear trend in increased tumor incidence, especially mammary tumors in female animals, in a number of the treatment groups. Our data highlight the inadequacy of 90-day feeding studies and the need to conduct long-term (2 years) investigations to evaluate the life-long impact of GM food consumption and exposure to complete pesticide formulations.

Tumors are reported in line with the requirements of OECD chronic toxicity protocols 452 and 453, which require all 'lesions' (which by definition include tumors) to be reported. These findings are summarized in Figure 4. The results are presented in the form of real-time cumulative curves (each step corresponds to an additional tumor in the group). Only the growing largest palpable growths (above a diameter of 17.5 mm in females and 20 mm in males) are presented (for example, see Figure 5A, B, C). These were found to be in 95% of cases non-regressive tumors (Figure 5D, E, F, G, H, I, J) and were not infectious nodules. These arose from time to time; then, most often disappeared and were not different from controls after bacterial analyses. The real tumors were recorded independently of their grade, but dependent on their morbidity, since non-cancerous tumors can be more lethal than those of cancerous nature, due to internal hemorrhaging or compression and obstruction of the function of vital organs, or toxins or hormone secretions. These tumors progressively increased in size and number, but not proportionally to the treatment dose, over the course of the experiment (Figure 4). As in the case of rates of mortality (Figure 6), this suggests that a threshold in effect was reached at the lower doses. Tumor numbers were rarely equal but almost always more than in controls for all treated groups, often with a two- to threefold increase for both sexes. Tumors began to reach a large size on average 94 days before controls in treated females and up to 600 days earlier in two male groups fed with GM maize (11 and 22% with or without R).

Glyphosate formulations induce apoptosis and necrosis in human umbilical, embryonic, and placental cells.

We have evaluated the toxicity of four glyphosates *(G)-based herbicides in Roundup formulations, from 10(5) times dilutions, on three different human cell types. This dilution level is far below agricultural recommendations and corresponds to low levels of residues in food or feed. The formulations have been compared to G alone and with its main metabolite AMPA or with one known adjuvant of R formulations, POEA. HUVEC primary neonate umbilical cord vein cells have been tested with 293 embryonic kidney and JEG3 placental cell lines. All R formulations cause total cell death within 24 h, through an inhibition of the mitochondrial succinate dehydrogenase activity, and necrosis, by the release of cytosolic adenylate kinase measuring membrane damage. They also induce apoptosis via activation of enzymatic caspases 3/7 activity. This is confirmed by characteristic DNA fragmentation, nuclear shrinkage (pyknosis), and nuclear fragmentation (karyorrhexis), which is demonstrated by DAPI in apoptotic round cells. G provokes only apoptosis, and HUVEC is 100 times more sensitive overall at this level. The deleterious effects are not proportional to G concentrations but rather depend on the nature of the adjuvants. AMPA and POEA separately and synergistically damage cell membranes like R but at different concentrations. Their mixtures are generally even more harmful to G. In conclusion, the R adjuvants like POEA change human cell permeability and amplify toxicity induced already by G, through apoptosis and necrosis. The real threshold of G toxicity must take into account the presence of adjuvants but also G metabolism and time-amplified effects or bioaccumulation. This should be discussed when analyzing the in vivo toxic actions of R. This work clearly confirms that the adjuvants in Roundup formulations are not inert. Moreover, the proprietary mixtures available on the market could cause cell damage and even death around residual levels to be expected, especially in food and feed derived from R formulation-treated crops.*

This poses a major question in my mind; can the target in this ruse, be you and your money? It's obvious what the end result is and that's displayed in the record profits of the pharmaceutical industry. The more disease caused by this herbicide, the more medicine the pharmaceutical industry sells. Monsanto owns the crop seed companies. They own the chemical company that produces the herbicide, and they used to own the pharmaceutical corporations, so they're profiting much more than two or three times in this ruse. It's that simple. They're making money off of your ignorance of the facts. They've withheld information that's vital to your health. They've outright lied to you to keep you in the dark. They don't want you to know this information. The only blessing here is that we don't have to eat it. We can say no to glyphosate by not eating any grains, including sugar.

Only you can control this transformation of your health, this travesty of justice. Only you can say no to the grains that this herbicide poisons. It's your choice to remain a slave to Monsanto or be free. All you have to do is to give up the grains.

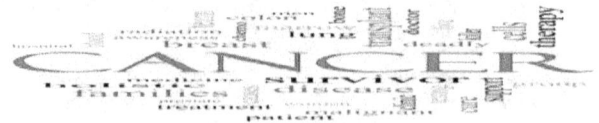

Your Carb Diet Brings This Destruction,

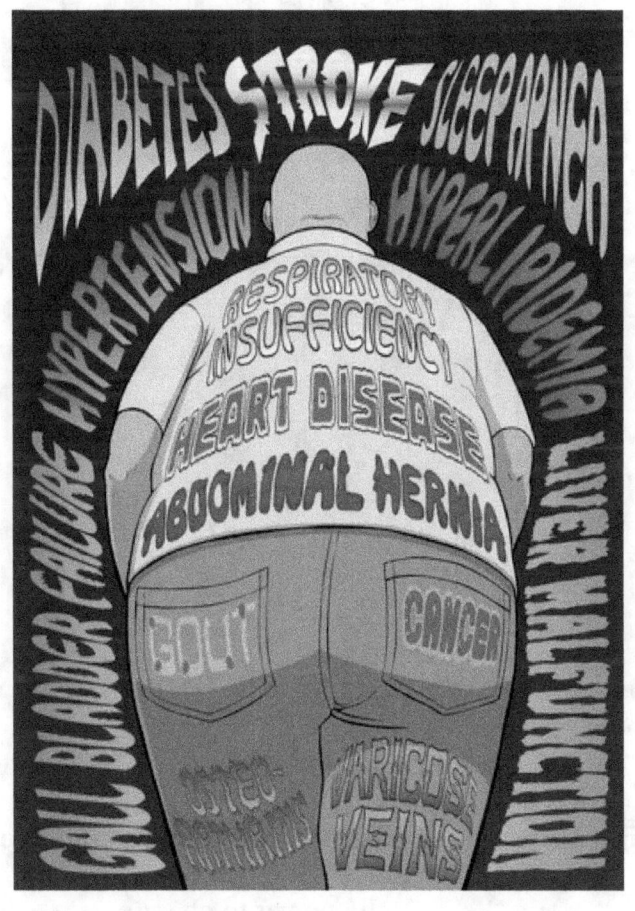

Unless You Change the Pattern,

Your Poison Will Pick You

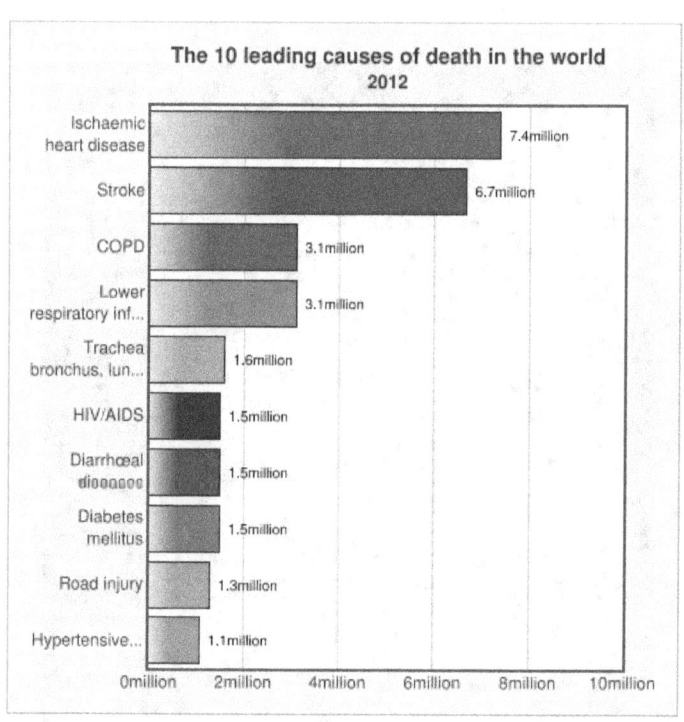

The 10 leading causes of death in the world 2012

Ischaemic heart disease	7.4million
Stroke	6.7million
COPD	3.1million
Lower respiratory inf...	3.1million
Trachea bronchus, lun...	1.6million
HIV/AIDS	1.5million
Diarrhœal diseases	1.5million
Diabetes mellitus	1.5million
Road injury	1.3million
Hypertensive...	1.1million

0million   2million   4million   6million   8million   10million

7 of the above 10 causes of death are a direct result of ECC, Excessive Carbohydrate Consumption, something you have the power to change.

CHAPTER 6

THE GRAIN INDUSTRY'S RUSE TO FEED YOU DISEASE

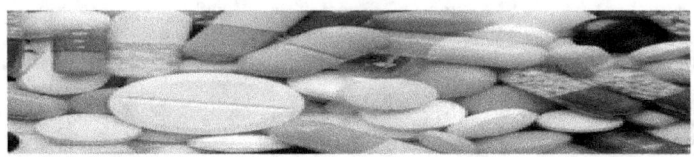

My father disposed of a 1 gallon Ziploc bag full of these drugs after my mother died - $921,324.83 worth.

This is a matter of your health being engineered without your knowledge or consent. The engineering, in this case, is not good. Actually, it's creating pain where none should exist. Our food supply industry may be the most important industry concerned when it comes to our health. As everyone knows, 'you are what you eat', so it's vital that what you eat won't make you sick. Unfortunately, for those who still masturbate their taste buds with their addiction to sugar, this couldn't be further from the truth. Our food supply has been hijacked by the same industry that treats you for the illness their food supplies. Granted the healthcare industry is vital to our health, but I submit that it wouldn't be as important as it is today if we paid more attention to what we eat.

Because I now watch what I eat, I can change the "we" to "you", meaning "you" have to watch what you eat. (All that means is that you still have an addiction to break, I don't, I broke mine three years ago.) Because of this addiction, you've doomed yourself unwittingly to a lifetime of medications. That is unless you're one of the .05% who shows no ill effects from glycation. I have yet to meet one of them. If you eat at a restaurant or buy groceries at a grocery store, you're subject to this addiction. It's in their food everywhere you look. You actually look for it because you love to eat it. You love their advertising. What's not to love, it's full of attractive people selling you what appears to provide health, but in all reality provides nothing but the opposite, as it's responsible for most all pain, most all disease, all brain damage, all atherosclerosis, all diseases affiliated with inflammation, and this is just for starters.

Monsanto has politically engineered their dominance of your food supply and subsequent health by forcing as many farmers as they can to use Monsanto's seed companies' GMO seed to grow their crops. Monsanto has many seed companies. Their control over the seed industry was mirrored by their control over the pharmaceutical industry because they could use the seed companies to influence the profits of their drug companies. Monsanto owns 15 crop seed companies all selling GMO seed for their contracted farmers to grow. Five of these companies sell seed for wheat crops. That's the seed that grows the wheat that's ground into flour for your bread and crackers.

Their contracted farmers have to grow Monsanto's GMO seed at risk of facing legal action if caught growing anything else. This is how Monsanto controls what goes on your table to eat. This is also how Monsanto forces you into purchasing the ***CELEBREX***, made by Searle Pharmaceuticals. Searle had been part of Monsanto from 1985 – 2003 when it was sold to Pfizer along with the rest of Pharmacia. The Celebrex is what your doctor prescribes for your arthritis that's caused by the glycation set up from the grain diet you've been on all your life. After you get arthritis that you will inevitably get from eating their GMO grains, you'll be begging your doctor for that prescription for the Celebrex.

Then you'll get to deal with the side effects of the Celebrex that it inevitably presents to the body. That's the damage to your body from the drug side of their industry. The damage from the crop seed side includes crops that are not only GMO seed, they are laden with Roundup, the glyphosate herbicide that works by inhibiting enzymes from doing what they supposed to do by instructing cells how to operate. Even though Monsanto claims that these enzyme inhibitors affect only targeted enzymes, the rise in cancer alone, that the nation has seen since the mid to late 80's, has told a completely different story.

The rise in these disorders is directly caused by an increase in the glycation that occurs in the blood by the high glucose laden grains this company forces their farmers to grow. That means that the food going on your table is engineered to make you need the medications that the pharmaceutical companies sell. This makes me wonder if a hidden clause in their merger is forcing Monsanto to provide customers for their old pharmaceutical companies. I know you haven't considered the possibility, but I would suggest that you do, your health is at risk. (It's probably many clauses in many contracts involving stock options.) That's the only thing I can think of that could drive this behavior for the USDA and the FDA.

According to Wikipedia; *"In December 1997 Monsanto merged with Pharmacia and Upjohn. The agricultural division became a wholly owned subsidiary of the "new" Pharmacia; Monsanto's medical research division, which included products such as Celebrex."*

Searle and Pharmacia were the other sides of Monsanto's multinational chemical companies that includes Upjohn as well. Searle merged with Monsanto in 1985 two years after Monsanto started dabbling in GMO crops. In 1993 Searle filed for a patent for Celebrex, its widely used arthritis drug. I'll bet you didn't know that it is Monsanto's seed companies that force their contracted farmers to grow GMO seed designed to make you need their Celebrex. Is this what you thought you were buying when you bought those corn chips last time? Was this what you thought you were buying when you purchased those pretzels?

Whether or not it was, that's what you got. You also got all the rest of the damage that glycation does to the body, which includes atherosclerosis, cancer, and dementia as well. You're also subjecting yourself to the hunger cycle, probably the worst manifestation of a carb diet. The more carbs you eat, the hungrier you get. That's a cycle that can't be broken if you don't stop the fuel that feeds it. Stopping the fuel is the only way to stop the glycation. That means that it's the only way to stop the inflammation, which means it's the only way to stop the illness and disorder that glycation is responsible for.

The following studies are available on the National Library of Medicine's *PubMed.gov*, out of 11,750 studies at last check.

This study done on glycative effects and Alzheimer's disease was completed in 2005. Glycation of cholesterol into amyloid plaque was researched in this study. It showed that the plaque was responsible for Alzheimer's disease. Where were the warnings then? It's now 15 years later and millions of people have died from Alzheimer's disease. The question I ask is why? Why weren't we notified of this revelation 14 years ago? It's been in the archives of PubMed since then. Why the delay? How much more must die before this news of the glycative effects of glucose, is publicized so that the FDA and the USDA have to recognize its dangers?

This report from Sep 20, 2005, explains how the plaques from glycation contribute to Alzheimer's disease;

- **5-aminoimidazole-4-carboxamide-1-beta-4-ribofuranoside (AICAR) attenuates the expression of LPS- and Aβ peptide-induced inflammatory mediators in astroglia. J Biol Chem. 1985 Sep 5;260(19):10629-36.**

Alzheimer's disease (AD) pathology shows characteristic 'plaques' rich in amyloid beta (Aβ) peptide deposits. Inflammatory process-related proteins such as pro-inflammatory cytokines have been detected in AD brain suggesting that an inflammatory immune reaction also plays a role in the pathogenesis of AD.

Alzheimer's disease (AD) is a neurological disorder and the brain pathology is characterized by the presence of senile plaques rich in insoluble aggregates of beta-amyloid (1–40) and (1–42) peptides, degradation products of the larger amyloid precursor protein. All major pro-inflammatory cytokines with the exception of IFN-γ (TNF-α, IL-1, and IL-6) have been detected in AD brain suggesting that an inflammatory immune reaction also plays a role in the pathogenesis of AD. The deposited Aβ peptides have also been implicated in oxidative stress-induced responses, via NADPH oxidase activation and superoxide anion generation.

This has been known for more than 11 years, yet nobody knows about it except for a few researchers. Fewer are trying to disseminate this info.

This study done on the effects of glucose on glycation was done in September 1985. Have you seen or heard of any part of this report prior to today? I haven't. I had to search for it. The question I have is why wasn't the public notified of this revelation? Were the research results suppressed so as to hide the truth from the public? I have to wonder.

- *Glycation of amino groups in protein. Studies on the specificity of modification of RNase by glucose.*

Watkins NG, Thorpe SR, Baynes JW.

Ribonuclease A has been used as a model protein for studying the specificity of glycation of amino groups in protein under physiological conditions (phosphate buffer, pH 7.4, 37 degrees C). Incubation of RNase with glucose led to an enhanced rate of inactivation of the enzyme relative to the rate of modification of lysine residues, suggesting a preferential modification of active site lysine residues...Both the equilibrium Schiff base concentration and the rate of the Amadori rearrangement at each site were found to be important in determining the specificity of glycation of RNase.

This means that around 1985, they were learning about the effects of glycation, yet an industry that depends on this action to feed their customer base in the pharmaceutical industry, was doing what it could to keep these reports from becoming public information.

About this same time, according to Wikipedia;

In 1985, Monsanto acquired G. D. Searle & Company, a life sciences company focusing on pharmaceuticals, agriculture and animal health. In 1993, its Searle division filed a patent application for Celebrex, which is 1998 became the first selective COX-2 inhibitor to be approved by the U.S. Food and Drug Administration (FDA). Celebrex became a blockbuster drug and was often mentioned as a key reason for Pfizer's acquisition of Monsanto's pharmaceutical business in 2002.

Was it coincidence? I have to wonder. Since then, Monsanto has made moves to control all of the grain industry in America, by contracting farmers to grow no other seed than their own GMO seed. This allows the farmers who do this to spray massive amounts of herbicides on those crops. The herbicide they spray is Monsanto's Roundup, a glyphosate herbicide that works by inhibiting the actions of enzymes. Enzymes are important proteins and peptides in the body as they're cell signaling proteins that instruct cells how to operate. This is important because it's that instruction that the cells need to *NOT BECOME GLYCATION.*

Otherwise, without that enzyme, you create glycation and inflammation. Inflammation is the foundation of all modern diseases. This is why grains are slowly killing those who eat them, cutting their lives short, to the tune of 2,684 deaths every day can be attributed to these killing field grains. These signaling cells are cells like hormones and polypeptides that affect your body's functions. If these aren't working because of an enzyme inhibitor floating around in your blood, it's going to lead to glycation and disease. This is the scary part of this story if you eat bread or anything flour is used in, you're eating this herbicide along with your bread. If you use canola oil or eat corn chips when you go out for Mexican food, you're putting this glyphosate herbicide in your body. It's used on **ALL** corn products, **ALL** soy products. Monsanto removed GMO wheat seeds from the European market due to restrictions on GMO foods there. One this side of the pond, there are no restrictions. Pretty much everything you eat is grown from GMO, Roundup ready seed.

This study was completed in September 1985. That was about the same time Monsanto acquired G.D. Searle Pharmaceuticals. 8 years later they filed for a patent for Celebrex their arthritis painkiller drug. Celebrex is a Cox 2 NSAID with the following side effects and concerns, according to Searle, and I'm listing all of them. (16 pages worth); If you take this drug, read this disclaimer well.

CONTRAINDICATIONS

NSAIDS MAY BE USED WITH CAUTION BY PEOPLE WITH THE FOLLOWING CONDITIONS:

IRRITABLE BOWEL SYNDROME

- *PERSONS WHO ARE OVER AGE 50, AND WHO HAVE A FAMILY HISTORY OF GI (GASTROINTESTINAL) PROBLEMS*
- *PERSONS WHO HAVE HAD PAST GI PROBLEMS FROM NSAID USE*

NSAIDS SHOULD USUALLY BE AVOIDED BY PEOPLE WITH THE FOLLOWING CONDITIONS:

- *PEPTIC ULCER STOMACH BLEEDING*
- *UNCONTROLLED HYPERTENSION*
- *KIDNEY DISEASE*
- *PEOPLE THAT SUFFER FROM INFLAMMATORY BOWEL DISEASE (CROHN'S DISEASE OR ULCERATIVE COLITIS)[6]*
- *PAST TRANSIENT ISCHEMIC ATTACK(EXCLUDING IBUPROFEN)*
- *PAST STROKE(EXCLUDING IBUPROFEN)*
- *PAST MYOCARDIAL INFARCTION(EXCLUDING IBUPROFEN)[6]*
- *CORONARY ARTERY DISEASE(EXCLUDING IBUPROFEN)[6]*
- *UNDERGOING CORONARY ARTERY BYPASS SURGERY[6]*
- *TAKING IBUPROFEN FOR HEART*
- *CONGESTIVE HEART FAILURE(EXCLUDING LOW-DOSE IBUPROFEN)*
- *IN THE THIRD TRIMESTER OF PREGNANCY*
- *PERSONS WHO HAVE UNDERGONE GASTRIC BYPASS SURGERY*

- *PERSONS WHO HAVE A HISTORY OF ALLERGIC OR ALLERGIC-TYPE NSAID HYPERSENSITIVITY REACTIONS, E.G. ASPIRIN-INDUCED ASTHMA*

ADVERSE EFFECTS

THE WIDESPREAD USE OF NSAIDS HAS MEANT THAT THE ADVERSE EFFECTS OF THESE DRUGS HAVE BECOME INCREASINGLY COMMON. USE OF NSAIDS INCREASES RISK OF HAVING A RANGE OF GASTROINTESTINAL(GI) PROBLEMS. WHEN NSAIDS ARE USED FOR PAIN MANAGEMENT AFTER SURGERY THEY CAUSE INCREASED RISK OF KIDNEY PROBLEMS. AN ESTIMATED 10–20% OF NSAID PATIENTS EXPERIENCE DYSPEPSIA. IN THE 1990S HIGH DOSES OF PRESCRIPTION NSAIDS WERE ASSOCIATED WITH SERIOUS UPPER GASTROINTESTINAL ADVERSE EVENTS, INCLUDING BLEEDING. OVER THE PAST DECADE, DEATHS ASSOCIATED WITH GASTRIC BLEEDING HAVE DECLINED.

NSAIDS, LIKE ALL DRUGS, MAY INTERACT WITH OTHER MEDICATIONS. FOR EXAMPLE, CONCURRENT USE OF NSAIDS AND QUINOLONES MAY INCREASE THE RISK OF QUINOLONES' ADVERSE CENTRAL NERVOUS SYSTEM EFFECTS, INCLUDING SEIZURE.

THERE IS ARGUMENT OVER THE BENEFITS AND RISKS OF NSAIDS FOR TREATING CHRONIC MUSCULOSKELETAL PAIN. EACH DRUG HAS A BENEFIT-RISK PROFILE AND BALANCING THE RISK OF NO TREATMENT WITH THE COMPETING POTENTIAL RISKS OF VARIOUS THERAPIES IS THE CLINICIAN'S RESPONSIBILITY.

COMBINATIONAL RISK

IF A COX-2 INHIBITOR IS TAKEN, A TRADITIONAL NSAID (PRESCRIPTION OR OVER-THE-COUNTER) SHOULD NOT BE TAKEN AT THE SAME TIME. IN ADDITION, PEOPLE ON DAILY ASPIRIN THERAPY (E.G., FOR REDUCING CARDIOVASCULAR RISK) MUST BE CAREFUL IF THEY ALSO USE OTHER NSAIDS, AS THESE MAY INHIBIT THE CARDIOPROTECTIVE EFFECTS OF ASPIRIN.

ROFECOXIB (VIOXX) WAS SHOWN TO PRODUCE SIGNIFICANTLY FEWER GASTROINTESTINAL ADVERSE DRUG REACTIONS (ADRS) COMPARED WITH NAPROXEN. THIS STUDY, THE VIGOR TRIAL, RAISED THE ISSUE OF THE CARDIOVASCULAR SAFETY OF THE COXIBS. A STATISTICALLY SIGNIFICANT INCREASE IN THE INCIDENCE OF MYOCARDIAL INFARCTIONS WAS OBSERVED IN PATIENTS ON ROFECOXIB. FURTHER DATA, FROM THE APPROVE TRIAL, SHOWED A STATISTICALLY SIGNIFICANT RELATIVE RISK OF CARDIOVASCULAR EVENTS OF 1.97 VERSUS PLACEBO WHICH CAUSED A WORLDWIDE WITHDRAWAL OF ROFECOXIB IN OCTOBER 2004.

USE OF METHOTREXATE TOGETHER WITH NSAIDS IN RHEUMATOID ARTHRITIS IS SAFE IF ADEQUATE MONITORING IS DONE.

CARDIOVASCULAR

NSAIDS ASIDE FROM ASPIRIN, BOTH NEWER SELECTIVE COX-2 INHIBITORS AND TRADITIONAL ANTI-INFLAMMATORIES, INCREASE THE RISK OF MYOCARDIAL INFARCTION AND STROKE. THEY ARE NOT RECOMMENDED IN THOSE WHO HAVE

HAD A PREVIOUS HEART ATTACK AS THEY INCREASE THE RISK OF DEATH AND/OR RECURRENT MI. EVIDENCE INDICATES THAT NAPROXEN MAY BE THE LEAST HARMFUL OUT OF THESE.

NSAIDS ASIDE FROM (LOW-DOSE) ASPIRIN ARE ASSOCIATED WITH A DOUBLED RISK OF HEART FAILURE IN PEOPLE WITHOUT A HISTORY OF CARDIAC DISEASE. FOR PEOPLE WITH SUCH A HISTORY, USE OF NSAIDS (ASIDE FROM LOW-DOSE ASPIRIN) WAS ASSOCIATED WITH A MORE THAN 10-FOLD INCREASE IN HEART FAILURE. IF THIS LINK IS PROVEN CAUSAL, RESEARCHERS ESTIMATE THAT NSAIDS WOULD BE RESPONSIBLE FOR UP TO 20 PERCENT OF HOSPITAL ADMISSIONS FOR CONGESTIVE HEART FAILURE. FOR PEOPLE WITH HEART FAILURE, NSAIDS INCREASE MORTALITY RISK (HAZARD RATIO) BY APPROXIMATELY 1.2–1.3 FOR NAPROXEN AND IBUPROFEN, 1.7 FOR ROFECOXIB AND CELECOXIB, AND 2.1 FOR DICLOFENAC.

ON 9 JULY 2015, THE FDA TOUGHENED WARNINGS OF INCREASED HEART ATTACK AND STROKE RISK ASSOCIATED WITH NONSTEROIDAL ANTI-INFLAMMATORY DRUGS (NSAID). ASPIRIN IS AN NSAID BUT IS NOT AFFECTED BY THE NEW WARNINGS.

POSSIBLE ERECTILE DYSFUNCTION RISK

A 2005 FINNISH STUDY LINKED LONG TERM (OVER 3 MONTHS) USE OF NSAIDS WITH AN INCREASED RISK OF ERECTILE DYSFUNCTION. THIS STUDY WAS CORRELATIONAL ONLY AND DEPENDED SOLELY ON SELF-REPORTS (QUESTIONNAIRES).

A 2011 PUBLICATION IN THE JOURNAL OF UROLOGY RECEIVED WIDESPREAD PUBLICITY. ACCORDING TO THIS STUDY, MEN WHO USED NSAIDS REGULARLY WERE AT SIGNIFICANTLY INCREASED RISK OF ERECTILE DYSFUNCTION. A LINK BETWEEN NSAID USE AND ERECTILE DYSFUNCTION STILL EXISTED AFTER CONTROLLING FOR SEVERAL CONDITIONS. HOWEVER, THE STUDY WAS OBSERVATIONAL AND NOT CONTROLLED, WITH LOW ORIGINAL PARTICIPATION RATE, POTENTIAL PARTICIPATION BIAS, AND OTHER UNCONTROLLED FACTORS. THE AUTHORS WARNED AGAINST DRAWING ANY CONCLUSION REGARDING CAUSE.

GASTROINTESTINAL

THE MAIN ADVERSE DRUG REACTIONS (ADRS) ASSOCIATED WITH NSAID USE RELATE TO DIRECT AND INDIRECT IRRITATION OF THE GASTROINTESTINAL (GI) TRACT. NSAIDS CAUSE A DUAL ASSAULT ON THE GI TRACT: THE ACIDIC MOLECULES DIRECTLY IRRITATE THE GASTRIC MUCOSA, AND INHIBITION OF COX-1 AND COX-2 REDUCES THE LEVELS OF PROTECTIVE PROSTAGLANDINS. INHIBITION OF PROSTAGLANDIN SYNTHESIS IN THE GI TRACT CAUSES INCREASED GASTRIC ACID SECRETION, DIMINISHED BICARBONATE SECRETION, DIMINISHED MUCUS SECRETION AND DIMINISHED TROPHIC [EFFECTS ON EPITHELIAL MUCOSA. COMMON GASTROINTESTINAL ADRS INCLUDE

- *NAUSEA/VOMITING*
- *DYSPEPSIA*
- *GASTRIC ULCERATION/BLEEDING*

- *DIARRHEA*

CLINICAL NSAID ULCERS ARE RELATED TO THE SYSTEMIC EFFECTS OF NSAID ADMINISTRATION. SUCH DAMAGE OCCURS IRRESPECTIVE OF THE ROUTE OF ADMINISTRATION OF THE NSAID (E.G., ORAL, RECTAL, OR PARENTERAL) AND CAN OCCUR EVEN IN PATIENTS WITH ACHLORHYDRIA.

ULCERATION RISK INCREASES WITH THERAPY DURATION, AND WITH HIGHER DOSES. TO MINIMISE GI ADRS, IT IS PRUDENT TO USE THE LOWEST EFFECTIVE DOSE FOR THE SHORTEST PERIOD OF TIME—A PRACTICE THAT STUDIES SHOW IS OFTEN NOT FOLLOWED. RECENT STUDIES SHOW THAT OVER 50% OF PATIENTS WHO TAKE NSAIDS HAVE SUSTAINED SOME MUCOSAL DAMAGE TO THEIR SMALL INTESTINE.

THERE ARE ALSO SOME DIFFERENCES IN THE PROPENSITY OF INDIVIDUAL AGENTS TO CAUSE GASTROINTESTINAL ADRS. INDOMETHACIN, KETOPROFEN, AND PIROXICAM APPEAR TO HAVE THE HIGHEST PREVALENCE OF GASTRIC ADRS, WHILE IBUPROFEN (LOWER DOSES) AND DICLOFENAC, APPEAR TO HAVE LOWER RATES.

CERTAIN NSAIDS, SUCH AS ASPIRIN, HAVE BEEN MARKETED IN ENTERIC-COATED FORMULATIONS THAT MANUFACTURERS CLAIM REDUCE THE INCIDENCE OF GASTROINTESTINAL ADRS. SIMILARLY, SOME BELIEVE THAT RECTAL FORMULATIONS MAY REDUCE GASTROINTESTINAL ADRS. HOWEVER, CONSISTENT WITH THE SYSTEMIC MECHANISM OF SUCH ADRS, AND IN CLINICAL PRACTICE, THESE FORMULATIONS HAVE NOT DEMONSTRATED A REDUCED RISK OF GI ULCERATION.

COMMONLY, GASTRIC (BUT NOT NECESSARILY INTESTINAL) ADVERSE EFFECTS CAN BE REDUCED THROUGH SUPPRESSING ACID PRODUCTION, BY CONCOMITANT USE OF A PROTON PUMP INHIBITOR, E.G., OMEPRAZOLE, ESOMEPRAZOLE; OR THE PROSTAGLANDIN ANALOGUE MISOPROSTOL. MISOPROSTOL IS ITSELF ASSOCIATED WITH A HIGH INCIDENCE OF GASTROINTESTINAL ADRS (DIARRHEA). WHILE THESE TECHNIQUES MAY BE EFFECTIVE, THEY ARE EXPENSIVE FOR MAINTENANCE THERAPY.

INFLAMMATORY BOWEL DISEASE

NSAIDS SHOULD BE USED WITH CAUTION IN INDIVIDUALS WITH INFLAMMATORY BOWEL DISEASE (E.G., CROHN'S DISEASE OR ULCERATIVE COLITIS) DUE TO THEIR TENDENCY TO CAUSE GASTRIC BLEEDING AND FORM ULCERATION IN THE GASTRIC LINING. PAIN RELIEVERS SUCH AS PARACETAMOL (ALSO KNOWN AS ACETAMINOPHEN) OR DRUGS CONTAINING CODEINE (WHICH SLOWS DOWN BOWEL ACTIVITY) ARE SAFER MEDICATIONS FOR PAIN RELIEF IN IBD.

RENAL

NSAIDS ARE ALSO ASSOCIATED WITH A FAIRLY HIGH INCIDENCE OF RENAL ADVERSE DRUG REACTIONS (ADRS). THE MECHANISM OF THESE RENAL ADRS IS DUE TO CHANGES IN RENAL HAEMODYNAMICS (KIDNEY BLOOD FLOW), ORDINARILY MEDIATED BY PROSTAGLANDINS, WHICH ARE AFFECTED BY NSAIDS. PROSTAGLANDINS NORMALLY CAUSE VASODILATION OF THE AFFERENT

ARTERIOLES OF THE GLOMERULI. THIS HELPS MAINTAIN NORMAL GLOMERULAR PERFUSION AND GLOMERULAR FILTRATION RATE (GFR), AN INDICATOR OF RENAL FUNCTION. THIS IS PARTICULARLY IMPORTANT IN RENAL FAILURE WHERE THE KIDNEY IS TRYING TO MAINTAIN RENAL PERFUSION PRESSURE BY ELEVATED ANGIOTENSIN II LEVELS. AT THESE ELEVATED LEVELS, ANGIOTENSIN II ALSO CONSTRICTS THE AFFERENT ARTERIOLE INTO THE GLOMERULUS IN ADDITION TO THE EFFERENT ARTERIOLE IT NORMALLY CONSTRICTS. PROSTAGLANDINS SERVE TO DILATE THE AFFERENT ARTERIOLE; BY BLOCKING THIS PROSTAGLANDIN-MEDIATED EFFECT, PARTICULARLY IN RENAL FAILURE, NSAIDS CAUSE UNOPPOSED CONSTRICTION OF THE AFFERENT ARTERIOLE AND DECREASED RPF (RENAL PERFUSION PRESSURE).

COMMON ADRS ASSOCIATED WITH ALTERED RENAL FUNCTION INCLUDE:

- SALT (SODIUM) AND FLUID RETENTION
- HYPERTENSION(HIGH BLOOD PRESSURE)

THESE AGENTS MAY ALSO CAUSE RENAL IMPAIRMENT, ESPECIALLY IN COMBINATION WITH OTHER NEPHROTOXIC AGENTS. RENAL FAILURE IS ESPECIALLY A RISK IF THE PATIENT IS ALSO CONCOMITANTLY TAKING AN ACE INHIBITOR (WHICH REMOVES ANGIOTENSIN II'S VASOCONSTRICTION OF THE EFFERENT ARTERIOLE) AND A DIURETIC (WHICH DROPS PLASMA VOLUME, AND THEREBY RPF)—THE SO-CALLED "TRIPLE WHAMMY" EFFECT.

IN RARER INSTANCES NSAIDS MAY ALSO CAUSE MORE SEVERE RENAL CONDITIONS:

- INTERSTITIAL NEPHRITIS
- NEPHROTIC SYNDROME
- ACUTE RENAL FAILURE
- ACUTE TUBULAR NECROSIS
- RENAL PAPILLARY NECROSIS

NSAIDS IN COMBINATION WITH EXCESSIVE USE OF PHENACETINAND/OR PARACETAMOL (ACETAMINOPHEN) MAY LEAD TO ANALGESIC NEPHROPATHY.

PHOTOSENSITIVITY

PHOTOSENSITIVITY IS A COMMONLY OVERLOOKED ADVERSE EFFECT OF MANY OF THE NSAIDS. THE 2-ARYLPROPIONIC ACIDS ARE THE MOST LIKELY TO PRODUCE PHOTOSENSITIVITY REACTIONS, BUT OTHER NSAIDS HAVE ALSO BEEN IMPLICATED INCLUDING PIROXICAM, DICLOFENAC, AND BENZYDAMINE.

BENOXAPROFEN, SINCE WITHDRAWN DUE TO ITS HEPATOTOXICITY, WAS THE MOST PHOTOACTIVE NSAID OBSERVED. THE MECHANISM OF PHOTOSENSITIVITY, RESPONSIBLE FOR THE HIGH PHOTOACTIVITY OF THE 2-ARYLPROPIONIC ACIDS, IS THE READY DECARBOXYLATION OF THE CARBOXYLIC ACID MOIETY. THE SPECIFIC ABSORBANCE CHARACTERISTICS OF THE DIFFERENT CHROMOPHORIC 2-ARYL SUBSTITUENTS, AFFECTS THE DECARBOXYLATION MECHANISM.

WHILE IBUPROFEN HAS WEAK ABSORPTION, IT HAS BEEN REPORTED AS A WEAK PHOTOSENSITISING AGENT.

DURING PREGNANCY

NSAIDS ARE NOT RECOMMENDED DURING PREGNANCY, PARTICULARLY DURING THE THIRD TRIMESTER. WHILE NSAIDS AS A CLASS IS NOT DIRECT TERATOGENS, THEY MAY CAUSE PREMATURE CLOSURE OF THE FETAL DUCTUS ARTERIOSUS AND RENAL ADRS IN THE FETUS. ADDITIONALLY, THEY ARE LINKED TO PREMATURE BIRTH AND MISCARRIAGE. ASPIRIN, HOWEVER, IS USED TOGETHER WITH HEPARIN IN PREGNANT WOMEN WITH ANTIPHOSPHOLIPID ANTIBODIES. ADDITIONALLY, INDOMETHACIN IS USED IN PREGNANCY TO TREAT POLYHYDRAMNIOS BY REDUCING FETAL URINE PRODUCTION VIA INHIBITING FETAL RENAL BLOOD FLOW.

BY CONTRAST, PARACETAMOL (ACETAMINOPHEN) IS REGARDED AS BEING SAFE AND WELL-TOLERATED DURING PREGNANCY, BUT LEFFERS ET AL. RELEASED A STUDY IN 2010 INDICATING THAT THERE MAY BE ASSOCIATED MALE INFERTILITY IN THE UNBORN. DOSES SHOULD BE TAKEN AS PRESCRIBED, DUE TO RISK OF HEPATOTOXICITY WITH OVERDOSES. IN FRANCE, THE COUNTRY'S HEALTH AGENCY CONTRAINDICATES THE USE OF NSAIDS, INCLUDING ASPIRIN, AFTER THE SIXTH MONTH OF PREGNANCY.

ALLERGY/ALLERGY-LIKE HYPERSENSITIVITY REACTIONS

A VARIETY OF ALLERGIC OR ALLERGIC-LIKE NSAID HYPERSENSITIVITY REACTIONS FOLLOW THE INGESTION OF NSAIDS. THESE HYPERSENSITIVITY REACTIONS DIFFER FROM THE OTHER ADVERSE REACTIONS LISTED HERE WHICH ARE TOXICITY REACTIONS, I.E. UNWANTED REACTIONS THAT RESULT FROM THE PHARMACOLOGICAL ACTION OF A DRUG, ARE DOSE-RELATED, AND CAN OCCUR IN ANY TREATED INDIVIDUAL; HYPERSENSITIVITY REACTIONS ARE IDIOSYNCRATIC REACTIONS TO A DRUG.[51] SOME NSAID HYPERSENSITIVITY REACTIONS ARE TRULY ALLERGIC IN ORIGIN: 1) REPETITIVE IGE-MEDIATED URTICARIAL SKIN ERUPTIONS, ANGIOEDEMA, AND ANAPHYLAXIS FOLLOWING IMMEDIATELY TO HOURS AFTER INGESTING ONE STRUCTURAL TYPE OF NSAID BUT NOT AFTER INGESTING STRUCTURALLY UNRELATED NSAIDS; AND 2) COMPARATIVELY MILD TO MODERATELY SEVERE T CELL-MEDIATED DELAYED ONSET (USUALLY MORE THAN 24 HOUR), SKIN REACTIONS SUCH AS MACULOPAPULAR RASH, FIXED DRUG ERUPTIONS, PHOTOSENSITIVITY REACTIONS, DELAYED URTICARIA, AND CONTACT DERMATITIS; OR 3) FAR MORE SEVERE AND POTENTIALLY LIFE-THREATENING T-CELL MEDIATED DELAYED SYSTEMIC REACTIONS SUCH AS THE DRESS SYNDROME, ACUTE GENERALIZED EXANTHEMATOUS PUSTULOSIS, THE STEVENS–JOHNSON SYNDROME, AND TOXIC EPIDERMAL NECROLYSIS. OTHER NSAID HYPERSENSITIVITY REACTIONS ARE ALLERGY-LIKE SYMPTOMS BUT DO NOT INVOLVE TRUE ALLERGIC MECHANISMS; RATHER, THEY APPEAR DUE TO THE ABILITY OF NSAIDS TO ALTER THE METABOLISM OF ARACHIDONIC ACID IN FAVOR OF FORMING METABOLITES THAT PROMOTE ALLERGIC SYMPTOMS. AFFLICTED INDIVIDUALS MAY BE ABNORMALLY SENSITIVE TO THESE PROVOCATIVE METABOLITES AND/OR OVERPRODUCE THEM AND TYPICALLY ARE SUSCEPTIBLE TO A WIDE RANGE OF STRUCTURALLY DISSIMILAR NSAIDS, PARTICULARLY THOSE THAT INHIBIT COX1. SYMPTOMS, WHICH DEVELOP IMMEDIATELY TO HOURS AFTER INGESTING ANY OF VARIOUS NSAIDS THAT INHIBIT COX-1, ARE: 1) EXACERBATIONS OF ASTHMATIC AND RHINITIS (SEE ASPIRIN-INDUCED ASTHMA) SYMPTOMS IN

INDIVIDUALS WITH A HISTORY OF ASTHMA OR RHINITIS AND 2) EXACERBATION OR FIRST-TIME DEVELOPMENT OF WHEALS AND/OR ANGIOEDEMA IN INDIVIDUALS WITH OR WITHOUT A HISTORY OF CHRONIC URTICARIAL LESIONS OR ANGIOEDEMA.

CONTRAINDICATIONS

NSAIDS MAY BE USED WITH CAUTION BY PEOPLE WITH THE FOLLOWING CONDITIONS

- *IRRITABLE BOWEL SYNDROME*
- *PERSONS WHO ARE OVER AGE 50, AND WHO HAVE A FAMILY HISTORY OF GI (GASTROINTESTINAL) PROBLEMS*
- *PERSONS WHO HAVE HAD PAST GI PROBLEMS FROM NSAID USE*

NSAIDS SHOULD USUALLY BE AVOIDED BY PEOPLE WITH THE FOLLOWING CONDITIONS

- *PEPTIC ULCER OR STOMACH BLEEDING*
- *UNCONTROLLED HYPERTENSION*
- *KIDNEY DISEASE*
- *PEOPLE THAT SUFFER FROM INFLAMMATORY BOWEL DISEASE (CROHN'S DISEASE OR ULCERATIVE COLITIS)*
- *PAST TRANSIENT ISCHEMIC ATTACK (EXCLUDING IBUPROFEN)*
- *PAST STROKE (EXCLUDING IBUPROFEN)*
- *PAST MYOCARDIAL INFARCTION (EXCLUDING IBUPROFEN)*
- *CORONARY ARTERY DISEASE(EXCLUDING IBUPROFEN)*
- *UNDERGOING CORONARY ARTERY BYPASS SURGERY*
- *TAKING IBUPROFEN FOR HEART*
- *CONGESTIVE HEART FAILURE(EXCLUDING LOW-DOSE IBUPROFEN)*
- *IN THE THIRD TRIMESTER OF PREGNANCY*
- *PERSONS WHO HAVE UNDERGONE GASTRIC BYPASS SURGERY*
- *PERSONS WHO HAVE A HISTORY OF ALLERGIC OR ALLERGIC-TYPE NSAID HYPERSENSITIVITY REACTIONS, E.G. ASPIRIN-INDUCED ASTHMA*

ADVERSE EFFECTS

THE WIDESPREAD USE OF NSAIDS HAS MEANT THAT THE ADVERSE EFFECTS OF THESE DRUGS HAVE BECOME INCREASINGLY COMMON. USE OF NSAIDS INCREASES RISK OF HAVING A RANGE OF GASTROINTESTINAL(GI) PROBLEMS. WHEN NSAIDS ARE USED FOR PAIN MANAGEMENT AFTER SURGERY THEY CAUSE INCREASED RISK OF KIDNEY PROBLEMS.

AN ESTIMATED 10–20% OF NSAID PATIENTS EXPERIENCE DYSPEPSIA. IN THE 1990S HIGH DOSES OF PRESCRIPTION NSAIDS WERE ASSOCIATED WITH SERIOUS UPPER GASTROINTESTINAL ADVERSE EVENTS, INCLUDING BLEEDING. OVER THE PAST DECADE, DEATHS ASSOCIATED WITH GASTRIC BLEEDING HAVE DECLINED.

NSAIDS, LIKE ALL DRUGS, MAY INTERACT WITH OTHER MEDICATIONS. FOR EXAMPLE, CONCURRENT USE OF NSAIDS AND QUINOLONES MAY INCREASE THE

RISK OF QUINOLONES' ADVERSE CENTRAL NERVOUS SYSTEM EFFECTS, INCLUDING SEIZURE.

THERE IS ARGUMENT OVER THE BENEFITS AND RISKS OF NSAIDS FOR TREATING CHRONIC MUSCULOSKELETAL PAIN. EACH DRUG HAS A BENEFIT-RISK PROFILE AND BALANCING THE RISK OF NO TREATMENT WITH THE COMPETING POTENTIAL RISKS OF VARIOUS THERAPIES IS THE CLINICIAN'S RESPONSIBILITY.

COMBINATIONAL RISK

IF A COX-2 INHIBITOR IS TAKEN, A TRADITIONAL NSAID (PRESCRIPTION OR OVER-THE-COUNTER) SHOULD NOT BE TAKEN AT THE SAME TIME. IN ADDITION, PEOPLE ON DAILY ASPIRIN THERAPY (E.G., FOR REDUCING CARDIOVASCULAR RISK) MUST BE CAREFUL IF THEY ALSO USE OTHER NSAIDS, AS THESE MAY INHIBIT THE CARDIOPROTECTIVE EFFECTS OF ASPIRIN.

ROFECOXIB (VIOXX) WAS SHOWN TO PRODUCE SIGNIFICANTLY FEWER GASTROINTESTINAL ADVERSE DRUG REACTIONS (ADRS) COMPARED WITH NAPROXEN. THIS STUDY, THE VIGOR TRIAL, RAISED THE ISSUE OF THE CARDIOVASCULAR SAFETY OF THE COXIBS. A STATISTICALLY SIGNIFICANT INCREASE IN THE INCIDENCE OF MYOCARDIAL INFARCTIONS WAS OBSERVED IN PATIENTS ON ROFECOXIB. FURTHER DATA, FROM THE APPROVE TRIAL, SHOWED A STATISTICALLY SIGNIFICANT RELATIVE RISK OF CARDIOVASCULAR EVENTS OF 1.97 VERSUS PLACEBO WHICH CAUSED A WORLDWIDE WITHDRAWAL OF ROFECOXIB IN OCTOBER 2004.

 USE OF METHOTREXATE TOGETHER WITH NSAIDS IN RHEUMATOID ARTHRITIS IS SAFE IF ADEQUATE MONITORING IS DONE.

CARDIOVASCULAR

NSAIDS ASIDE FROM ASPIRIN, BOTH NEWER SELECTIVE COX-2 INHIBITORS AND TRADITIONAL ANTI-INFLAMMATORIES, INCREASE THE RISK OF MYOCARDIAL INFARCTION AND STROKE. THEY ARE NOT RECOMMENDED IN THOSE WHO HAVE HAD A PREVIOUS HEART ATTACK AS THEY INCREASE THE RISK OF DEATH AND/OR RECURRENT MI. EVIDENCE INDICATES THAT NAPROXEN MAY BE THE LEAST HARMFUL OUT OF THESE.

NSAIDS ASIDE FROM (LOW-DOSE) ASPIRIN ARE ASSOCIATED WITH A DOUBLED RISK OF HEART FAILURE IN PEOPLE WITHOUT A HISTORY OF CARDIAC DISEASE. FOR PEOPLE WITH SUCH A HISTORY, USE OF NSAIDS (ASIDE FROM LOW-DOSE ASPIRIN) WAS ASSOCIATED WITH A MORE THAN 10-FOLD INCREASE IN HEART FAILURE. IF THIS LINK IS PROVEN CAUSAL, RESEARCHERS ESTIMATE THAT NSAIDS WOULD BE RESPONSIBLE FOR UP TO 20 PERCENT OF HOSPITAL ADMISSIONS FOR CONGESTIVE HEART FAILURE. FOR PEOPLE WITH HEART FAILURE, NSAIDS INCREASE MORTALITY RISK (HAZARD RATIO) BY APPROXIMATELY 1.2–1.3 FOR NAPROXEN AND IBUPROFEN, 1.7 FOR ROFECOXIB AND CELECOXIB, AND 2.1 FOR DICLOFENAC.

ON 9 JULY 2015, THE FDA TOUGHENED WARNINGS OF INCREASED HEART ATTACK AND STROKE RISK ASSOCIATED WITH NONSTEROIDAL ANTI-

INFLAMMATORY DRUGS (NSAID). ASPIRIN IS AN NSAID BUT IS NOT AFFECTED BY THE NEW WARNINGS.

POSSIBLE ERECTILE DYSFUNCTION RISK

A 2005 FINNISH STUDY LINKED LONG TERM (OVER 3 MONTHS) USE OF NSAIDS WITH AN INCREASED RISK OF ERECTILE DYSFUNCTION. THIS STUDY WAS CORRELATIONAL ONLY AND DEPENDED SOLELY ON SELF-REPORTS (QUESTIONNAIRES).

A 2011 PUBLICATION IN THE JOURNAL OF UROLOGY RECEIVED WIDESPREAD PUBLICITY. ACCORDING TO THIS STUDY, MEN WHO USED NSAIDS REGULARLY WERE AT SIGNIFICANTLY INCREASED RISK OF ERECTILE DYSFUNCTION. A LINK BETWEEN NSAID USE AND ERECTILE DYSFUNCTION STILL EXISTED AFTER CONTROLLING FOR SEVERAL CONDITIONS. HOWEVER, THE STUDY WAS OBSERVATIONAL AND NOT CONTROLLED, WITH LOW ORIGINAL PARTICIPATION RATE, POTENTIAL PARTICIPATION BIAS, AND OTHER UNCONTROLLED FACTORS. THE AUTHORS WARNED AGAINST DRAWING ANY CONCLUSION REGARDING CAUSE.

GASTROINTESTINAL

THE MAIN ADVERSE DRUG REACTIONS (ADRS) ASSOCIATED WITH NSAID USE RELATE TO DIRECT AND INDIRECT IRRITATION OF THE GASTROINTESTINAL (GI) TRACT. NSAIDS CAUSE A DUAL ASSAULT ON THE GI TRACT: THE ACIDIC MOLECULES DIRECTLY IRRITATE THE GASTRIC MUCOSA, AND INHIBITION OF COX-1 AND COX-2 REDUCES THE LEVELS OF PROTECTIVE PROSTAGLANDINS. INHIBITION OF PROSTAGLANDIN SYNTHESIS IN THE GI TRACT CAUSES INCREASED GASTRIC ACID SECRETION, DIMINISHED BICARBONATE SECRETION, DIMINISHED MUCUS SECRETION AND DIMINISHED TROPHIC EFFECTS ON EPITHELIAL MUCOSA.

COMMON GASTROINTESTINAL ADRS INCLUDE:

- *NAUSEA/VOMITING*
- *DYSPEPSIA*
- *GASTRIC ULCERATION/BLEEDING*
- *DIARRHEA*

CLINICAL NSAID ULCERS ARE RELATED TO THE SYSTEMIC EFFECTS OF NSAID ADMINISTRATION. SUCH DAMAGE OCCURS IRRESPECTIVE OF THE ROUTE OF ADMINISTRATION OF THE NSAID (E.G., ORAL, RECTAL, OR PARENTERAL) AND CAN OCCUR EVEN IN PATIENTS WITH ACHLORHYDRIA."

ULCERATION RISK INCREASES WITH THERAPY DURATION, AND WITH HIGHER DOSES. TO MINIMISE GI ADRS, IT IS PRUDENT TO USE THE LOWEST EFFECTIVE DOSE FOR THE SHORTEST PERIOD OF TIME—A PRACTICE THAT STUDIES SHOW IS OFTEN NOT FOLLOWED. RECENT STUDIES SHOW THAT OVER 50% OF PATIENTS WHO TAKE NSAIDS HAVE SUSTAINED SOME MUCOSAL DAMAGE TO THEIR SMALL INTESTINE.

THERE ARE ALSO SOME DIFFERENCES IN THE PROPENSITY OF INDIVIDUAL AGENTS TO CAUSE GASTROINTESTINAL ADRS. INDOMETHACIN, KETOPROFEN, AND PIROXICAM APPEAR TO HAVE THE HIGHEST PREVALENCE OF GASTRIC ADRS, WHILE IBUPROFEN (LOWER DOSES) AND DICLOFENAC, APPEAR TO HAVE LOWER RATES.

CERTAIN NSAIDS, SUCH AS ASPIRIN, HAVE BEEN MARKETED IN ENTERIC-COATED FORMULATIONS THAT MANUFACTURERS CLAIM REDUCE THE INCIDENCE OF GASTROINTESTINAL ADRS. SIMILARLY, SOME BELIEVE THAT RECTAL FORMULATIONS MAY REDUCE GASTROINTESTINAL ADRS. HOWEVER, CONSISTENT WITH THE SYSTEMIC MECHANISM OF SUCH ADRS, AND IN CLINICAL PRACTICE, THESE FORMULATIONS HAVE NOT DEMONSTRATED A REDUCED RISK OF GI ULCERATION.

COMMONLY, GASTRIC (BUT NOT NECESSARILY INTESTINAL) ADVERSE EFFECTS CAN BE REDUCED THROUGH SUPPRESSING ACID PRODUCTION, BY CONCOMITANT USE OF A PROTON PUMP INHIBITOR, E.G., OMEPRAZOLE, ESOMEPRAZOLE; OR THE PROSTAGLANDIN ANALOGUE MISOPROSTOL. MISOPROSTOL IS ITSELF ASSOCIATED WITH A HIGH INCIDENCE OF GASTROINTESTINAL ADRS (DIARRHEA). WHILE THESE TECHNIQUES MAY BE EFFECTIVE, THEY ARE EXPENSIVE FOR MAINTENANCE THERAPY.

INFLAMMATORY BOWEL DISEASE

NSAIDS SHOULD BE USED WITH CAUTION IN INDIVIDUALS WITH INFLAMMATORY BOWEL DISEASE (E.G., Crohn's disease OR ULCERATIVE COLITIS) DUE TO THEIR TENDENCY TO CAUSE GASTRIC BLEEDING AND FORM ULCERATION IN THE GASTRIC LINING. PAIN RELIEVERS SUCH AS PARACETAMOL (ALSO KNOWN AS ACETAMINOPHEN) OR DRUGS CONTAINING CODEINE (WHICH SLOWS DOWN BOWEL ACTIVITY) ARE SAFER MEDICATIONS FOR PAIN RELIEF IN IBD.

RENAL

NSAIDS ARE ALSO ASSOCIATED WITH A FAIRLY HIGH INCIDENCE OF RENAL ADVERSE DRUG REACTIONS (ADRS). THE MECHANISM OF THESE RENAL ADRS IS DUE TO CHANGES IN RENAL HAEMODYNAMICS (KIDNEY BLOOD FLOW), ORDINARILY MEDIATED BY PROSTAGLANDINS, WHICH ARE AFFECTED BY NSAIDS. PROSTAGLANDINS NORMALLY CAUSE VASODILATION OF THE AFFERENT ARTERIOLES OF THE GLOMERULI. THIS HELPS MAINTAIN NORMAL GLOMERULAR PERFUSION AND GLOMERULAR FILTRATION RATE (GFR), AN INDICATOR OF RENAL FUNCTION. THIS IS PARTICULARLY IMPORTANT IN RENAL FAILURE WHERE THE KIDNEY IS TRYING TO MAINTAIN RENAL PERFUSION PRESSURE BY ELEVATED ANGIOTENSIN II LEVELS. AT THESE ELEVATED LEVELS, ANGIOTENSIN II ALSO CONSTRICTS THE AFFERENT ARTERIOLE INTO THE GLOMERULUS IN ADDITION TO THE EFFERENT ARTERIOLE IT NORMALLY CONSTRICTS. PROSTAGLANDINS SERVE TO DILATE THE AFFERENT ARTERIOLE; BY BLOCKING THIS PROSTAGLANDIN-MEDIATED EFFECT, PARTICULARLY IN RENAL FAILURE, NSAIDS CAUSE UNOPPOSED CONSTRICTION OF THE AFFERENT ARTERIOLE AND DECREASED RPF (RENAL PERFUSION PRESSURE). COMMON ADRS ASSOCIATED WITH ALTERED RENAL FUNCTION INCLUDE:

- SALT (SODIUM) AND FLUID RETENTION

- *HYPERTENSION(HIGH BLOOD PRESSURE)*

THESE AGENTS MAY ALSO CAUSE RENAL IMPAIRMENT, ESPECIALLY IN COMBINATION WITH OTHER NEPHROTOXIC AGENTS. RENAL FAILURE IS ESPECIALLY A RISK IF THE PATIENT IS ALSO CONCOMITANTLY TAKING AN ACE INHIBITOR (WHICH REMOVES ANGIOTENSIN II'S VASOCONSTRICTION OF THE EFFERENT ARTERIOLE) AND A DIURETIC (WHICH DROPS PLASMA VOLUME, AND THEREBY RPF)—THE SO-CALLED "TRIPLE WHAMMY" EFFECT.

IN RARER INSTANCES NSAIDS MAY ALSO CAUSE MORE SEVERE RENAL CONDITIONS:

- *INTERSTITIAL NEPHRITIS*
- *NEPHROTIC SYNDROME*
- *ACUTE RENAL FAILURE*
- *ACUTE TUBULAR NECROSIS*
- *RENAL PAPILLARY NECROSIS*

NSAIDS IN COMBINATION WITH EXCESSIVE USE OF PHENACETINAND/OR PARACETAMOL (ACETAMINOPHEN) MAY LEAD TO ANALGESIC NEPHROPATHY.

PHOTOSENSITIVITY

PHOTOSENSITIVITY IS A COMMONLY OVERLOOKED ADVERSE EFFECT OF MANY OF THE NSAIDS. THE 2-ARYLPROPIONIC ACIDS ARE THE MOST LIKELY TO PRODUCE PHOTOSENSITIVITY REACTIONS, BUT OTHER NSAIDS HAVE ALSO BEEN IMPLICATED INCLUDING PIROXICAM, DICLOFENAC, AND BENZYDAMINE.

BENOXAPROFEN, SINCE WITHDRAWN DUE TO ITS HEPATOTOXICITY, WAS THE MOST PHOTOACTIVE NSAID OBSERVED. THE MECHANISM OF PHOTOSENSITIVITY, RESPONSIBLE FOR THE HIGH PHOTOACTIVITY OF THE 2-ARYLPROPIONIC ACIDS, IS THE READY DECARBOXYLATION OF THE CARBOXYLIC ACID MOIETY. THE SPECIFIC ABSORBANCE CHARACTERISTICS OF THE DIFFERENT CHROMOPHORIC 2-ARYL SUBSTITUENTS, AFFECTS THE DECARBOXYLATION MECHANISM. WHILE IBUPROFEN HAS WEAK ABSORPTION, IT HAS BEEN REPORTED AS A WEAK PHOTOSENSITISING AGENT.

DURING PREGNANCY

NSAIDS ARE NOT RECOMMENDED DURING PREGNANCY, PARTICULARLY DURING THE THIRD TRIMESTER. WHILE NSAIDS AS A CLASS IS NOT DIRECT TERATOGENS, THEY MAY CAUSE PREMATURE CLOSURE OF THE FETAL DUCTUS ARTERIOSUS AND RENAL ADRS IN THE FETUS. ADDITIONALLY, THEY ARE LINKED TO PREMATURE BIRTH AND MISCARRIAGE. ASPIRIN, HOWEVER, IS USED TOGETHER WITH HEPARIN IN PREGNANT WOMEN WITH ANTIPHOSPHOLIPID ANTIBODIES. ADDITIONALLY, INDOMETHACIN IS USED IN PREGNANCY TO TREAT POLYHYDRAMNIOS BY REDUCING FETAL URINE PRODUCTION VIA INHIBITING FETAL RENAL BLOOD FLOW.

BY CONTRAST, PARACETAMOL (ACETAMINOPHEN) IS REGARDED AS BEING SAFE AND WELL-TOLERATED DURING PREGNANCY, BUT LEFFERS ET AL. RELEASED A STUDY IN 2010 INDICATING THAT THERE MAY BE ASSOCIATED MALE INFERTILITY IN THE UNBORN. DOSES SHOULD BE TAKEN AS PRESCRIBED, DUE TO RISK OF HEPATOTOXICITY WITH OVERDOSES.

IN FRANCE, THE COUNTRY'S HEALTH AGENCY CONTRAINDICATES THE USE OF NSAIDS, INCLUDING ASPIRIN, AFTER THE SIXTH MONTH OF PREGNANCY.

ALLERGY/ALLERGY-LIKE HYPERSENSITIVITY REACTIONS

A VARIETY OF ALLERGIC OR ALLERGIC-LIKE NSAID HYPERSENSITIVITY REACTIONS FOLLOW THE INGESTION OF NSAIDS. THESE HYPERSENSITIVITY REACTIONS DIFFER FROM THE OTHER ADVERSE REACTIONS LISTED HERE WHICH ARE TOXICITY REACTIONS, I.E. UNWANTED REACTIONS THAT RESULT FROM THE PHARMACOLOGICAL ACTION OF A DRUG, ARE DOSE-RELATED, AND CAN OCCUR IN ANY TREATED INDIVIDUAL; HYPERSENSITIVITY REACTIONS ARE IDIOSYNCRATIC REACTIONS TO A DRUG. SOME NSAID HYPERSENSITIVITY REACTIONS ARE TRULY ALLERGIC IN ORIGIN:

1) REPETITIVE IGE-MEDIATED URTICARIAL SKIN ERUPTIONS, ANGIOEDEMA, AND ANAPHYLAXIS FOLLOWING IMMEDIATELY TO HOURS AFTER INGESTING ONE STRUCTURAL TYPE OF NSAID BUT NOT AFTER INGESTING STRUCTURALLY UNRELATED NSAIDS;

AND 2)COMPARATIVELY MILD TO MODERATELY SEVERE T CELL-MEDIATED DELAYED ONSET (USUALLY MORE THAN 24 HOUR), SKIN REACTIONS SUCH AS MACULOPAPULAR RASH, FIXED DRUG ERUPTIONS, PHOTOSENSITIVITY REACTIONS, DELAYED URTICARIA, AND CONTACT DERMATITIS;

OR 3) FAR MORE SEVERE AND POTENTIALLY LIFE-THREATENING T-CELL MEDIATED DELAYED SYSTEMIC REACTIONS SUCH AS THE DRESS SYNDROME, ACUTE GENERALIZED EXANTHEMATOUS PUSTULOSIS, THE STEVENS-JOHNSON SYNDROME, AND TOXIC EPIDERMAL NECROLYSIS. OTHER NSAID HYPERSENSITIVITY REACTIONS ARE ALLERGY-LIKE SYMPTOMS BUT DO NOT INVOLVE TRUE ALLERGIC MECHANISMS; RATHER, THEY APPEAR DUE TO THE ABILITY OF NSAIDS TO ALTER THE METABOLISM OF ARACHIDONIC ACID IN FAVOR OF FORMING METABOLITES THAT PROMOTE ALLERGIC SYMPTOMS. AFFLICTED INDIVIDUALS MAY BE ABNORMALLY SENSITIVE TO THESE PROVOCATIVE METABOLITES AND/OR OVERPRODUCE THEM AND TYPICALLY ARE SUSCEPTIBLE TO A WIDE RANGE OF STRUCTURALLY DISSIMILAR NSAIDS, PARTICULARLY THOSE THAT INHIBIT COX1. SYMPTOMS, WHICH DEVELOP IMMEDIATELY TO HOURS AFTER INGESTING ANY OF VARIOUS NSAIDS THAT INHIBIT COX-1, ARE:

1)EXACERBATIONS OF ASTHMATIC AND RHINITIS (SEE ASPIRIN-INDUCED ASTHMA) SYMPTOMS IN INDIVIDUALS WITH A HISTORY OF ASTHMA OR RHINITIS AND

2) EXACERBATION OR FIRST-TIME DEVELOPMENT OF WHEALS AND/OR ANGIOEDEMA IN INDIVIDUALS WITH OR WITHOUT A HISTORY OF CHRONIC URTICARIAL LESIONS OR ANGIOEDEMA.

Other

COMMON ADVERSE DRUG REACTIONS (ADR), OTHER THAN LISTED ABOVE, INCLUDE RAISED LIVER ENZYMES, HEADACHE, DIZZINESS. UNCOMMON ADRS INCLUDE HYPERKALAEMIA, CONFUSION, BRONCHOSPASM, RASH. RAPID AND SEVERE SWELLING OF THE FACE AND/OR BODY. IBUPROFEN MAY ALSO RARELY CAUSE IRRITABLE BOWEL SYNDROME SYMPTOMS. NSAIDS ARE ALSO IMPLICATED IN SOME CASES OF STEVENS-JOHNSON SYNDROME. MOST NSAIDS PENETRATE POORLY INTO THE CENTRAL NERVOUS SYSTEM (CNS). HOWEVER, THE COX ENZYMES ARE EXPRESSED CONSTITUTIVELY IN SOME AREAS OF THE CNS, MEANING THAT EVEN LIMITED PENETRATION MAY CAUSE ADVERSE EFFECTS SUCH AS SOMNOLENCE AND DIZZINESS. IN VERY RARE CASES, IBUPROFEN CAN CAUSE ASEPTIC MENINGITIS. AS WITH OTHER DRUGS, ALLERGIES TO NSAIDS MIGHT EXIST. WHILE MANY ALLERGIES ARE SPECIFIC TO ONE NSAID, UP TO 1 IN 5 PEOPLE MAY HAVE UNPREDICTABLE CROSS-REACTIVE ALLERGIC RESPONSES TO OTHER NSAIDS AS WELL.

DRUG INTERACTIONS

NSAIDS REDUCE RENAL BLOOD FLOW AND THEREBY DECREASE THE EFFICACY OF DIURETICS, AND INHIBIT THE ELIMINATION OF LITHIUM AND METHOTREXATE. NSAIDS CAUSE HYPOCOAGULABILITY, WHICH MAY BE SERIOUS WHEN COMBINED WITH OTHER DRUGS THAT ALSO DECREASE BLOOD CLOTTING, SUCH AS WARFARIN. NSAIDS MAY AGGRAVATE HYPERTENSION (HIGH BLOOD PRESSURE) AND THEREBY ANTAGONIZE THE EFFECT OF ANTIHYPERTENSIVES, SUCH AS ACE INHIBITORS. NSAIDS MAY INTERFERE AND REDUCE EFFICIENCY OF SSRI ANTIDEPRESSANTS. VARIOUS WIDELY USED NONSTEROIDAL ANTI-INFLAMMATORY DRUGS (NSAIDS) ENHANCE ENDOCANNABINOID SIGNALING BY BLOCKING THE ANANDAMIDE-DEGRADING MEMBRANE ENZYME FATTY ACID AMIDE HYDROLASE (FAAH).

HOW'S THAT FOR A WARNING LABEL? Did it have enough side effects for you? Think you might need more meds after taking this one? That label was 4094 words long. How many of those did you read? How do you know what you're doing to your body if you don't know what you're putting into it? Do you think it a coincidence that Monsanto started their GMO seed about the same time that glycation started being researched? Since much of this kind of research is funded by the industry it affects, I wouldn't doubt that Monsanto had a hand in this research. This would allow them to immediately file these studies on glycation so that doctors and other scientists couldn't find them to review. It would also allow them to genetically modify their food to make it more fattening by allowing it to stand up to glyphosate herbicide. Yet each and every one of these 17,000+ studies has been vetted and examined by the NIH and PubMed. What I'd like to know is, why weren't warnings about glycation revealed then? Did Monsanto have anything to do with that?

The above list is the warning label for the adverse effects of Celebrex. Do you take Celebrex? Have you read the above warnings? Use of this drug can only lead to the use of more and more drugs. What do you think that would do for the profits for Monsanto and Pfizer? Do you still think this is a coincidence? From renal failure to the increased risk of **myocardial infarction** and **stroke**, this drug brings on more drug use, simply so people can get away from their pain. This pain is directly caused by the consumption of Monsanto's grains. To me, this is completely an unsustainable cycle. It's a cycle of hunger, dependence, disease, and death, leaving only people in pain. Where is the sense in keeping this addiction?

I propose that we tell Monsanto how we feel about this, not with our voices, but with our mouths in what we eat. All you have to do is quit eating grains. They're responsible for nearly all the pain you experience (with the exception of a few physical injuries).Grains and the glycation they bring, bring all inflammation that influences all diseases. Stop buying bread, crackers, cookies, anything that flour is used in, stop using it, forever. That's the only way you can start to free yourself from the addiction. You have to stop buying their junk food. Their comfort food is making you sick. It's making you sicker by the day.

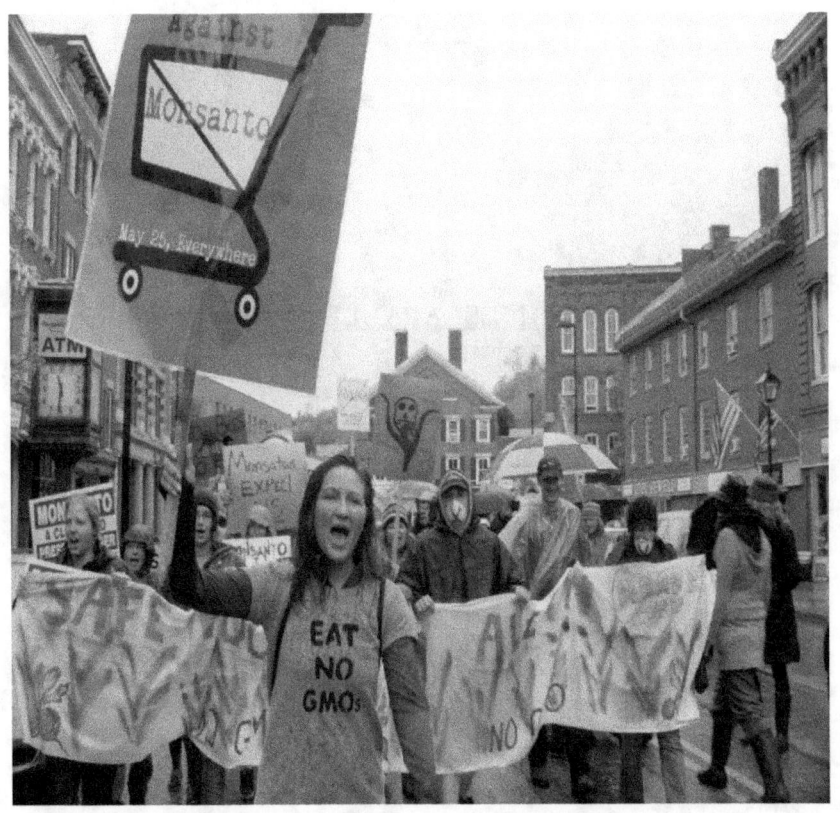

IT'S TIME TO TAKE OUR LIVES BACK!

PART III

THE INESCAPABLE DAMAGE

THE DESTINY OF GRAINS IN THE DIET

CHAPTER 7

Disorders Influenced By the Formation of Plaque in Your Body

Plaque is arguably the worst manifestation of glycation from sugar and carbs in the diet. It happens when a sugar molecule combines with any fat or protein molecule, (including hemoglobin) without a cell signaling protein (hormone) to tell it what to do. It besets the true destructive force of glucose on your body. This is why insulin is so important. It's that cell signaling protein, a hormone, in this case, that tells glucose to turn into fat, so it can be used as fuel. Without the insulin, the glucose is free to attach its polymer base molecule to any protein or lipid (usually an LDL particle or hemoglobin protein in your blood), to start the process of glycation.

Whether the glycation is of a lipid or a protein, which is always the case when it comes in contact with cholesterol (especially LDL particles), the resulting glycation usually ends up in the form of plaque, macrophages, and cytokines. There are several forms of plaque. According to Wikipedia, there are seven different kinds of plaque, Amyloid Plaque, Atheroma Plaque, Dental plaque, Mucoid plaque, Pleural plaque, Senile plaques, Viral plaque.

By far the worst of the plaques caused by digesting wheat and gluten is amyloid plaque, because of all the diseases it has a role in. According to Wikipedia;

*"Amyloids are insoluble fibrous protein aggregates sharing specific structural traits. They are insoluble and arise from at least 18 inappropriately folded versions of proteins and polypeptides present naturally in the body. These misfolded structures alter their proper configuration such that they erroneously interact with one another or other cell components forming insoluble fibrils. They have been associated with the pathology of more than 20 serious human diseases in that abnormal accumulation of amyloid fibrils in organs may lead to amyloidosis, and may play a role in various neurodegenerative disorders. "*The list of diseases caused by amyloid plaque is quite extensive, ranging from Alzheimer's disease to Diabetes, Parkinson's and Huntington's diseases and more.

The list on Wikipedia is 21 diseases and disorders or conditions associated with amyloid plaque. In my opinion, amyloid plaque is caused by the digestion of gluten from any source, whether it's wheat, barley or rye.

Wikipedia also says;

"Studies have shown that amyloid deposition is associated with mitochondrial dysfunction and a resulting generation of reactive oxygen species (ROS), which can initiate a signaling pathway leading to apoptosis." In short amyloid plaque is caused by oxidative stress and cell death, both of which are caused by consumption of gluten and other high starch products.

ATHEROMATOUS Plaques are basically plaques from fats and is the type of plaque that clogs up your artery walls. This is the type of plaque that causes atherosclerosis and leads to heart and cardiovascular disease. It is the root cause of high blood pressure.

Dental plaque is caused by the excessive amount of sugar on the teeth, creating bacteria, causing decay. Although I think that bread plays a larger role in Dental Plaque.

Remember, carbs = sugar, and saliva is a major enzyme for digestion called α-amylase, an important enzyme for breaking down starches. This is the enzyme that starts glycation. If plaque from glycation can accumulate on your teeth, this is a sign of glycation starting even before you can swallow.

"Senile plaques (also known as neuritic plaques, senile druse and brain druse) are extracellular deposits of amyloid beta in the grey matter of the brain. They're responsible for diseases such as Alzheimer's disease and dementia, and play a role in most every other cognitive disorder due to the way this plaque gums up the neurons in your brain.

"Mucoid plaque (or mucoid cap or rope) is a pseudoscientific term used by some alternative medicine advocates to describe what is claimed to be a combination of allegedly harmful mucus-like material and food residue that they say coats the gastrointestinal tract of most people. The term was coined by Richard Anderson, a naturopath, and entrepreneur, who sells a range of products that claim to "cleanse" the body of such purported plaques."

Pleural plaques are indicators of asbestos exposure and the most common asbestos-induced lesion. They usually appear after 20 years or more of exposure and degenerate into mesothelioma. They appear as fibrous plaques on the parietal pleura, usually on both sides, and at the posterior and inferior part of the chest wall as well as the diaphragm.

With atherosclerosis being arguably the worst of these manifestations as it's at the root of most heart disease and cardiovascular disease, the plaque that creates this atherosclerosis earns itself #1 in the death and destruction category. Since this comes mostly from sugar and grains, both products of Monsanto's farmers, you can thank Monsanto for your cancers and CVDs, your arthritis and IBS, your diabetes and your pancreatitis. The list can keep going on and on and on. It's the gluten that breaks down into glucose to create that glycation. This was shown in a 1984 study, yet the practice continued and even escalated to the point of where it is today. With all this plaque caused by glycation, I have to wonder why this food hasn't been condemned yet.

According to Wikipedia; *"The formation and accumulation of advanced glycation endproducts (AGEs) have been implicated in the progression of age-related diseases. AGEs have been implicated in Alzheimer's disease, cardiovascular disease, and stroke. The mechanism by which AGEs induce damage is through a process called cross-linking that causes intracellular damage and apoptosis. They form photosensitizers in the crystalline lens, which has implications for cataract development. Reduced muscle function is also associated with AGEs."*

What it boils down to is this;

- sugar creates glycation
- Glycation creates inflammation
- inflammation is responsible for most pain in your body as well as
- most disease in your body
- Hypertension
- hyperlipidemia
- atherosclerosis
- Inflammatory heart disease
- Inflammatory Bowel syndrome
- Every form of cancer
- Alzheimer's disease
- Parkinson's disease

- Schizophrenia
- Depression
- Bipolar disorder
- arthritis
- *CHRONIC PAIN*
- *HEADACHES*

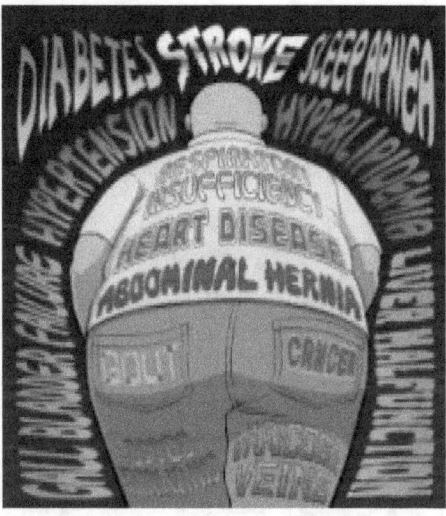

If you could eliminate all of the above disorders by limiting the amount of cholesterol that's glycated into plaque, wouldn't you consider that at least a step toward a cure? By that logic, wouldn't limit the amount of glucose you put in your body limit the amount of glycation and plaque in your blood since it's the glucose that does the glycating? This is something that you have full control over how it affects your body.

Failure to Control Your Glucose Intake Brings You to

Your Destiny;

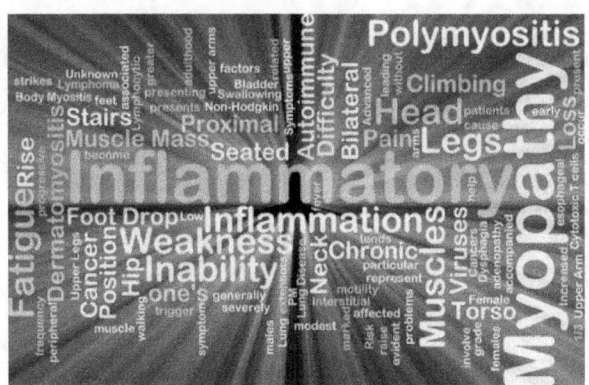

Rampant Glycation

Chapter 8

Glycation - The Real Poisoning of America

Of the causes of death below from Wikipedia, Ischemic heart disease @ 7.4 million ranks right at the top. This is the result of glycation, 5 of the following 8 are also caused by non-enzymatic glycation. Hence my proposal, control the glycation and you control all modern diseases.

According to Wikipedia;

Leading causes of preventable death worldwide as of the year 2001, according to researchers working with the Disease Control Priorities Network (DCPN) and the World Health Organization (WHO). (THE WHO'S 2008 statistics SHOW VERY SIMILAR TRENDS.) IMAGINE WHAT THEY ARE RIGHT NOW, 8 YEARS LATER AND WHAT THEY WILL BE EIGHT YEARS FROM NOW IF NOTHING IS DONE ABOUT IT. THINK IT MIGHT BE TIME FOR A CURE?

The top 10 causes of preventable death, ones influenced by glycation are in red. Although it may be difficult to stop all glycation in the body, due to its commonality, you can control a major portion of it. Excessive Carbohydrate Consumption, the primary cause of glycation is controllable. Failure to control your consumption leads directly to any of the following disorders in red ;

1. Ischaemic heart disease @ 7.4 mil
2. Stroke@ 6.7 mil
3. COPD @ 3.1 mil
4. Lower Respiratory infection @ 3.1mil
5. Trachea bronchus, lung infection@ 1.8 mil
6. HIV/AIDS@1.5 mil
7. Diarrheal diseases@1.5 mil
8. Diabetes mellitus@1.5 mil
9. Road injury@1.3 mil
10. Hypertension@1.1 mil

85% of these deaths or 24.5 million are directly linked to **ECC,** Excessive Carbohydrate Consumption, making them the most preventable causes of death. 24.5 million deaths each and every year amounts to over 67,123 people each and every day. That includes approximately 2684 Americans each and every day. We have full control of this. All it would take is to say no to the sugar and grain industries. This one response would allow over 2680 more Americans to stay alive, every day. The cessation of carb consumption could add an additional 10-20 years to their lives, simply by eliminating the primary cause of inflammation, glucose. The continuation of carb consumption will, by contrast, prove the destructive power of sugar, by eventually killing all of its hosts.

Glycation is a common everyday experience that you accelerate with a carbohydrate diet. The more carbs you eat, the more glycation you'll get to deal with. Glycation is controllable by controlling what you put in your mouth to eat. Although not totally responsible for some of these cancers, they would not exist if the glycation didn't exist. This is the basis of my contention that if you eliminate the reason for the glycation, you eliminate the reason for inflammation, which in turn will eliminate the reason for these diseases, thereby eliminating the disease. It's really not hard to see, once you take a good look at it; carb consumption is responsible for the inflammation that builds in the blood that is responsible for 90% of all modern diseases. Remove the inflammation by removing the sugar, which means removing the carbs. A simpler solution doesn't exist and this cure can be yours.

THESE ARE SOME OF THE SMOKING GUN ARTICLES OF EVIDENCE

THAT THE FDA AND THE USDA ARE IGNORING.

THEY PUT YOUR HEALTH AND LIFE AT RISK, BY DOING SO.

50 of the 17676 studies done on glycation are below. These research studies were chosen from 281 studies that I examined for evidence of what glycation does to the body. By going through only 2% of these studies, I was able to find enough damning evidence to condemn this food 31 times over. By this ratio, I'll end up finding at the least 1950 more studies showing damage that glycation does.

I chose to search glycation because I know that it's at the root of all modern diseases from cancer to CVDs to arthritis to dementia including Alzheimer disease. The following studies are the proof of what glycation does, and with sugar being the primary instigator of glycation, removal of sugar from the diet will eliminate everything it's responsible for. **These AGEs are responsible for all modern diseases and thus, are the reason for this book. When you eat carbs, you need to know what those carbs do to your body.**

The study that piqued my interest initially was the report on RAGEs, this report dated Jun 5, 2011, can be found in PubMed at *Receptor for advanced glycation end-products-mediated inflammation and diabetic vascular complications*. It explains how glycation turns your body's fuel (cholesterol) and proteins (hemoglobin) into AGEs before they can be used for fuel and body repair.

- *Receptor for advanced glycation end products*

"Exposure of amino residue of proteins to reducing sugars, such as glucose, glucose phosphate, fructose, ribose and intermediate aldehydes, results in nonenzymatic glycation, which forms reversible Schiff bases and Amadori compounds. A series of further complex molecular rearrangements then yield irreversible advanced glycation endproducts (AGE). The aldehydes, highly reactive AGE precursors, are produced by both enzymatic and nonenzymatic pathways. The enzymatic pathways include a route of myeloperoxidase in inflammatory cells, such as activated macrophages, which produces hypochlorite, then reacting with serine to generate glycolaldehyde." Study Link

The following report from Oct 27, 2016, is the evidence of glucose's involvement in arthritis. By being responsible for glycation, the glucose from broken down carbs, again, is directly responsible for arthritis, just like it was in the 4,000 yr old ice mummy recovered from a receding glacier.

- *"Protein oxidation, nitration and glycation biomarkers for early-stage diagnosis of osteoarthritis of the knee and typing and progression of arthritic disease"*

"Glycated, oxidized and nitrated proteins and amino acids were detected in synovial fluid and plasma of arthritic patients with characteristic patterns found in early and advanced OA and RA, and non-RA, with respect to healthy controls. In early-stage disease, two algorithms for

consecutive use in diagnosis were developed: (1) disease versus healthy control, and (2) classification as OA, RA, and non-RA." Study Link

The following report from Sep 23, 2016, shows the effects that AGEs have on the body in the diseases it promotes.

- "EFFECT OF GLYCATION INHIBITORS ON AGING AND AGE-RELATED DISEASES"

"Vast evidence supports the view that glycation of proteins is one of the main factors contributing to aging and is an important element of etiopathology of age-related diseases, especially type 2 diabetes mellitus, cataract, and neurodegenerative diseases. Counteracting glycation can, therefore, be a means of increasing both the lifespan and health span. In this review, accumulation of glycation products during aging is presented, pathophysiological effects of glycation are discussed and ways of attenuation of the effects of glycation are described, concentrating on prevention of glycation. The effects of glycation and glycation inhibitors on the course of selected age-related diseases, such as Alzheimer's disease, Parkinson's disease, and cataract are also reviewed." Study Link

This study from Oct 21, 2016, looks at the damaging effects of glycation along with the protective effects of certain phytochemicals (anti-oxidant producing agents).

- *"Phytochemicals against advanced glycation end products (AGEs) and the receptor system"*

"Reducing sugars can react non-enzymatically with amino groups of proteins and lipids to form irreversibly cross-linked macro protein derivatives called as advanced glycation end products (AGEs). Cross-linking modification of extracellular matrix proteins by AGEs deteriorate their tertiary structural integrity and function, contributing to aging-related organ damage and diabetes-associated complications, such as cardiovascular disease (CVD). Moreover, engagement of receptor for AGEs, RAGE with the ligands evoke oxidative stress generation and inflammatory, thrombotic and fibrotic reactions in various kinds of tissues, further exacerbating the deleterious effects of AGEs on multiple organ systems. So the AGE-RAGE axis is a novel therapeutic target for numerous devastating disorders. Several observational studies have shown the association of dietary consumption of fruits and vegetables with the reduced risk of CVD in a general population. Although beneficial effects of fruits and vegetables against CVD could mainly be ascribed to its anti-oxidative properties, blockade of the AGE-RAGE axis by phytochemicals may also contribute to cardiovascular event protection. Therefore, in this review, we focus on 4 phytochemicals (quercetin, sulforaphane, iridoids, and curcumin) and summarize their effects on AGE formation as well as RAGE-mediated signaling pathway in various cell types and organs, including endothelial cells, vessels, and heart."

This report from Sep 16, 2016, examines the nature of amyloid plaque and glyoxal *(Glyoxal is an inflammatory compound formed when cooking oils and fats are heated to high temperatures). It's also made in your body when your body breaks down glucose.*

- *"Glyoxal administration induces formation of high molecular weight aggregates of hemoglobin exhibiting amyloidal nature in experimental rats: An in vivo study"*

"Glyoxal, a highly reactive α-oxoaldehyde, increases in diabetic condition and reacts with proteins to form advanced glycation end products (AGEs). In the present study, we have investigated the effect of glyoxal on experimental rat hemoglobin in vivo after external administration of the α-dicarbonyl compound in animals. Gel electrophoretic profile of hemolysate collected from glyoxal-treated rats (32mg/kg body wt. dose) after one week exhibited the presence of some high molecular weight protein bands that were found to be absent for control, untreated rats. Mass spectrometric and absorption studies indicated that

the bands represented hemoglobin. Further studies revealed that the fraction exhibited the presence of intermolecular cross β-sheet structure. Thus glyoxal administration induces the formation of high molecular weight aggregates of hemoglobin with amyloid characteristics in rats. Aggregated hemoglobin fraction was found to exhibit higher stability compared to glyoxal-untreated hemoglobin. As evident from mass spectrometric studies, glyoxal was found to modify Arg-30β and Arg-31α of rat hemoglobin to hydroimidazolone adducts. The modifications thus appear to induce amyloid-like aggregation of hemoglobin in rats. Considering the increased level of glyoxal in diabetes mellitus as well as its high reactivity, the above findings may be physiologically significant.

In view of its inflammatory function in innate immunity and its ability to detect a class of ligands through a common structural motif, rage is often referred to as a pattern recognition receptor." Study link

This report from Oct 18, 2016, examines the relationship of high mobility group box 1 (HMGB1) and the effects it has on the body. HMGB1 is one of the most prevalent RAGE's, as near as I can tell. It comes up in more studies...

- *"HMGB1 ACTIVATES PROINFLAMMATORY SIGNALING VIA TLR5 LEADING TO ALLODYNIA"*

"Infectious and sterile inflammatory diseases are correlated with increased levels of high mobility group box 1 (HMGB1) in tissues and serum. Extracellular HMGB1 is known to activate Toll-like receptors (TLRs) 2 and 4 and RAGE (receptor for advanced glycation end products) in inflammatory conditions. Here, we find that TLR5 is also an HMGB1 receptor that was previously overlooked due to lack of functional expression in the cell lines usually used for studying TLR signaling. HMGB1 binding to TLR5 initiates the activation of an NF-κB signaling pathway in a MyD88-dependent manner, resulting in pro-inflammatory cytokine production and pain enhancement in vivo. Biophysical and in vitro results highlight an essential role for the C-terminal tail region of HMGB1 in facilitating interactions with TLR5. These results suggest that HMGB1-modulated TLR5 signaling is responsible for pain hypersensitivity." Study Link

I see HMGB1 come up in almost all modern diseases. This must be the most popular RAGEs.

The proof that carb consumption also contributes to lung cancer is in the following report from Oct 18, 2016, also. The underlying cause is inflammation.

- *The Ser82 RAGE Variant Affects Lung Function and Serum RAGE in Smokers and sRAGE Production In Vitro*

*"**Abstract***
INTRODUCTION:

Genome-Wide Association Studies have identified associations between lung function measures and Chronic Obstructive Pulmonary Disease (COPD) and chromosome region 6p21 containing the gene for the Advanced Glycation End Product Receptor (AGER, encoding RAGE). We aimed to (i) characterize RAGE expression in the lung, (ii) identify AGER transcripts, (iii) ascertain if SNP rs2070600 (Gly82Ser C/T) is associated with lung function and serum sRAGE levels and (iv) identify whether the Gly82Ser variant is functionally important in altering sRAGE levels in an airway epithelial cell model.
METHODS:

Immunohistochemistry was used to identify RAGE protein expression in 26 human tissues and qPCR was used to quantify AGER mRNA in lung cells. Gene expression array data was used to identify AGER expression during lung development in 38 fetal lung samples. RNA-Seq was used to identify AGER transcripts in lung cells. sRAGE levels were assessed in cells and patient serum by ELISA. BEAS2B-R1 cells were transfected to overexpress RAGE

protein with either the Gly82 or Ser82 variant and sRAGE levels identified.
RESULTS:

Immunohistochemical assessment of 6 adult lung samples identified high RAGE expression in the alveoli of healthy adults and individuals with COPD. AGER/RAGE expression increased across developmental stages in the human fetal lung at both the mRNA (38 samples) and protein levels (20 samples). Extensive AGER splicing was identified. The rs2070600T (Ser82) allele is associated with higher FEV1, FEV1/FVC and lower serum sRAGE levels in UK smokers. Using an airway epithelium model overexpressing the Gly82 or Ser82 variants we found that HMGB1 activation of the RAGE-Ser82 receptor results in lower sRAGE production.

CONCLUSIONS:

This study provides new information regarding the expression profile and potential role of RAGE in the human lung and shows a functional role of the Gly82Ser variant. These findings advance our understanding of the potential mechanisms underlying COPD particularly for carriers of this AGER polymorphism." _Study Link

I wonder if the ACS, American Cancer Society will take this information and realize what foods are responsible for this report showing how RAGEs have a role in COPD and ultimately lung cancer? Will it provoke a response from the ACS on the consumption of the foods responsible for this RAGE? Will they issue a warning or are they more concerned with an industry that depends on this disorder, the pharmaceutical industry, or maybe an industry that provokes this disorder, the grain industry?

You may ask though, shouldn't smoking play a larger role in this equation? I submit that if the glycation never existed in the first place, the smoking wouldn't play as large of a role as it does with the inflammation in the body. It takes the glycation to create the RAGE responsible for lung cancer, yet no one knows of glycation or its effects from the FDA, the USDA or the CDC. Who are they trying to protect? Why isn't glycation considered a disease?

In the following from an April 19, 2016, study, the emergence of the HMGB1 RAGE in head and the skin cancer, neck squamous cell carcinoma,

- *"Clinical Value of High Mobility Group Box 1 and the Receptor for Advanced Glycation End-products in Head and Neck Cancer: A Systematic Review"*

"Introduction   High mobility group box 1 is a versatile protein involved in gene transcription, extracellular signaling, and response to inflammation. Extracellularly, high mobility group box 1 binds to several receptors, notably the receptor for advanced glycation end-products. Expression of high mobility group box 1 and the receptor for advanced glycation end-products has been described in many cancers.

Objectives   To systematically review the available literature using PubMed and Web of Science to evaluate the clinical value of high mobility group box 1 and the receptor for advanced glycation end-products in head and neck squamous cell carcinomas.

Data Synthesis   A total of eleven studies were included in this review. High mobility group box 1 overexpression is associated with poor prognosis and many clinical and pathological characteristics of head and neck squamous cell carcinomas patients. Additionally, the receptor for advanced glycation end-products demonstrates potential value as a clinical indicator of tumor angiogenesis and advanced staging. In diagnosis, high mobility group box 1 demonstrates low sensitivity.

Conclusion   High mobility group box 1 and the receptor for advanced glycation end-products are associated with clinical and pathological characteristics of head and neck squamous cell carcinomas. Further investigation of the prognostic and diagnostic value of these molecules is warranted." Study Link

Although the study above was published in Oct 2016, this kind of evidence has been around for over 20 years. These reports started showing up in 1984;

- *Nonenzymatic* glycation *of human lens crystallin. Effect of aging and diabetes mellitus*

We have examined the nonenzymatic glycation of human lens crystallin, an extremely long-lived protein, from 16 normal human ocular lenses 0.2-99 yr of age, and from 11 diabetic lenses 52-82-yr-old…the nonenzymatic glycation of nondiabetic lens crystallin may be regarded as a biological clock…The glucitol-lysine (Glc-Lys) content of soluble and insoluble crystallin was determined after reduction with H-borohydride followed by acid hydrolysis, boronic acid affinity chromatography, and high-pressure cation exchange chromatography…Over an age range comparable to that of the control samples, the diabetic crystallin samples contained about twice as much Glc-Lys.

More on cataracts is found later in this chapter. This study from Oct 6, 2016, shows glycations implication in cardiovascular disease;

- *"Therapeutic interventions for Advanced Glycation-End Products and its Receptor-Mediated Cardiovascular Disease"*

"Advanced glycation end products (AGEs) are a heterogeneous group of molecules formed from the non-enzymatic reaction of reducing sugars with the amino group of proteins, lipids, and nucleic acid. Interaction of AGEs with its cell-bound receptor (RAGE) results in the generation of oxygen radicals, nuclear factor kappa-β, pro-inflammatory cytokines and cell adhesion molecules, and is involved in the pathophysiology of cardiovascular diseases (CVD). Circulating soluble forms of RAGE (sRAGE) and endo-secretory RAGE (esRAGE) compete with RAGE for ligand binding and function as a decoy. This paper describes the endogenous and exogenous (high dietary AGEs, cooking food under high dry heat, elevated pH, and long period) sources of AGEs. AGE-RAGE-mediated CVD includes atherosclerosis, coronary artery disease, carotid artery disease, hypertension, peripheral vascular diseases, heart failure, cardiomyopathy, and microangiopathy. The therapeutic intervention with a reduction in AGEs and RAGE and elevation in sRAGE has been reported for the treatment of AGE-RAGE-mediated CVD. Reduction in levels of AGEs can be achieved by a reduction in consumption of food containing or creating the low amount of AGEs, cooking food at low temperature, moist heat, and shorter duration. AGE formation can be reduced with drugs, vitamins, and stoppage of cigarette smoking. Statins, telmisartan, and curcumin have been used for suppression of RAGE. Statins, ACE-inhibitors, Rosiglitazone and vitamin D have been used to increase levels of sRAGE. Finally, exogenous administration of sRAGE can be helpful in amelioration of CVD. In conclusion, AGE-RAGE-mediated CVD could be attenuated with a reduction in consumption of AGEs, suppression of RAGE and elevation of sRAGE."

Instead of looking at eliminating the glycating factor, their resolution to this problem is contained in more drugs. They think that creating more drugs to counteract the glycation is going to solve the problem of glycation. Is that because more drugs will ultimately lead to more drugs?

Statins are the most dangerous in the above equation as they unbalance your cholesterol which puts everything in your body out of balance. It's your cholesterol that regulates a good portion of your hormones. You should already know how much your hormones affect your emotions, energy, intelligence, aging, and basic proper functioning of your body, right down to digesting carbs (insulin). Granted insulin is made in the pancreas, although other more influential hormones are made in your fat which is what statins reduce.

Side effects of statins; Common statin-related side effects (headaches, stomach upset, abnormal liver function tests and muscle cramps)… Side effects of statins include muscle pain, increased risk of diabetes mellitus, and abnormalities in liver enzyme tests. Additionally, they have rare but severe adverse effects, particularly muscle damage. As of 2010, a number of statins are on the market: atorvastatin, fluvastatin, lovastatin, pitavastatin, pravastatin, rosuvastatin, and simvastatin. Several combination preparations of a statin and another agent, such as ezetimibe/simvastatin, are also available. In 2005 sales were estimated at $18.7

billion in the United States.

Side effects ultimately lead to other drugs down the road. It's inevitable. This is how the pharmaceutical corporations make as much money as they do. And you gladly give it to them, simply to keep up your addiction and later to fight your CVD or cancer. How much sense this makes to you? What concerns me more than anything else is the fact the atorvastatin is the best selling pharmaceutical in history, with sales of $12.4 billion in 2008. With all of the side effects listed above, how many patients taking these drugs will not ever have to use any more pharmaceuticals. This is the way they guarantee a return consumer. I know. (I was one of them. I won't be anymore due to my keto diet.)

The best-selling statin is atorvastatin, which in 2003 became the best-selling pharmaceutical in history. The manufacturer Pfizer reported sales of US$12.4 billion in 2008. Pfizer and Monsanto were under one roof at in 2003. That was the year Pfizer started their divestiture of Monsanto. (Maybe it was the lawsuits that were starting to pile up, that they didn't appreciate.) I wonder how many lawsuits Pfizer has against itself for its pharmaceutical statins. Below are the contraindications for atorvastatin (Lipitor).

Contraindications

Active liver disease: **cholestasis, hepatic encephalopathy, hepatitis,** and **jaundice**

Unexplained elevations in **AST** or **ALT** levels

Pregnancy: Atorvastatin may cause fetal harm by affecting serum cholesterol and triglyceride levels, which are essential for fetal development.

Breastfeeding: Small amounts of other statin drugs have been found to pass into breast milk, although atorvastatin has not been studied, specifically.

Markedly elevated **CPK** levels or if a **myopathy** is suspected or diagnosed after dosing of atorvastatin has begun. Very rarely, atorvastatin may cause **rhabdomyolysis,** and it may be very serious leading to acute renal failure due to **myoglobinuria**. If rhabdomyolysis is suspected or diagnosed, atorvastatin therapy should be discontinued immediately. The likelihood of developing a **myopathy** is increased by the co-administration of **cyclosporine, fibric acid derivatives, erythromycin, niacin,** and **azole antifungals.**

Adverse effects

Major

Diabetes mellitus type 2, an uncommon class effect of all statins.

Myopathy with elevation of creatinine kinase (CK) and **rhabdomyolysis** are the most serious side effects, occurring rarely at a rate of 2.3 to 9.1 per 10,000 person-years among patients taking atorvastatin. As mentioned previously, atorvastatin should be discontinued immediately if this occurs.

Persistent liver enzyme abnormalities occurred in 0.7% of patients who received atorvastatin in clinical trials. It is recommended that hepatic function is assessed with laboratory tests before beginning atorvastatin treatment and repeated as clinically indicated thereafter. If evidence of serious liver injury occurs while a patient is taking atorvastatin, it should be discontinued and not restarted until the etiology of the patient's liver dysfunction is defined. If no other cause is found, atorvastatin should be discontinued permanently.

Common

The following have been shown to occur in 1–10% of patients taking atorvastatin in clinical trials.

Arthralgia,

Diarrhea,

Dyspepsia,

Myalgia,

Nausea

High-dose atorvastatin has also been associated with worsening glycemic control.

Other

In 2014 the FDA reported memory loss, forgetfulness, and confusion with all statin products including atorvastatin. The symptoms were not serious, and they were rare and reversible on cessation of drug treatment.

Interactions

Interactions with clofibrate, fenofibrate, gemfibrozil, which are fibrates used in accessory therapy in many forms of **hypercholesterolemia***, usually in combination with statins, increase the risk of* **myopathy** *and* **rhabdomyolysis***.*

Co-administration of atorvastatin with one of **CYP3A4** *inhibitors such as* **itraconazole***,* **telithromycin***, and* **voriconazole***, may increase serum concentrations of atorvastatin, which may lead to adverse reactions. This is less likely to happen with other CYP3A4 inhibitors such as* **diltiazem***,* **erythromycin***,* **fluconazole***,* **ketoconazole***,* **clarithromycin***,* **cyclosporine***,* **pr otease inhibitors***, or* **verapamil***, and only rarely with other CYP3A4 inhibitors, such as* **amiodarone** *and* **aprepitant***. Often,* **bosentan***,* **fosphenytoin***, and* **phenytoin***, which are CYP3A4 inducers, can decrease the plasma concentrations of atorvastatin. Only rarely, though,* **barbiturates***,* **carbamazepine***,* **efavirenz***,* **nevirapine***,* **oxcarbazepine***,* **rifampin***, and* **rifamycin***, which are also CYP3A4 inducers, can decrease the plasma concentrations of atorvastatin.* **Oral contraceptives** *increased AUC values for* **norethisterone** *and* **ethinylestradiol***; these increases should be considered when selecting an oral contraceptive for a woman taking atorvastatin.*

Antacids *can rarely decrease the plasma concentrations of statin drugs, but do not affect the* **LDL-C***-lowering* **efficacy***.*

Niacin *also is proved to increase the risk of myopathy or rhabdomyolysis.*

Statins may also alter the concentrations of other drugs, such as **warfarin** *or* **digoxin***, leading to alterations in effect or a requirement for clinical monitoring.*

Vitamin D *supplementation lowers atorvastatin and active metabolite concentrations, yet* **synergistically** *reduces LDL and total* **cholesterol** *concentrations.* **Grapefruit juice** *components are known inhibitors of intestinal CYP3A4.*

Co-administration of grapefruit juice with atorvastatin may cause an increase in **Cmax** *and AUC, which can lead to adverse reactions or overdose toxicity.*

A few cases of myopathy have been reported when atorvastatin is given with **colchicine***.*

These are side effects of *Lipitor* and they include diarrhea, dyspepsia, myalgia, and nausea. Are you on statins? Did you read over your drug disclosure before you administered your dose? Do you fully know what this drug is doing to your body?

More importantly, were you told that you could cure this without drugs? Were you ever told that this disorder started with your diet of carbs? The earliest report in PMC I found was dated Jan 1974 and simply stated that weight reduction was important to controlling hyperlipoproteinemia, a fancy word for high amounts of apolipoproteins in the body which indicate levels of cholesterol. The apolipoprotein that's the most dangerous is apolipoprotein B. That's the one you get from carbs. This one is behind more disease than any of the other apolipoproteins.

With apolipoprotein B, an LDL particle being involved in more disorders than any of the other apolipoproteins, and apo α being the basis of HDL particles why isn't more attention devoted to balancing cholesterol than just lowering it? Were you aware that balancing your cholesterol was much more important to your body than lowering it? Lowering cholesterol is dangerous for the body as it's cholesterol that regulates your hormones, creates vitamin D in your skin to help usher in the LDL particles into your cells to use as fuel. Without the vitamin D, your cells couldn't operate properly and your LDL particles would build up in your bloodstream, waiting to be glycated or used as fuel, whichever comes first.

According to a study completed in 1995; *Population studies linking low cholesterol to noncoronary mortalities do not demonstrate cause-and-effect relations. In fact, based on current studies, the opposite is more likely to be the case. Drug intervention, however, should be used conservatively, particularly in young adults and the elderly. Drugs should be used only after diet and lifestyle interventions have failed. The evidence linking high blood cholesterol to coronary atherosclerosis and cholesterol-lowering to its prevention is broad-based and definitive. Concerns about cholesterol lowering and spontaneously low cholesterols should be pursued but should not interfere with the implementation of current public policies to reduce the still heavy burden of atherosclerosis in Western society.*

Another study from 1994 showed *the rethinking of the low-fat hi-carb diet that has been pushed for over 40 years (probably at the insistence of Monsanto). Since they owned GD Searle at the time it makes me wonder, was it their intent to hook us on more drugs? Even as recent Dec 31, 2016, the dept. of research at Kaiser Permanente Southern California, Pasadena came to this conclusion;*

From PMC, I found this report submitted Jun 17, 2013. It details the danger of statin use;

- *Statins in heart failure: do we need another trial?*

Two recent large randomized controlled trials, however, appear to suggest statins do not have beneficial effects on heart failure. In addition to lowering cholesterol, statins are believed to have many pleiotropic effects which could possibly influence the pathophysiology of heart failure. (Pleiotropic – one cause for many diseases)

Further, hyperuricemia is frequently present in chronic HF and has been attributed to increased production or decreased urinary excretion of uric acid (UA) or both in a compromised circulation.135 An elevated plasma level of UA is linked with a wide variety of injurious processes comprising increased inflammatory markers, cell apoptosis, and ED,139 which could cumulatively worsen HF. Serum UA is known to be a marker of HF prognosis and mortality140–142 and statins have been shown to decrease UA levels by increasing urate excretion.143,144

Our medical industry has had research for over 20 years on the benefits of cholesterol and the dangers of lowering it, yet because of our dependence on grains and sugar and Monsanto's influence in the FDA and USDA, the recommendations from the USDA's agency for food labeling to food safety to *MyPlate, the CCNP* and at least 3 other agencies in the USDA alone, the CDC, the ADA, the ACS still recommend that you keep whole grains in your diet, regardless of the studies completed that show their danger. Why?

Monsanto is in the crop seed industry owning over 15 crop seed companies, all wanting to sell

GMO seed, ready to handle Roundup herbicide to farmers contracted by Monsanto waiting to plant their next crop. They'll spray their crops according to their contract with Monsanto. It then goes on your table. Could Monsanto's old execs in the offices and agencies of the USDA and the FDA have anything to do with their decisions to ignore these facts? Or is this influence from Pfizer and Pharmacia? (I'm sure Monsanto stock is still in their portfolios.)

This article appeared 22 years ago in PubMed in Aug 1994. Even then low cholesterol was being questioned, yet in some corners, it's still promoted today;

- **The questionable wisdom of a low-fat diet and cholesterol reduction**

Although hypercholesterolemia is associated with increased liability to death from heart disease, it is as frequently associated with increased overall life expectancy as with decreased life expectancy. These findings are incompatible with labeling hypercholesterolemia an overall health hazard. Moreover, it is questionable if the cardiovascular liability associated with hypercholesterolemia is either causal or reversible. The complex relationships between diet, serum cholesterol, atherosclerosis, and mortality and their interactions with genetic and environmental factors suggest that the effects of simple dietary prescriptions are unlikely to be predictable, let alone beneficial. These cautions are borne out by numerous studies which have shown that multifactorial primary intervention to lower cholesterol levels is as likely to increase death from cardiovascular causes as to decrease it. Importantly, the only significant overall effect of a cholesterol-lowering intervention that has ever been shown is increased mortality.

With Monsanto's influence in the FDA, the USDA, the EPA and who knows what else, who's to protect our food supply? You have to protect yourself. Monsanto has proven they can't self-regulate their industry and keep us safe. The best way to start being safe is to not eat their food, which happens to include all grains. If you don't buy them, that may send the message.

More evidence, published Dec 18, 2016, of its influence in cancer is when this HMGB1 RAGE rears its ugly head again;

- *"Blockade of High Mobility Group Box 1 (HMGB1) augments anti-tumor T-cell response induced by peptide vaccination as a co-adjuvant"*

"High Mobility Group Box 1 (HMGB1) is a member of the damage-associated molecular patterns (DAMPs), which cause inflammation and trigger innate immunity through Toll-like receptors (TLRs) 2/4 and the receptor for advanced glycation end products (RAGE). We examined the effect of glycyrrhizin, a selective inhibitor of HMGB1, on the induction of cytotoxic T-lymphocytes (CTLs) in mice. B6 mice, either OT-1 spleen cell-transferred or untransferred, were immunized with an s.c. injection of the OVA257-264 peptide with topical imiquimod and glycyrrhizin was mixed with the antigen peptide. The proliferation of OT-1 cells after immunization was enhanced by glycyrrhizin. The effect of glycyrrhizin was confirmed in other adjuvant systems, such as CpG oligonucleotide and monophosphoryl lipid A (MPL), but glycyrrhizin was not effective in Freund's incomplete adjuvant system. The augmenting effects of glycyrrhizin were also observed in other synthetic HMGB1 inhibitors, i.e., gabexate mesylate, nafamostat, and sivelestat. Thus the effects are common to the HMGB1 inhibitors. Induction of CTLs detected by IFN-γ ELISPOT assay was similarly augmented by glycyrrhizin. In a therapeutic vaccine model, glycyrrhizin inhibited the growth of s.c. transplanted EG.7 tumors. Expression of inflammatory cytokines in the skin inoculation site was downregulated by glycyrrhizin. These results suggest that HMGB1 inhibitors might be useful as a co-adjuvant for peptide vaccination with an innate immunity receptor-related adjuvant. This article is protected by copyright. All rights reserved." Study Link

Were you ever told that this could happen if you continued your diet of bread, corn, soy and other carbs? (Neither was I.)

This is evidence of glycation's effect on the kidneys from this report dated Oct 6, 2016:

- *"AGEs/sRAGE, a novel risk factor in the pathogenesis of end-stage renal disease"*

"Interaction of advanced glycation end products (AGEs) with its cell-bound receptor (RAGE) results in cell dysfunction through activation of nuclear factor kappa-B, increase in expression and release of inflammatory cytokines, and generation of oxygen radicals. Circulating soluble receptors, soluble receptor (sRAGE), endogenous secretory receptor (esRAGE) and cleaved receptor (cRGAE) act as a decoy for RAGE ligands and thus have cytoprotective effects. Low levels of sRAGE and esRAGE have been proposed as biomarkers for many diseases. However sRAGE and esRAGE levels are elevated in diabetes and chronic renal diseases and still, tissue injury occurs. It is possible that increases in levels of AGEs are greater than increases in the levels of soluble receptors in these two diseases. Some new parameters have to be used which could be universal biomarkers for cell dysfunction. It is hypothesized that increases in serum levels of AGEs are greater than the increases in the soluble receptors, and that the levels of AGEs is correlated with soluble receptors and that the ratios of AGEs/sRAGE, AGEs/esRAGE, and AGEs/cRAGE are elevated in patients with end-stage renal disease (ESRD) and would serve as a universal risk marker for ESRD. The study subject comprised of 88 patients with ESRD and 20 healthy controls. AGEs, sRAGE and esRAGE were measured using commercially available enzyme-linked immune assay kits. cRAGE was calculated by subtracting esRAGE from sRAGE. The data show that the serum levels of AGEs, sRAGE, cRAGE are elevated and that the elevation of AGEs was greater than those of soluble receptors. The ratios of AGEs/sRAGE, AGEs/esRAGE, and AGEs/cRAGE were elevated and the elevation was similar in AGEs/sRAGE and AGEs/cRAGE but greater than AGEs/esRAGE. The sensitivity, specificity, accuracy, and positive and negative predictive value of AGEs/sRAGE and AGEs/cRAGE were 86.36 and 84.88%, 86.36 and 80.95%, 0.98 and 0.905, 96.2 and 94.8%, and 61.29 and 56.67% respectively. There was a positive correlation of sRAGE with esRAGE and cRAGE, and AGEs with esRAGE; and a negative correlation between sRAGE and AGEs/sRAGE, esRAGE and AGES/esRAGE, and cRAGE and AGES/cRAGE. In conclusion, AGEs/sRAGE, AGEs/cRAGE, and AGEs/esRAGE may serve as universal risk biomarkers for ESRD and that AGEs/sRAGE and AGEs/cRAGE are better risk biomarkers than AGEs/esRAGE." Study Link

This report from Sep15, 2016 is the evidence that breast cancer is influenced by glycation;

- *"Increased Expression of the Receptor for advanced glycation End-Products (RAGE) Is Associated with Advanced Breast Cancer Stage"*

"Abstract

BACKGROUND:

The receptor for advanced glycation end-products (RAGE) is a multiligand transmembrane receptor that is overexpressed in various pathological conditions including cancers. However, the expression pattern of RAGE in breast cancer tumors is still not completely clear.

METHODS:

In this study, we investigated the expression levels of RAGE in 25 fresh-frozen breast cancer samples and corresponding noncancerous tissue samples collected from breast cancer patients, by real-time polymerase chain reaction (PCR). Additionally, we performed immunohistochemistry on breast cancer specimens.

RESULTS:

The results indicate a high expression of the RAGE-encoding gene in the cancerous tissues. RAGE expression at the mRNA and protein levels was statistically significantly up-regulated in advanced-stage and triple-negative breast tumors and node-positive tissues compared with other tissues (p < 0.001). A significant association between RAGE expression and tumor size was observed (p = 0.029).

CONCLUSIONS:

Overexpression of RAGE in advanced-stage tumors may be a useful biomarker for diagnosis and the prediction of breast cancer progression." Study Link

I'm only sorry that I could include studies and reports for all forms of cancer, but with they're being so many of them, that's a virtually impossible task.

I'll bet you didn't realize that your bone mineral density was a result of your diet, did you? (Nobody does.) Evidence of bone density decline from glycation is in this report from Dec14, 2016;

- *"advanced glycation end Products, Diabetes, and Bone Strength"*

"Diabetic patients have a higher fracture risk than expected by their bone mineral density (BMD). Poor bone quality is the most suitable and explainable cause of the elevated fracture risk in this population. Advanced glycation end products (AGEs), which are diverse compounds generated via a non-enzymatic reaction between reducing sugars and amine residues, physically affect the properties of the bone material, one of a component of bone quality, through their accumulation in the bone collagen fibers. On the other hand, these compounds biologically act as agonists for these receptors for AGEs (RAGE) and suppress bone metabolism. The concentrations of AGEs and endogenous secretory RAGE, which acts as a "decoy receptor" that inhibits the AGEs-RAGE signaling axis, are associated with fracture risk in a BMD-independent manner. AGEs are closely associated with the pathogenesis of this unique clinical manifestation through physical and biological mechanisms in patients with diabetes mellitus." Study link

Evidence of Alzheimer's disease from glycation in this report from Oct 4, 2016;

- *"Genetic association between RAGE polymorphisms and Alzheimer's disease and Lewy body dementias in a Japanese cohort: a case-control study"*

"Abstract

BACKGROUND/AIMS:

Interaction of receptor for advanced glycation end products (RAGE) with amyloid-β increases amplification of oxidative stress and plays pathological roles in Alzheimer's disease (AD). Oxidative stress leads to α-synuclein aggregation and is also a major contributing factor in the pathogenesis of Lewy body dementias (LBDs). Therefore, we aimed to investigate whether RAGE gene polymorphisms were associated with AD and LBDs.

METHODS:

Four single nucleotide polymorphisms (SNPs)-rs1800624, rs1800625, rs184003, and rs2070600-of the gene were analyzed using a case-control study design comprising 288 AD patients, 76 LBDs patients, and 105 age-matched controls.

RESULTS:

Linkage disequilibrium (LD) examination showed strong LD from rs1800624 to rs2070600 on the gene (1.1 kb) in our cases in Japan. Rs184003 was associated with an increased risk of the AD. Although there were no statistical associations for the other three SNPs, haplotypic analyses detected genetic associations between AD and the RAGE gene. Although relatively few cases were studied, results from the SNPs showed that they did not modify the risk of developing LBDs in the Japanese population.

CONCLUSION: Our findings suggested that polymorphisms in the RAGE gene are involved in genetic susceptibility to the AD. Copyright © 2016 John Wiley & Sons, Ltd." Study Link

With the above evidence showing its involvement in brain diseases, how long will it take for this information to show up in the media? Doesn't anyone of authority examine these reports? More evidence below of cancer-causing agents from glycation leaving me to wonder; is anyone looking out for our benefit? This next report is from Oct 3, 2016;

- *"M2 macrophages do not fly into a "RAGE"*

"Tumor-associated macrophages (TAMs) are key elements in orchestrating host responses inside tumor stroma. This population may undergo a polarized activation process, thus rendering a heterogeneous spectrum of phenotypes, where the classically activated type 1 macrophages (M1) and the alternative activated type 2 macrophages (M2) represent two extreme phenotypes. In this commentary, based on very recent research findings, we intend to highlight how complex could be the crosstalk among all components of tumor stroma, where the coexistence of non-natural partners may even skew the canonical responses that we can expect." Study Link

This is where your addiction starts with this evidence of glycation causing agents in baby food. This is indicative of the glucose in the formula. Ask yourself why this is done if glucose is capable of doing this much harm;

- *"Protein breakdown and release of β-casomorphins during in vitro gastrointestinal digestion of sterilized model systems of liquid infant formula"*

"Protein modifications occurring during sterilization of infant formulas can affect protein digestibility and release of bioactive peptides. The effect of glycation and cross-linking on protein breakdown and release of β-casomorphins was evaluated during in vitro gastrointestinal digestion (GID) of six sterilized model systems of infant formula. Protein degradation during in vitro GID was evaluated by SDS-PAGE and by measuring the nitrogen content of ultrafiltration (3kDa) permeates before and after in vitro GID of model IFs. Glycation strongly hindered protein breakdown, whereas cross-linking resulting from β-elimination reactions had a negligible effect. Only β-casomorphin 7 (β-CM7) was detected (0.187-0.858mgL(-1)) at the end of the intestinal digestion in all untreated IF model systems. The level of β-CM7 in the sterilized model systems prepared without addition of sugars ranged from 0.256 to 0.655mgL(-1). The release of this peptide during GID was hindered by protein glycation." Study Link

Here's your proof that glucose and its glycative results are responsible for type 1 diabetes (the one thought to be an autoimmune disorder), this was just released Oct 15, 2010. Watch to ooo if you'll hear anything about it. If you don't, it's probably because Big Pharma has something to say about it;

- *"The Receptor for advanced glycation endproducts Drives T Cell Survival and Inflammation in Type 1 Diabetes Mellitus"*

"The ways in which environmental factors participate in the progression of autoimmune diseases are not known. After initiation, it takes years before hyperglycemia develops in patients at risk for type 1 diabetes (T1D). The receptor for advanced glycation endproducts (RAGE) is a scavenger receptor of the Ig family that binds damage-associated molecular patterns and advanced glycated end products and can trigger cell activation. We previously found constitutive intracellular RAGE expression in lymphocytes from patients with T1D. In this article, we show that there is increased RAGE expression in T cells from at-risk euglycemic relatives who progress to T1D compared with healthy control subjects, and in the CD8+ T cells in the at-risk relatives who do versus those who do not progress to T1D. Detectable levels of the RAGE ligand high mobility group box 1 were present in serum from at-risk subjects and patients with T1D. Transcriptome analysis of RAGE+ versus RAGE- T cells from patients with T1D showed differences in signaling pathways associated with increased cell activation and survival. Additional markers for effector memory cells and inflammatory function were elevated in the RAGE+ CD8+ cells of T1D patients and at-risk relatives of patients before disease onset. These studies suggest that expression of RAGE in T cells of subjects progressing to disease predates dysglycemia. These findings imply that RAGE expression enhances the inflammatory function of T cells, and its increased levels observed in T1D patients may account for the chronic autoimmune response when damage-

associated molecular patterns are released after cell injury and killing."

Study Link

Evidence of the role of AGEs in the process of neurodegenerative diseases in this study from Sep 21, 2016;

- *"Impact of Non-Enzymatic Glycation in Neurodegenerative Diseases: Role of Natural Products in Prevention"*

How long will it take for this information to be publicized? If it isn't, why not? Is it because there's no money in it?

The following is evidence of glycations role in cardiovascular disease from Sep 16, 2016;

- *"Advanced Glycation End-Products Induce Apoptosis of Vascular Smooth Muscle Cells: A Mechanism for Vascular Calcification"*

"Vascular calcification, especially medial artery calcification, is associated with cardiovascular death in patients with diabetes mellitus and chronic kidney disease (CKD). To determine the underlying mechanism of vascular calcification, we have demonstrated in our previous report that advanced glycation end-products (AGEs) stimulated calcium deposition in vascular smooth muscle cells (VSMCs) through excessive oxidative stress and phenotypic transition into osteoblastic cells. Since AGEs can induce apoptosis, in this study we investigated its role on VSMC apoptosis, focusing mainly on the underlying mechanisms. A rat VSMC line (A7r5) was cultured and treated with glycolaldehyde-derived AGE-bovine serum albumin (AGE3-BSA). Apoptotic cells were identified by Terminal deoxynucleotidyl transferase UTP nick end labeling (TUNEL) staining. To quantify apoptosis, an enzyme-linked immunosorbent assay (ELISA) for histone-complexed DNA fragments was employed. Real-time PCR was performed to determine the mRNA levels. Treatment of A7r5 cells with AGE3-BSA from 100 µg/mL concentration markedly increased apoptosis, which was suppressed by Nox inhibitors. AGE3-BSA significantly increased the mRNA expression of NAD (P)H oxidase components including Nox4 and p22(phox), and these findings were confirmed by protein levels using immunofluorescence. The dihydroethidium assay showed that compared with BSA, AGE3-BSA increased reactive oxygen species level in A7r5 cells. Furthermore, AGE3-induced apoptosis was significantly inhibited by siRNA-mediated knockdown of Nox4 or p22 (phox). Double knockdown of Nox4 and p22 (phox) showed a similar inhibitory effect on apoptosis as single gene silencing. Thus, our results demonstrated that NAD (P)H oxidase-derived oxidative stress is involved in AGEs-induced apoptosis of VSMCs. These findings might be important to understand the pathogenesis of vascular calcification in diabetes and CKD."

Evidence of glycation from this study completed last year on mental disorders like schizophrenia;

- *"The regulation of soluble receptor for AGEs contributes to carbonyl stress in schizophrenia"*

"Our previous study showed that enhanced carbonyl stress is closely related to schizophrenia. The endogenous secretory receptor for advanced glycation end-products (esRAGE) is a splice variant of the AGER gene and is one of the soluble forms of RAGE. esRAGE is considered to be a key molecule for alleviating the burden of carbonyl stress by entrapping advanced glycation end-products (AGEs). In the current study, we conducted genetic association analyses focusing on AGER, in which we compared 212 schizophrenic patients to 214 control subjects. We also compared esRAGE levels among a subgroup of 104 patients and 89 controls and further carried out measurements of total circulating soluble RAGE (sRAGE) in 25 patients and 49 healthy subjects. Although the genetic association study yielded inconclusive results, multiple regression analysis indicated that a specific haplotype composed of rs17846798, rs2071288, and a 63 bp deletion, which were in perfect linkage disequilibrium (r2 = 1), and rs2070600 (Gly82Ser) were significantly associated with a marked

decrease in serum esRAGE levels. Furthermore, compared to healthy subjects, schizophrenia showed significantly lower esRAGE (p = 0.007) and sRAGE (p = 0.03) levels, respectively. This is the first study to show that serum esRAGE levels are regulated by a newly identified specific haplotype in AGER and that a subpopulation of schizophrenic patients is more vulnerable to carbonyl stress. Copyright © 2016 The Authors. Published by Elsevier Inc. All rights reserved." Study Link

Methylglyoxal is what makes up pyruvic acid which is a foundation for energy expenditure. It comes from glycogen which comes from glucose and can be made into lipids to be used for cholesterol or glucose to be used by your brain when the ketones aren't enough to power all lobes in the brain. This the link from glucose to disease through its conversion to AGEs, advanced glycation endproducts as explained by this study published Sep 2016;

- *"Methylglyoxal in Metabolic Disorders: Facts, Myths, and Promises"*

"Glucose and fructose metabolism originates the highly reactive by-product methylglyoxal (MG), which is a strong precursor of advanced glycation end products (AGE). The MG has been implicated in classical diabetic complications such as retinopathy, nephropathy, and neuropathy, but has also been recently associated with cardiovascular diseases and central nervous system disorders such as cerebrovascular diseases and dementia. Recent studies even suggested its involvement in insulin resistance and beta-cell dysfunction, contributing to the early development of type2 diabetes and creating a vicious circle between glycation and hyperglycemia. Despite several drugs and natural compounds have been identified in the last years in order to scavenge MG and inhibit AGE formation, we are still far from having an effective strategy to prevent MG-induced mechanisms. This review summarizes the endogenous and exogenous sources of MG, also addressing the current controversy about the importance of exogenous MG sources. The mechanisms by which MG changes cell behavior and its involvement in type2 diabetes development and complications and the pathophysiological implication are also summarized. Particular emphasis will be given to the pathophysiological relevance of studies using higher MG doses, which may have produced biased results. Finally, we also overview the current knowledge about detoxification strategies, including modulation of endogenous enzymatic systems and exogenous compounds able to inhibit MG effects on biological systems." Study Link

Evidence of glycations influence in pancreatic complications was detailed in this report dated Aug 22, 2016;

- *"advanced glycation end Products Impair Glucose-Stimulated Insulin Secretion of a Pancreatic β-Cell Line INS-1-3 by Disturbance of Microtubule Cytoskeleton via p38/MAPK Activation"*

Advanced glycation end products (AGEs) are believed to be involved in diverse complications of diabetes mellitus. Overexposure to AGEs of pancreatic β-cells leads to decreased insulin secretion and cell apoptosis. Here, to understand the cytotoxicity of AGEs to pancreatic β-cells, we used INS-1-3 cells as a β-cell model to address this question, which was a subclone of INS-1 cells and exhibited a high level of insulin expression and high sensitivity to glucose stimulation. Exposed to a large dose of AGEs, even though more insulin was synthesized, its secretion was significantly reduced from INS-1-3 cells. Further, AGEs treatment led to a time-dependent increase of depolymerized microtubules, which was accompanied by an increase of activated p38/MAPK in INS-1-3 cells. Pharmacological inhibition of p38/MAPK by SB202190 reversed microtubule depolymerization to a stabilized polymerization status but could not rescue the reduction of insulin release caused by AGEs. Taken together, these results suggest a novel role of AGEs-induced impairment of insulin secretion, which is partially due to a disturbance of microtubule dynamics that resulted from an activation of the p38/MAPK pathway." Study Link

In my estimation, this is the worst manifestation of bread in the diet. Amyloid plaque is at the root of most modern diseases, ranging from cancer to heart disease to arthritis to Alzheimer's disease and Parkinson's disease. This report is from Aug22, 2016;

- *"Glycation induced generation of amyloid fibril structures by glucose metabolites"*

"The non-enzymatic reaction (glycation) of reducing sugars with proteins has received increased interest in dietary and therapeutic research lately. In the present work, the impact of glycation on structural alterations of camel serum albumin (CSA) by different glucose metabolites was studied. Glycation of CSA was evaluated by specific fluorescence of advanced glycation end-products (AGEs) and determination of available amino groups. Further, conformational changes in CSA during glycation were also studied using 8-analino 1-naphthalene sulfonic acid (ANS) binding assay, circular dichroism (CD) and thermal analysis. Intrinsic fluorescence measurement of CSA showed a 22 nm red shift after methylglyoxal treatment, suggesting glycation induced denaturation of CSA. Rayleigh scattering analysis showed glycation induced turbidity and aggregation in CSA. Furthermore, ANS binding to native and glycated-CSA reflected perturbation in the environment of hydrophobic residues. However, CD spectra did not reveal any significant modifications in the secondary structure of the glycated-CSA. Thioflavin T (ThT) fluorescence of CSA increased after glycation, illustrated cross β-structure and amyloid formation. Transmission electron microscopy (TEM) analysis further reaffirms the formation of aggregate and amyloid. In summary, glucose metabolites induced conformational changes in CSA and produced aggregate and amyloid structures."

This is more evidence of glycation's involvement in Alzheimer's disease. This report was submitted on Aug 24, 2016, have you heard anything about this yet? Who doesn't want you to know? Who have interests in selling your medication for memory loss? How would you learn this information if you didn't see it here? Do you know where to look for it? Do you even know to look for it? Am I fishing or can this be a conspiracy?

- *"HMGB1 and thrombin mediate the blood-brain barrier dysfunction acting as biomarkers of neuroinflammation and progression to neurodegeneration in Alzheimer's disease"*

"BACKGROUND:

The blood-brain barrier (BBB) dysfunction represents an early feature of Alzheimer's disease (AD) that precedes the hallmarks of amyloid beta (amyloid β) plaque deposition and neuronal neurofibrillary tangle (NFT) formation. A damaged BBB correlates directly with neuroinflammation involving microglial activation and reactive astrogliosis, which is associated with increased expression and/or release of high-mobility group box protein 1 (HMGB1) and thrombin. However, the link between the presence of these molecules, BBB damage, and progression to neurodegeneration in the AD is still elusive. Therefore, we aimed to profile and validate non-invasive clinical biomarkers of BBB dysfunction and neuroinflammation to assess the progression to neurodegeneration in mild cognitive impairment (MCI) and AD patients.

METHODS:

We determined the serum levels of various proinflammatory damage-associated molecules in aged control subjects and patients with MCI or AD using validated ELISA kits. We then assessed the specific and direct effects of such molecules on BBB integrity in vitro using human primary brain microvascular endothelial cells or a cell line.

RESULTS:

We observed a significant increase in serum HMGB1 and soluble receptor for advanced glycation end products (sRAGE) that correlated well with amyloid beta levels in AD patients (vs. control subjects). Interestingly, serum HMGB1 levels were significantly elevated in MCI patients compared to controls or AD patients. In addition, as a marker of BBB damage, soluble thrombomodulin (TM) antigen, and activity were significantly (and distinctly) increased in MCI and AD patients. Direct in vitro BBB integrity assessment further revealed a significant and concentration-dependent increase in paracellular permeability to dextrans by HMGB1 or α-thrombin, possibly through disruption of zona occludins-1 bands. Pre-treatment with anti-HMGB1 monoclonal antibody blocked HMGB1 effects and leaving BBB integrity intact.

CONCLUSIONS:

Our current studies indicate that thrombin and HMGB1 are causal proximate proinflammatory mediators of BBB dysfunction, while STM levels may indicate BBB endothelial damage; HMGB1 and sRAGE might serve as clinical biomarkers for progression and/or therapeutic efficacy along the AD spectrum." Study Link

With the previous study being completed last year, I'm curious to learn how long it will take for this information to be publicized. (If it ever is.)

More evidence of the damaging effects of glycation was submitted July 15, 2016. Have you heard anything about this report yet?

- *"The false alarm hypothesis: Food allergy is associated with high dietary advanced glycation end-products and proglycating dietary sugars that mimic alarmins."*

"The incidence of food allergy has increased dramatically in the last few decades in westernized developed countries. We propose that the Western lifestyle and diet promote innate danger signals and immune responses through production of "alarmins. Alarmins are endogenous molecules secreted from cells undergoing nonprogrammed cell death that signal tissue and cell damage. High molecular group S (HMGB1) is a major alarmin that binds to the receptor for advanced glycation end-products (RAGE). Advanced glycation end-products (AGEs) are also present in foods. We propose the "false alarm" hypothesis, in which AGEs that are present in or formed from the food in our diet are predisposing to food allergy. The Western diet is high in AGEs, which are derived from cooked meat, oils, and cheese. AGEs are also formed in the presence of a high concentration of sugars. We propose that a diet high in AGEs and AGE-forming sugars results in misinterpretation of a threat from dietary allergens, promoting the development of food allergy. AGEs and other alarmins inadvertently prime innate signaling through multiple mechanisms, resulting in the development of allergic phenotypes. Current hypotheses and models of food allergy do not adequately explain the dramatic increase in food allergy in Western countries. Dietary AGEs and AGE-forming sugars might be the missing link, a hypothesis supported by a number of convincing epidemiologic and experimental observations, as discussed in this article." Study Link

Again no alert about this evidence of the influence of glycation in dementia submitted in Aug 2016 from the Oxford Journal of Gerontology;

- *"Inflammatory Biomarkers Predict Domain-Specific Cognitive Decline in Older Adults"*

"BACKGROUND:

Vascular risk factors, including inflammation, may contribute to dementia development. We investigated the associations between peripheral inflammatory biomarkers and cognitive decline in five domains (memory, construction, language, psychomotor speed, and executive function).

METHODS:

Community-dwelling older adults from the Ginkgo Evaluation of Memory Study (n = 1,159, aged 75 or older) free of dementia at baseline were included and followed for up to 7 years. Ten biomarkers were measured at baseline representing different sources of inflammation: vascular inflammation (pentraxin 3 and serum amyloid P), endothelial function (endothelin-1), metabolic function (adiponectin, resistin, and plasminogen activating inhibitor-1), oxidative stress (receptor for advanced glycation end products), and general inflammation (interleukin-

6, interleukin-2, and interleukin-10). A combined z-score was created from these biomarkers to represent total inflammation across these sources. We utilized generalized estimating equations that included an interaction term between z-scores and time to assess the effect of inflammation on cognitive decline, adjusting for demographics (such as age, race/ethnicity, and sex), cardiovascular risk factors, and apolipoprotein E ε4 carrier status. A Bonferroni-adjusted significance level of .01 was used. We explored associations between individual biomarkers and cognitive decline without adjustment for multiplicity.

RESULTS:

The combined inflammation z-score was significantly associated with memory and psychomotor speed ($p < .01$). Pentraxin 3, serum amyloid P, endothelin-1, and interleukin-2 were associated with a change in at least one cognitive domain ($p < .05$).

CONCLUSION:

Our results suggest that total inflammation is associated with memory and psychomotor speed. In particular, systemic inflammation, vascular inflammation, and altered endothelial function may play roles in the domain-specific cognitive decline of nondemented individuals. © The Author 2016. Published by Oxford University Press on behalf of The Gerontological Society of America. All rights reserved." Study Link

Are you beginning to wonder why we've never been informed of these dangers? Evidence below of glycation in lung cancer was submitted on Aug 9, 2016. I've not heard anything about this. Doesn't the ACS care? They're still recommending carbs in the diet, so they must not;

- "advanced glycation end-Products Enhance Lung Cancer Cell Invasion and Migration"

"Effects of carboxymethyl-lysine (CML) and pentosidine, two advanced glycation end-products (AGEs), upon invasion and migration in A549 and Calu-6 cells, two non-small cell lung cancer (NSCLC) cell lines were examined. CML or pentosidine at 1, 2, 4, 8 or 16 µmol/L were added into cells. Proliferation, invasion, and migration were measured. CML or pentosidine at 4-16 µmol/L promoted invasion and migration in both cell lines and increased the production of reactive oxygen species, tumor necrosis factor-α, interleukin-6 and transforming growth factor-β1. CML or pentosidine at 2-16 µmol/L up-regulated the protein expression of AGE receptor, p47(phox), intercellular adhesion molecule-1 and fibronectin in test NSCLC cells. Matrix metalloproteinase-2 protein expression in A549 and Calu-6 cells was increased by CML or pentosidine at 4-16 µmol/L. These two AGEs at 2-16 µmol/L enhanced nuclear factor κ-B (NF-κ B) p65 protein expression and p38 phosphorylation in A549 cells. However, CML or pentosidine at 4-16 µmol/L up-regulated NF-κB p65 and p-p38 protein expression in Calu-6 cells. These findings suggest that CML and pentosidine, by promoting the invasion, migration, and production of associated factors, benefit NSCLC metastasis." Study Link

This is the evidence of your back problems being caused by glycation. This study shows how the inflammatory responses to glycation causing vertebral disk degeneration;

- "IL-1β/HMGB1 signaling promotes the inflammatory cytokines release via TLR signaling in human intervertebral disc cells"

"Inflammation and cytokines have been recognized to correlate with intervertebral disc (IVD) degeneration (IDD), via mediating the development of clinical signs and symptoms. However, the regulation mechanism remains unclear. We aimed at investigating the regulatory role of interleukin (IL)β and high mobility group box 1 (HMGB1) in the inflammatory response in human IVD cells and then explored the signaling pathways mediating such regulatory effect. Firstly, the promotion of inflammatory cytokines in IVD cells was examined with ELISA method. And then western blot and real-time quantitative PCR were performed to analyze the expression of toll-like receptors (TLRs), receptors for advanced glycation endproducts (RAGE) and NF-κB signaling markers in the IL-1β- or (and) HMGB1-treated IVD cells. Results demonstrated that either IL-1β or HMGB1 promoted the release of the inflammatory cytokines such as prostaglandin E2 (PGE2), TNF-α, IL-6 and IL-8 in human IVD cells. And the expression of matrix metalloproteinases (MMPs) such as MMP-1, -3 and -9 was also additively up-regulated by IL-1β and HMGB1. We also found such additive promotion to the expression of TLR-2, TLR-4 and RAGE, and the NF-κB signaling in intervertebral disc cells. In summary, our study demonstrated that IL-1β and HMGB1 additively promote the release of inflammatory cytokines and the expression of MMPs in human IVD cells. The TLRs and RAGE and the NF-κB signaling were also additively promoted by IL-1β and HMGB1. Our study implied that the additive promotion by IL-1β and HMGB1 to inflammatory cytokines and MMPs might aggravate the progression of IDD." Study Link

That study was submitted on Sep 16, 2016. I would have thought that I would have heard something about this by now, but I guess there's not enough money in curing. There's only enough money in treatment, as in continuous treatment.

It has to do with supply and demand. In this case, it's the pharmaceutical industry supplying its own demand...for customers, that is. They must think that the crop seed industry isn't sending them enough. If that isn't greed, I don't know what it.

Even unborn babies are not immune to the effects of what this industry is intent on putting as many Americans as they can, though. The damage they choose to ignore is in the glycation that's evidenced by this report dated Aug 10, 2016. How long do you think it will take for this information to be publicized? My estimate: never. (No money in it);

- "Accumulation of advanced glycation end Products Involved in Inflammation and Contributing to Severe Preeclampsia, in Maternal Blood, Umbilical Blood, and Placental Tissues"

Abstract

OBJECTIVE:

To investigate the expression of advanced glycation end products (AGEs) and the receptor for AGE (RAGEs) in maternal blood, umbilical blood and placental tissues in women with severe preeclampsia (PE) as well as any association with inflammatory processes.

METHODS:

The expressions of AGEs, RAGE, tumor necrosis factor-alpha (TNF)-α and vascular cell adhesion molecule-1 (VCAM)-1 in placental tissues were measured using immunohistochemistry. The levels of AGEs, RAGE, TNF-α and VCAM-1 in maternal blood, umbilical blood and placental extracts were assessed using enzyme-linked immunosorbent assays. Placental RAGE, TNF-α, and VCAM-1 mRNA expression levels were determined by PCR. Placental AGEs, RAGE, TNF-α and VCAM-1 protein levels were determined by western blotting.

RESULTS:

The levels of AGEs, TNF-α, and VCAM-1 in the maternal tissues and umbilical blood were significantly higher in the SPE group than in the normal pregnancy (NP) controls ($p < 0.05$). The serum level of sRAGE in the umbilical blood was lower in the SPE group than in the NP controls ($p < 0.05$), while sRAGE was higher in the maternal blood of SPE than in the NP ($p < 0.05$). The maternal serum levels of AGEs were positively correlated with that of TNF-α and VCAM-1 in the maternal blood. There were no correlations between the levels of RAGE, TNF-α or VCAM-1 in maternal blood or umbilical serum. There were no correlations between the levels of sRAGE and TNF-α or VCAM-1 in maternal blood or umbilical serum. The levels of AGEs were positively correlated with those of TNF-α and VCAM-1 in placental lysates.

CONCLUSION:

AGEs and RAGE appear to act as important mediators in regulating the inflammatory pathways of preeclampsia.

From this report from Aug 9, 2016, ovarian cancer is a consequence of glycation;

- *S100B Mediates Stemness of Ovarian Cancer Stem-like Cells Through Inhibiting p53*

"S100B is one of the members of the S100 protein family and is involved in the progression of a variety of cancers. Ovarian cancer is driven by cancer stem-like cells (CSLCs) that are involved in tumor genesis, metastasis, chemoresistance and relapse. We then hypothesized that S100B might exert pro-tumor effects by regulating ovarian CSLCs stemness, a key characteristic of CSLCs. First, we observed the high expression of S100B in ovarian cancer specimens when compared to that in normal ovary. The S100B upregulation associated with more advanced tumor stages, poorer differentiation and poorer survival. In addition, elevated S100B expression correlated with increased expression of stem cell markers including CD133, Nanog and Oct4. Then, we found that S100B was preferentially expressed in CD133+ ovarian CSLCs derived from both ovarian cancer cell lines and primary tumors of patients. More importantly, we revealed that S100B knockdown suppressed the in vitro self-renewal and in vivo tumorigenicity of ovarian CSLCs and decreased their expression of stem cell markers. S100B ectopic expression endowed non-CSLCs with stemness, which has been demonstrated with both in vitro and in vivo experiments. Mechanically, we demonstrated that the underlying mechanism of S100B-mediated effects on CSLCs stemness was not dependent on its binding with a receptor for advanced glycation end products (RAGE), but might be through intracellular regulation, through the inhibition of p53 expression and phosphorylation. In conclusion, our results elucidate the importance of S100B in maintenance of ovarian CSLCs stemness, which might provide a promising therapeutic target for ovarian cancer. Stem Cells 2016." Study Link

HMGB1 is a label that's been assigned to a type of AGE or RAGE. It's importance lies in its ability to create pain in your body. This is one of over 11,851 warnings and notices of what glycation does to the body that available for your perusal on the effects of glycation on PubMed;

- *The Emerging Role of HMGB1 in Neuropathic Pain: A Potential Therapeutic Target for Neuroinflammation*

Neuropathic pain (NPP) is intolerable, persistent, and specific type of long-term pain. It is considered to be a direct consequence of pathological changes affecting the somatosensory system and can be debilitating for affected patients. Despite recent progress and growing interest in understanding the pathogenesis of the disease, NPP still presents a major diagnostic and therapeutic challenge. High mobility group box 1 (HMGB1) mediates inflammatory and immune reactions in nervous system and emerging evidence reveals that HMGB1 plays an essential role in neuroinflammation through receptors such as Toll-like receptors (TLR), receptor for advanced glycation end products (RAGE), C-X-X motif chemokines receptor 4 (CXCR4), and N-methyl-D-aspartate (NMDA) receptor. In this review, we present evidence from studies that address the role of HMGB1 in NPP. First, we review studies aimed at determining the role of HMGB1 in NPP and discuss the possible mechanisms underlying HMGB1-mediated NPP progression where receptors for HMGB1 are involved. Then we review studies that address HMGB1 as a potential therapeutic target for NPP.   Study Link

The following study was completed in July 2010, explaining the health benefits of calorie restriction. This is what was being researched over 120 years ago, as ketonuria was noticed in the urine of fasting patients, giving them ketonemia. This is a condition that best serves healing in the body for multiple reasons and has been shown to heal many diseases, simply from fasting. Since 500BC fasting has been used to cure many diseases with astonishing success. This is what's known as ketosis today and is what your body goes through as a healing, fat burning type of metabolism. It uses your own fat to provide everything from hormones to glucose, through gluconeogenesis, the perfect glucose for the body as it made from your fat, making it a clean glucose source;

- *Dietary Interventions to Extend Life Span and Health Span Based on Calorie Restriction*

The societal impact of obesity, diabetes, and other metabolic disorders continues to rise despite increasing evidence of their negative long-term consequences on health span, longevity, and aging. Unfortunately, dietary management and exercise frequently fail as remedies, underscoring the need for the development of alternative interventions to successfully treat metabolic disorders and enhance lifespan and health span. Using calorie restriction (CR)—which is well known to improve both health and longevity in controlled studies—as their benchmark, gerontologists are coming closer to identifying dietary and pharmacological therapies that may be applicable to aging humans. This review covers some of the more promising interventions targeted to affect pathways implicated in the aging process as well as variations on classical CR that may be better suited to human adaptation.

Another report submitted Nov, 08 to the *Official Journal of the International League Against Epilepsy*, basically said the same thing while they were looking for the best way to approach putting the body into ketosis;

The ketogenic diet (KD) is a 90% fat diet that is an effective treatment for intractable epilepsy. Rapid initiation of the KD requires hospital admission because of the complexity of the protocol and frequent mild and moderate adverse events. The purpose of the study was to compare the efficacy of a gradual KD initiation with the standard KD initiation preceded by a 24- to 48-h fast.

Perhaps the most damning report against aging was issued in January of 1984, yet nothing was mentioned about this report; it was one of the first indications of what glycation does to the body and with a major cause of glycation being glucose or sugar, I have to wonder why the FDA didn't say anything about it then. Why weren't we, at least, informed about this study? Industry concerns?

- *Collagen aging in vitro by nonenzymatic glycosylation and browning*

Aging and diabetes mellitus are associated with cross-linking and nonenzymatic glycosylation of collagen. Incubation of tendon fibers with reducing sugars results in increased breaking time in urea similar to that seen in aging, and in nonenzymatic glycosylation and browning. Effect of a sugar is proportional to the amount of sugar available in the open chain form. The increase in breaking time correlates with the appearance of chromophores characteristic of cross-linked browning products. Collagen altered by nonenzymatic browning may play a role in some age-like major complications of diabetes.   Study Link

This evidence of glycation's role in atherosclerosis was in this study submitted in May 1988. Was this publicized? Did you hear about this? Did the FDA know?

Diminished adhesion of endothelial aortic cells on fibronectin and collagen layers after nonenzymatic glycation

Adhesion of bovine endothelial cells on fibronectin and collagen before and after nonenzymatic glycation in vitro has been studied. Nonenzymatic glycation of these proteins reduced their ability to bind endothelial cells. Furthermore, nonenzymatically glycated fibronectin failed to bind to normal and nonenzymatically glycated gelatin and to fibrin. So gelatin and fibrin Sepharoses can be used to separate highly glycated fibronectins from fibronectins with a low degree of nonenzymatic glucose substitution. Sodium dodecyl sulfate-polyacrylamide gel electrophoresis did not demonstrate a covalent cross-link between nonenzymatically glycated fibronectins. These results present further evidence for the role of nonenzymatic glycation of proteins in the development of vascular complications in long-term diabetes and of atherosclerosis.   Study Link

This shows the damage done by glycation on the blood. I posted this study because I wanted to note what the first sentence states, that this damage, at the time of publication, had been known for 20 years. The date of this study is marked on July 29, 1988. That means that his damage was discovered in 1968, 48 years ago.

- *Glycated haemoglobins*

The association between elevated levels of glycated hemoglobins and diabetes mellitus has been known for twenty years [92]. Since then the determination of glycated hemoglobins has become a valuable tool for the objective assessment of long-term glycemia in diabetic patients. The marked clinical interest in reliable measurements of glycated hemoglobins has stimulated the development and perfection of the necessary methodology. Limitations of the techniques have led to an investigation of the underlying causes. Some of them led to the recognition of processes that were not known to occur in vivo before, such as glycation at sites other than the amino terminus of the beta-chains, modification of hemoglobin by reactants other than glucose or the existence of labile hemoglobin adducts. With ideal methodology, these features would have gone unnoticed. Furthermore, the determination of glycated hemoglobin in large populations of diabetic patients has to lead to the discovery of new, clinically silent mutant hemoglobins. Today, the routine determination of glycated hemoglobins in diabetic patients probably represents the broadest screening for mutant hemoglobins. The experience with glycated hemoglobins shows that overcoming difficulties in their determination, and progress in biomedical research, are closely intertwined.

This study shows how proteins exposed to glucose undergoes oxidative stress, the basis of aging;

- *"Autoxidative glycosylation": free radicals and glycation theory.*

Studies have shown that glycation in vitro is complicated by the ability of glucose to oxidise, in the presence of trace amounts of a transition metal, generating protein-reactive ketoaldehydes, hydrogen peroxide, and diverse free radicals. Protein exposed to glucose undergoes fragmentation and conformational alterations, and these, as well as thiol oxidation, appear to be caused by hydroxyl radicals. Glycofluorophore formation is dependent upon ketoaldehyde formation. It is suggested that glucose autoxidation contributes to oxidative stress in pathophysiology associated with diabetes and aging via this newly described process of "autoxidative glycosylation".

The following report from Oct 30, 1981, shows the effects of glycation on cholesterol, LDL particles particularly and how it leads to atherosclerosis ;

- *Nonenzymatic glycosylation of low-density lipoproteins in vitro. Effects on cell-interactive properties*

Atherosclerosis occurs at an accelerated rate in patients with diabetes mellitus. Since some proteins undergo nonenzymatic glycosylation in diabetic patients and because certain chemical modifications of low-density lipoproteins produced alterations in their interactions with certain cultured cells, a fact that may be relevant to atherogenesis, we investigated the effect of in vitro glycosylation on cell-related properties of low-density lipoproteins. Glycosylation was carried out by incubating LDL (1-10 mg LDL-protein/ml) with glucose (0-100 mM) in 0.5 M phosphate buffer, pH 8.0, at 37 degrees C. The amount of glucose incorporated into LDL after 1-2 wk of incubation was estimated to be in the range of 1-10 mol/mol LDL-protein. Amino acid analysis of glycosylated LDL showed that glucose was covalently bound to lysine residues. In studies with cultured human fibroblasts, glycosylated LDL was internalized and degraded significantly less than control LDL, in proportion to the estimated degree of glycosylation (12% of control for the most extensively glycosylated LDL). Glycosylation of LDL also impaired significantly its ability to stimulate cholesteryl ester synthesis in cultured fibroblasts. Glycosylated LDL did not stimulate cholesteryl ester synthesis in rat peritoneal macrophages. If glycosylation of LDL occurs in diabetic patients, some pathophysiologic consequences related to the increased incidence of atherosclerosis in *these patients may result.*

Study Link

In 1981 this was discovered, yet it's been 35 years since then and yet few people are aware of this. My question is, why? Maybe I should ask the sugar industry.

The following study shows the how the adhesive qualities of glucose creates fibrinogen, which becomes a target for glycation;

- *Polymerisation and crosslinking of fibrin monomers in diabetes mellitus*

Polymerisation and crosslinking of fibrin monomers were studied in 35 healthy volunteers and in 42 poorly controlled diabetic patients. Polymerisation did not show any difference between control subjects (n = 10) and diabetic patients (n = 11) (p greater than 0.1), although fibrinogen was 35% more glycated in the diabetic patients (p less than 0.001). Alpha chain crosslinking in the diabetic patients, however, was impaired as is shown from an increase in intermediate alpha polymers with a concomitant decrease in alpha monomer disappearance. A significant positive correlation was found between the degree of glycation of fibrinogen and the defective alpha chain polymerization (r = 0.86, p less than 0.005). These results were consistent with the results of thrombin and reptilase experiments. The reaction rate with reptilase did not show any difference between the two groups (p greater than 0.1), whereas the reaction rate with thrombin was significantly slower in the diabetic group compared to the control subjects (p less than 0.001). Purified fibrin clots obtained from the diabetic patients were more susceptible to plasmin than clots obtained from control subjects. It is concluded that in poorly controlled diabetic patients polymerization of fibrin monomers is normal, but crosslinking of the alpha chains is impaired, leading to a higher susceptibility of the clots to plasmin degradation.

FROM WIKIPEDIA ON FIBRINOGEN;

Fibrinogen (factor I) is a glycoprotein in vertebrates that helps in the formation of blood clots. It consists of a linear array of three nodules held together by a very thin thread which is estimated to have a diameter between 8 and 15 Angstrom (Å). The two end nodules are alike but the center one is slightly smaller. Measurements of shadow lengths indicate that nodule diameters are in the range 50 to 70 Å. The length of the dried molecule is 475 ± 25 Å.[2]

- *Effect of-of low-density lipoprotein on the immunological determination glycation of apolipoprotein B*

Non-enzymatic glycation of low-density lipoprotein (LDL) may contribute to the premature atherogenesis of patients with diabetes mellitus. To assess whether glycation of apolipoprotein B, the predominant protein of LDL, interferes with the ability to immunologically quantify this protein, we prepared and purified glycated LDL by incubating normal plasma samples with high concentrations of glucose. Although both the plasma and the LDL specimens incubated with glucose contained significantly more glycated protein than control specimens, the quantitative interaction of an apolipoprotein B-specific antibody with glycated vs nonglycated LDL was not significantly different. We conclude that apolipoprotein B can be accurately quantified immunologically despite the presence of clinically excessive degrees of LDL glycation.

Study Link

I included the following study from November 1989 because of its explanation of how glycation is responsible for inflammation;

- *Changes in concanavalin A-reactive proteins in inflammatory disorders*

Quantitative changes of concanavalin A (Con A)-reactive proteins in serum samples obtained from rats with induced inflammation and from patients with inflammatory and autoimmune diseases were examined by use of lectin blots. Treatment of rats with a single dose of fermented yeast to induce inflammation caused an extensive increase in Con A-reactivity. These changes were time-dependent and were similar in both sexes of the animals. When we examined serum samples obtained from patients with various inflammatory disorders for their Con A-reactive proteins as compared with normal donors, we noted that the Con A-reactivity increased in patients with rheumatoid arthritis and systemic lupus erythematosus. Among all the glycoproteins examined by lectin blots with use of Con A, a set of five proteins was selected for detailed analysis by densitometric scanning. These included alpha 2-macroglobulin, P-150, P-95, P-40, and P-35, of Mr 180,000, 150,000, 95,000, 40,000, and 35,000, respectively, by sodium dodecyl sulfate-polyacrylamide gel electrophoresis under reducing conditions. Densitometric scanning analysis of the lectin blots revealed that the Con A-reactivity of these proteins increased during inflammation. Because alpha 2-macroglobulin is not an acute-phase protein in humans, an increase in Con A staining of this protein suggested that altered glycation is associated with autoimmune diseases. Thus, the study of changes in Con A-reactive proteins in human sera may facilitate our understanding of the etiology and pathophysiology of autoimmune diseases.   Study Link

- *Clinical Value of High Mobility Group Box 1 and the Receptor for **Advanced Glycation End-products** in Head and Neck Cancer: A Systematic **Review***

"Abstract Introduction   High mobility group box 1 is a versatile protein involved in gene transcription, extracellular signaling, and response to inflammation. Extracellularly, high mobility group box 1 binds to several receptors, notably the receptor for advanced glycation end-products. Expression of high mobility group box 1 and the receptor for advanced glycation end-products has been described in many cancers. Objectives To systematically review the available literature using PubMed and Web of Science to evaluate the clinical value of high mobility group box 1 and the receptor for advanced glycation end-products in head and neck squamous cell carcinomas. Data Synthesis A total of eleven studies were included in this review. High mobility group box 1 overexpression is associated with poor prognosis and many clinical and pathological characteristics of head and neck squamous cell carcinomas patients. Additionally, the receptor for advanced glycation end-products demonstrates potential value as a clinical indicator of tumor angiogenesis and advanced staging. In diagnosis, high mobility group box 1 demonstrates low sensitivity. Conclusion   High mobility group box 1 and the receptor for advanced glycation end-products are associated with clinical and pathological characteristics of head and neck squamous cell carcinomas. Further investigation of the prognostic and diagnostic value of these molecules is warranted."

- *[Glycosylated lipoprotein]*

"Diabetes is frequently associated with cardiovascular diseases (coronary heart disease, cerebrovascular disease, peripheral vascular disease), and several risk factors have been proposed. Recent studies have strengthened the importance of chronic hyperglycemia because this modifies a variety of circulating substances including lipoproteins, and the glycosylated ones can be involved in the process of accelerating atherosclerosis. In this review, previous studies indicating the significance of glycosylated lipoproteins in the progression of atherosclerosis were overviewed. We also discussed AGE (advanced glycation end products) which may play an important role of atherogenesis in diabetes."The most recent study, submitted in October 2016 reveals some of the known damage that glycation is responsible for;

- *The relationship between plasma glycation with membrane modification, oxidative stress and expression of glucose transporter-1 in type 2 diabetes patients with vascular complications.*

BACKGROUND OF STUDY:

Enhanced protein glycation in diabetes causes irreversible cellular damage through membrane modifications. Erythrocytes are persistently exposed to plasma glycated proteins;

however, little is known about its consequences on the membrane. The aim of this study was to examine the relationship between plasma protein glycation with erythrocyte membrane modifications in type 2 diabetes patients with and without vascular complications.

METHOD:

We recruited 60 healthy controls, 85 type 2 diabetic mellitus (DM) and 75 type 2 diabetic patients with complications (DMC). Levels of plasma glycation adduct with antioxidants (fructosamine, protein carbonyl, β-amyloids, thiol groups, total antioxidant status), erythrocyte membrane modifications (protein carbonyls, β-amyloids, free amino groups, erythrocyte fragility), antioxidant profile (GSH, catalase, lipid peroxidation) and Glut-1 expression were quantified.

RESULT:

Compared with controls, DM and DMC patients had significantly higher level of glycation adducts, erythrocyte fragility, lipid peroxidation and Glut-1 expression whereas declined levels of plasma and cellular antioxidants. Correlation studies revealed the positive association of membrane modifications with erythrocyte sedimentation rate, fragility, peroxidation whereas the negative association with free amino groups, glutathione, and catalase.

CONCLUSION:

Our data suggest that plasma glycation is associated with oxidative stress, Glut-1 expression and erythrocyte fragility in DM patients. This may further contribute to the progression of vascular complications.

More evidence of the role glucose plays in brain degradation;

- *Glycation potentiates neurodegeneration in models of Huntington's disease.*

Protein glycation is an age-dependent posttranslational modification associated with several neurodegenerative disorders, including Alzheimer's and Parkinson's diseases. By modifying amino-groups, glycation interferes with the folding of proteins, increasing their aggregation potential. Here, we studied the effect of pharmacological and genetic manipulation of glycation on huntingtin (HTT), the causative protein in Huntington's disease (HD). We observed that glycation increased the aggregation of mutant HTT exon 1 fragments associated with HD (HTT72Q and HTT103Q) in yeast and mammalian cell models. We found that glycation impairs HTT clearance thereby promoting its intracellular accumulation and aggregation. Interestingly, under these conditions autophagy increased and the levels of mutant HTT released to the culture medium decreased. Furthermore, increased glycation enhanced HTT toxicity in human cells and neurodegeneration in fruit flies, impairing eclosion and decreasing lifespan. Overall, our study provides evidence that glycation modulates HTT exon-1 aggregation and toxicity, and suggests it may constitute a novel target for therapeutic intervention in HD.

Brain development hinges on the cholesterol as well, as cholesterol is your brain's neuronal-connectors. It couldn't operate without it. This report illustrates the importance of cholesterol in the brain;

- *Cholesterol in brain disease: sometimes determinant and frequently implicated*

Cholesterol is essential for neuronal physiology, both during development and in the adult life: as a major component of cell membranes and precursor of steroid hormones, it contributes to the regulation of ion permeability, cell shape, cell-cell interaction, and transmembrane signaling. Consistently, hereditary diseases with mutations in cholesterol-related genes result in impaired brain function during early life. In addition, defects in brain cholesterol metabolism may contribute to neurological syndromes, such as Alzheimer's disease (AD), Huntington's disease (HD), and Parkinson's disease (PD), and even to the cognitive deficits typical of the old age. In these cases, brain cholesterol defects may be secondary to disease-causing elements and contribute to the functional deficits by altering synaptic functions. In the first part of this review, we will describe hereditary and non-hereditary causes of cholesterol dyshomeostasis and the relationship to brain diseases. In the second part, we will focus on the mechanisms by which perturbation of cholesterol metabolism can affect synaptic function.

In summary, it is clear that a direct disturbance of cholesterol metabolism, for example, by defects in cholesterol synthesizing enzymes or transporters, impairs brain development and function. In addition, changes in cholesterol metabolism in the adult and during aging, and in several age-related neurodegenerative diseases, can directly impact on brain function.

Another report disputes the dangers of cholesterol in this report dated Feb 18, 2012;

- ***Is the use of cholesterol in mortality risk algorithms in clinical guidelines valid? Ten years prospective data from the Norwegian HUNT 2 study***

Many clinical guidelines for cardiovascular disease (CVD) prevention contain risk estimation charts/calculators. These have shown a tendency to overestimate risk, which indicates that there might be theoretical flaws in the algorithms. Total cholesterol is a frequently used variable in the risk estimates. Some studies indicate that the predictive properties of cholesterol might not be as straightforward as widely assumed. Our aim was to document the strength and validity of total cholesterol as a risk factor for mortality in a well-defined, general Norwegian population without known CVD at baseline.

Conclusions

Based on epidemiological analysis of updated and comprehensive population data, we found that the underlying assumptions regarding cholesterol in clinical guidelines for CVD prevention might be flawed: cholesterol emerged as an overestimated risk factor in our study, indicating that guideline information might be misleading, particularly for women with 'moderately elevated' cholesterol levels in the range of 5–7 mmol L−1. Our findings are in good accord with some previous studies. A potential explanation of the lack of accord between clinical guidelines and recent population data, including ours, is time trend changes for CVD/IHD and underlying causal (risk) factors.

Conclusion

Our study provides an updated epidemiological indication of possible errors in the CVD risk algorithms of many clinical guidelines. If our findings are generalizable, clinical and public health recommendations regarding the 'dangers' of cholesterol should be revised. This is especially true for women, for whom moderately elevated cholesterol (by current standards) may prove to be not only harmless but even beneficial.

The previous report disputes the often fatal assumption that high cholesterol is hazardous to your health. They're recommending a change, in the advice offered, on cholesterol. I contend that it's not the cholesterol, it's the glucose.

- *Extracellular HMGB1 promotes differentiation of nurse-like cells in chronic lymphocytic* LEUKEMIA

"Chronic lymphocytic leukemia (CLL) is a disease of an accumulation of mature B cells that are highly dependent on the microenvironment for maintenance and expansion. However, little is known regarding the mechanisms whereby CLL cells create their favorable microenvironment for survival. High-mobility group protein B-1 (HMGB1) is a highly conserved nuclear protein that can be actively secreted by innate immune cells and passively released by injured or dying cells. We found significantly increased HMGB1 levels in the plasma of CLL patients compared with healthy controls, and HMGB1 concentration is associated with absolute lymphocyte count. We, therefore, sought to determine potential roles of HMGB1 in modulating the CLL microenvironment. CLL cells passively released HMGB1, and the timing

and concentrations of HMGB1 in the medium were associated with differentiation of nurse-like cells (NLCs). Higher CD68 expression in CLL lymph nodes, one of the markers for NLCs, was associated with shorter overall survival of CLL patients. HMGB1-mediated NLC differentiation involved internalization of both receptors for advanced glycation end products (RAGE) and Toll-like receptor-9 (TLR9). Differentiation of NLCs can be prevented by blocking the HMGB1-RAGE-TLR9 pathway. In conclusion, this study demonstrates for the first time that CLL cells might modulate their microenvironment by releasing HMGB1." Free PMC Article

J Clin Invest. 1984 Nov;74(5):1742-9.

After searching these last few disorders I got a yen to search any disorder & glycation, and glycation turned up in everything except halitosis. The following report shows its involvement in stomach ulcers. I originally searched just ulcers and got back 30 studies showing involvement. The first few studies in the list were reports on foot ulcers, so I search stomach ulcers and found 3 studies, the following report was the first;

- *High-mobility group box 1 inhibits gastric ulcer healing through Toll-like receptor 4 and receptor for advanced glycation end products*

High-mobility group box 1 (HMGB1) was initially discovered as a nuclear protein that interacts with DNA as a chromatin-associated non-histone protein to stabilize nucleosomes and to regulate the transcription of many genes in the nucleus. Once leaked or actively secreted into the extracellular environment, HMGB1 activates inflammatory pathways by stimulating multiple receptors, including Toll-like receptor (TLR) 2, TLR4, and receptor for advanced glycation end products (RAGE), leading to tissue injury. Although HMGB1's ability to induce inflammation has been well documented, no studies have examined the role of HMGB1 in wound healing in the gastrointestinal field. The aim of this study was to evaluate the role of HMGB1 and its receptors in the healing of gastric ulcers. We also investigated which receptor among TLR2, TLR4, or RAGE mediates HMGB1's effects on ulcer healing. Gastric ulcers were induced by serosal application of acetic acid in mice, and gastric tissues were processed for further evaluation. The induction of ulcer increased the immunohistochemical staining of cytoplasmic HMGB1 and elevated serum HMGB1 levels. Ulcer size, myeloperoxidase (MPO) activity, and the expression of tumor necrosis factor α (TNFα) mRNA peaked on day 4. Intraperitoneal administration of HMGB1 delayed ulcer healing and elevated MPO activity and TNFα expression. In contrast, administration of anti-HMGB1 antibody promoted ulcer healing and reduced MPO activity and TNFα expression. TLR4 and RAGE deficiency enhanced ulcer healing and reduced the level of TNFα, whereas ulcer healing in TLR2 knockout (KO) mice was similar to that in wild-type mice. In TLR4 KO and RAGE KO mice, exogenous HMGB1 did not affect ulcer healing and TNFα expression. Thus, we showed that HMGB1 is a complicating factor in the gastric ulcer healing process, which acts through TLR4 and RAGE to induce excessive inflammatory responses. **Free PMC Article**

- *Nonenzymatic glycation of human lens crystallin, Effect of aging and diabetes mellitus*

We have examined the nonenzymatic glycation of human lens crystallin, an extremely long-lived protein, from 16 normal human ocular lenses 0.2-99 yr of age, and from 11 diabetic lenses 52-82-yr-old. The glucitol-lysine (Glc-Lys) content of soluble and insoluble crystallin was determined after reduction with H-borohydride followed by acid hydrolysis, boronic acid affinity chromatography, and high-pressure cation exchange chromatography. Normal lens crystallin, soluble and insoluble, had 0.028 +/- 0.011 nanomoles Glc-Lys per nanomole crystallin monomer. Soluble and insoluble crystallins had equivalent levels of glycation. The content of Glc-Lys in normal lens crystallin increased with age in a linear fashion. Thus, the nonenzymatic glycation of nondiabetic lens crystallin may be regarded as a biological clock. The diabetic lens crystallin samples (n = 11) had a higher content of Glc-Lys (0.070 +/- 0.034 nmol/nmol monomer). Over an age range comparable to that of the control samples, the diabetic crystallin samples contained about twice as much Glc-Lys. The Glc-Lys content of the *diabetic lens crystallin samples did not increase with lens age.*

This study looked at the effects of glycation on your eyes and cataracts it's responsible for. Yes, glycation and a glucose diet will buy you cataracts. My mother had two of them. A good friend who loved to eat her bread had cataracts in both of her eyes as well. What's interesting, this person was always complaining of headaches and stomach aches. Both of those manifestations are from an ECC diet. Again, here is more evidence of the glycative and addictive effects of a grain diet. In all, there were 3,629 studies on the effects of glucose glycating proteins, hemoglobin, and cholesterol dating back to March 1984. Incidentally, that was one month after I was released from the hospital after spending a month in a coma and suffering two strokes while comatose. I could have never come back this far without Dr. Perlmutter's help. Again, I have to thank you, Dr. Perlmutter.

They've had some of this evidence for over 30 years, why hasn't the public been told about glycation or the AGEs they create? It's those AGEs that are at the root of all modern diseases. If this was uncovered starting 30+ years ago, why have we just found out about it from the bestselling books from two doctors? Is someone trying to hide something? My guess is yes. This is Monsanto's path to power and freedom. They've politically engineered their freedom to wreak whatever havoc they can on your health by masturbating your taste buds with their glucose laden products, to grant them power by buying into their pharmaceutical cycle in the very near future. By near, I mean, it only takes a couple days before you're indebted. (That means addicted.) If you want true power and freedom, you can have it in two weeks to two months. That's how long it takes to break the addiction.

Each and every one of these 11,000+ studies has been vetted and examined by the NIH and PubMed for whom I thank immensely. It's clear that this *ruse/problem/pandemic* is not going to go away unless the consumer does something about it, them. The only way out of this dilemma leaves you with very limited options,

YOU HAVE TWO CHOICES;

1. Continue to masturbate your taste buds and collect these diseases and disorders in return.
2. Cut out as much as possible the starchy carbohydrates, (grains) and live free from dependence.

You need to realize that the comfort in comfort food, brings massive discomfort in the future, and the process starts immediately, with a process called glycation. This is the real poisoning of America and we can correct it. It lies within our power. Each and every one of us can correct this. I offer a cure, not a therapy or treatment, My cure simply involves removal of all glycating substances from the diet to eliminate this problem of glycation so that it never affects the body The glycating substances = carbs, sugar, glucose, fructose.

The above reports on the effects of glycation appeared in some cases, over 30 years ago in PubMed. Many of these reports were submitted just last year, as those are the first ones I come across.

I've only shown you a few of the reports out of 11,850 studies to date detailing the damaging effects of Excessive Carbohydrate Consumption, the primary cause of glycation, why doesn't the FDA or the USDA say anything about that? The 42nd study, submitted in November 1989 shows how it causes inflammation, and with inflammation a factor in so many diseases, it truly is a wonder that the FDA and USDA never even issued anything so simple as a warning. The **FDA'S INVOLVEMENT** in this issue is mostly explained by their influence from the one industry, where they get most of their management from, Monsanto.

From every form of cancer to Alzheimer's disease to heart disease and cardiovascular disease to arthritis to hypertension to high cholesterol these food sources (sugar and grains) are responsible for each and every one of these disorders. These studies are proof of exactly what sugar does to the body. To cure the glycation factor in these diseases, the best way is to eliminate it as much as possible. To do that you must eliminate its source and to eliminate the source, you have to eliminate the grains and sugar. Thank you, Dr. Davis and Dr. Perlmutter, for bringing this to my attention.

IN ALL, THERE WAS 3,629 STUDIES IN THE FDA'S DATABASE ON THE EFFECTS OF GLUCOSE GLYCATING PROTEINS, HEMOGLOBIN, AND CHOLESTEROL DATING BACK TO MARCH, 1984. INCIDENTALLY, THAT WAS ONE MONTH AFTER I WAS RELEASED FROM THE HOSPITAL AFTER SPENDING A MONTH IN A COMA AND SUFFERING TWO STROKES WHILE COMATOSE. I COULD HAVE NEVER COME BACK THIS FAR WITHOUT DR PERLMUTTER'S HELP. AGAIN, I HAVE TO THANK YOU, DR PERLMUTTER.

The above reports on the effects of glycation, appeared, in some cases over 30 years ago in PubMed or PMC. With 11,667 studies to date in PubMed, detailing the damaging effects of Excessive Carbohydrate Consumption, the primary cause of glycation, why doesn't the FDA say anything? There are roughly 6,000 more studies in PMC. The last study, submitted in November 1989 shows how it causes inflammation and with inflammation a factor in so many diseases, it truly is a wonder that the FDA never even issued anything as simple as a warning. The **FDA's involvement** in this issue is largely explained by the influence they receive from the one industry where they get a good portion of their execs from, Monsanto.

With having the evidence for over 30 years, why hasn't the public been told about glycation or the AGEs they create? It's those AGEs that are at the root of all modern diseases. If this was uncovered 30+ years ago, why have we just found out about it from the bestselling books from two doctors? Why did it take these two doctors to inform us of what's been going on? Why wasn't it the FDA or the USDA? Isn't that their job?

It would have been nice if someone could have warned me about this 20 or 30 years ago but the USDA and FDA had different ideas. For that, I thank Monsanto. Don't allow them to be in your driver's seat. As long as you remain on your carbohydrate diet, they're in the driver's seat for your health. Give up the carbs and put yourself back in the driver's seat. You are the only one who can change yourself. Enable yourself to do so.

Documentaries worth watching;

1. Food, Inc
2. Food Matters
3. Food Beware (French)
4. Genetically Modified Foods
5. David vs Monsanto
6. Of the Land
7. Hungry for Change
8. That Sugar Film
9. Fathead
10. Love Paleo
11. Heal Yourself
12. Fresh
13. Overfed and Undernourished
14. My Big Fat Body
15. Facing the Fat
16. Fat
17. Who Wants to Live Forever

Chapter 9

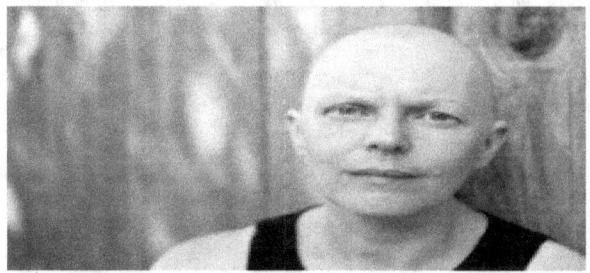

Can Your Cancer be Cured or Just Treated?

It's become evident to me that this problem of glycation goes much further than I previously thought when writing my second book, so it's important that I need to display a different chapter for the different types of damage that glycation induces. I'll list as many different types of cancer, here. All reports Of CVDs and other heart disorders will be located on the Atherosclerosis page. Dementias will be on a separate page as well, with all other diseases and disorders inflammation is responsible for. The third bout of breast cancer was what took my mother.

Listed below from PubMed or PMC or the FDA are reports of studies done on the effects of glycation and its influence in any cancer, which is a direct cause of glycation.

This report is dated Aug 9, 2016, and details AGEs role in lung cancer;

- *Advanced Glycation End-Products Enhance Lung Cancer Cell Invasion and Migration.*

Abstract

Effects of carboxymethyl-lysine (CML) and pentosidine, two advanced glycation end-products (AGEs), upon invasion and migration in A549 and Calu-6 cells, two non-small cell lung cancer (NSCLC) cell lines were examined. CML or pentosidine at 1, 2, 4, 8 or 16 µmol/L were added into cells. Proliferation, invasion, and migration were measured. CML or pentosidine at 4-16 µmol/L promoted invasion and migration in both cell lines and increased the production of reactive oxygen species, tumor necrosis factor-α, interleukin-6 and transforming growth factor-β1. CML or pentosidine at 2-16 µmol/L up-regulated the protein expression of AGE receptor, p47(phox), intercellular adhesion molecule-1 and fibronectin in test NSCLC cells. Matrix metalloproteinase-2 protein expression in A549 and Calu-6 cells was increased by CML or pentosidine at 4-16 µmol/L. These two AGEs at 2-16 µmol/L enhanced nuclear factor κ-B (NF-κ B) p65 protein expression and p38 phosphorylation in A549 cells. However, CML or pentosidine at 4-16 µmol/L up-regulated NF-κB p65 and p-p38 protein expression in Calu-6 cells. These findings suggest that CML and pentosidine, by promoting the invasion, migration, and production of associated factors, benefit NSCLC metastasis.

KEYWORDS: CML; invasion; migration; non-small cell lung cancer; pentosidine

I ran across this study on Polycystic Ovary Syndrome (PCOS). It details the influence that AGEs have on PCOS and how they contribute to the chronic inflammation and increased oxidative stress that is behind the disorder;

- *Do Advanced Glycation End Products (AGEs) Contribute to the comorbidities of Polycystic Ovary Syndrome (PCOS)?*

Advanced glycation end products (AGEs) are formed both during the endogenous and exogenous reactions and are implicated in the process of aging, pathogenesis of diabetes, atherosclerosis, female fertility, and cancers. Food and smoking are the most important sources of exogenous AGEs in daily life. The biochemical composition of the meal, cooking methods, time and temperature of food preparation may impact AGEs formation, therefore Western-type diet, rich in animal-derived products as well as in fast foods seems to be the main source of AGEs. Both, endogenous and exogenous AGEs can act intracellularly or during serum interaction with cell surface receptors called RAGE influencing a variety of molecular pathways. Polycystic ovary syndrome (PCOS) is the most common endocrinopathy in women of reproductive age. The etiology of this disorder remains unclear, however, the environmental and genetic factors may play an important role in its pathogenesis. Nevertheless, PCOS women have increased factors for reproductive and cardiometabolic comorbidities. AGEs can contribute to the pathogenesis of PCOS as well as its consequences. It has been shown that chronic inflammation and increased oxidative stress may be a link between the mechanisms of AGEs action and the metabolic and reproductive consequences of PCOS. This review highlights that high dietary AGEs intake promotes deteriorating biological effects in women with PCOS, whereas AGEs restriction seems to have a beneficial impact on women health. Better understanding AGEs formation and biochemistry as well as AGE-mediated pathophysiological mechanisms may open new therapeutic avenues converging to the achievement of the complete treatment of PCOS and its consequences.

This appears to be indicative of glucose's influence in ovarian cancer. Is this something you thought you were eating when you had your English muffin this morning?

The following report submitted Sept 1, 2008, was concerned about RAGEs correlation with cervical cancer;

- *Induction of receptor for advanced glycation end products by EBV latent membrane protein 1 and its correlation with angiogenesis and cervical lymph node metastasis in nasopharyngeal carcinoma.*

Abstract

PURPOSE:

The EBV oncoprotein, latent membrane protein 1 (LMP1), contributes to the metastasis of nasopharyngeal carcinoma (NPC) by inducing factors to promote tumor invasion and angiogenesis. The receptor for advanced glycation end products (RAGE) is associated with abnormal angiogenesis in diabetic microangiopathies. Moreover, some papers have suggested the association of RAGE overexpression with tumor metastasis; thus, the associations of RAGE with LMP1 and angiogenesis in NPC were examined.

EXPERIMENTAL DESIGN:

Forty-two patients with NPC were evaluated for expressions of LMP1, RAGE, and S100 proteins and for microvessel counts by immunohistochemistry. Then, the RAGE induction by LMP1 was examined with Western blotting and luciferase reporter assay.

RESULTS:

The microvessel counts were significantly higher in patients with high LMP1 expression or high RAGE expression compared with cases with low expressions (P=0.0049 and P<0.0001), respectively. Patients with advanced N classification were also significantly increased in these groups (P=0.0484 and P=0.0005). The expressions of LMP1 and RAGE proteins were clearly correlated in NPC tissues (P=0.0093). Transient transfection with an LMP1 expression plasmid induced RAGE protein in Ad-AH cells. The expression of LMP1 transactivated the RAGE promoter as shown by luciferase reporter assay. Mutation of the reporter at the nuclear factor-kappaB binding site (-671 to -663) abolished transactivation of the RAGE promoter by LMP1.

CONCLUSION:

These results suggest that LMP1-induced RAGE enhances lymph node metastasis through the induction of angiogenesis in NPC. The nuclear factor-kappaB binding site (-671 to -663) is essential for transactivation of the RAGE promoter by LMP1.

As of today January 10, 2017, this news still has not been spoken about in the media yet! No warnings about what causes glycation, only warnings against what doesn't cause it. That makes me wonder, is someone trying to hide this cure?

One wouldn't think that brain cancer would be affected by glycation, yet there's clear evidence of it in the following report, dated Mar 2008;

HMGB1 as an autocrine stimulus in human T98G glioblastoma cells: role in cell growth and migration.

Abstract

HMGB1 (high mobility group box 1 protein) is a nuclear protein that can also act as an extracellular trigger of inflammation, proliferation, and migration, mainly through RAGE (the receptor for advanced glycation end products); HMGB1-RAGE interactions have been found to be important in a number of cancers. We investigated whether HMGB1 is an autocrine factor in human glioma cells. Western blots showed HMGB1 and RAGE expression in human malignant glioma cell lines. HMGB1 induced a dose-dependent increase in cell proliferation, which was found to be RAGE-mediated and involved the MAPK/ERK pathway. Moreover, in a wounding model, it induced a significant increase in cell migration, and RAGE-dependent activation of Rac1 was crucial in giving the tumor cells a motile phenotype. The fact that blocking DNA replication with anti-mitotic agents did not reduce the distance migrated suggests the independence of the proliferative and migratory effects. We also found that glioma cells contain HMGB1 predominantly in the nucleus, and cannot secrete it constitutively or upon stimulation; however, necrotic glioma cells can release HMGB1 after it has translocated from the nucleus to cytosol. These findings provide the first evidence supporting the existence of HMGB1/RAGE signaling pathways in human glioblastoma cells and suggest that HMGB1 may play an important role in the relationship between necrosis and malignancy in glioma tumors by acting as an autocrine factor that is capable of promoting the growth and migration of tumor cells.

Even brain cancer is susceptible to glycation and its destructive effects. I can't seem to find cancer that isn't affected by glycation.

The following study was done in Sep 2013, and was concerned with the role of insulin and Insulin Growth Factor (IGF-1) signaling in cancer;

- ***The key role of growth hormone — insulin — IGF-1 signaling in aging and cancer***

Abstract

Studies in mammals have led to the suggestion that hyperglycemia and hyperinsulinemia are important factors in aging. GH/Insulin/insulin-like growth factor 1 (IGF-1) signaling molecules that have been linked to longevity include daf-2 and INR and their homologs in mammals, and inactivation of the corresponding genes increases lifespan in nematodes, fruit flies, and mice. The life-prolonging effects of caloric restriction are likely related to decreasing IGF-1 levels. Evidence has emerged that antidiabetic drugs are promising candidates for both lifespan extension and prevention of cancer. Thus, antidiabetic drugs postpone spontaneous carcinogenesis in mice and rats, as well as chemical and radiation carcinogenesis in mice, rats, and hamsters. Furthermore, metformin seems to decrease the risk for cancer in diabetic patients…

Research conducted during the last 15-20 years firmly established insulin, insulin-like and homologous signaling as key regulators of aging and longevity in organisms ranging from yeast to mammals.…dysregulation of insulin signaling and carbohydrate homeostasis in diabetes produces numerous aging-like symptoms including increased risk of cancer and other age-related diseases.

It's been over three years since that study was completed and no word has reached the media to tell the public about this finding. (I ask myself why.)

Published Oct 12, 2016, the following report acknowledges that diet plays a large role in the formation of AGEs the single most important factor in cancer, as AGEs are at the root of all cancers;

- *The Role of Advanced Glycation End-Products in Cancer Disparity.*

Abstract

While the socioeconomic and environmental factors associated with cancer disparity have been well documented, the contribution of biological factors is an emerging field of research. Established disparity factors such as low income, poor diet, drinking alcohol, smoking, and a sedentary lifestyle may have molecular effects on the inherent biological makeup of the tumor itself, possibly altering cell signaling events and gene expression profiles to profoundly alter tumor development and progression. Our understanding of the molecular and biological consequences of poor lifestyle is lacking, but such information may significantly change how we approach goals to reduce cancer incidence and mortality rates within minority populations. In this review, we will summarize the biological, socioeconomic, and environmental associations between a group of reactive metabolites known as advanced glycation end-products (AGEs) and cancer health disparity. Due to their links with lifestyle and the activation of disease-associated pathways, AGEs may represent both a biological consequence and a bio-behavioral indicator of poor lifestyle which may be targeted within specific populations to reduce disparities in cancer incidence and mortality.

Published at the end of last year was this report on the effects of HMGB1 on most all lung diseases;

- *Emerging role of HMGB1 in lung diseases: friend or foe.*

Abstract

Lung diseases remain a serious problem for public health. The immune status of the body is considered to be the main influencing factor for the progression of lung diseases. HMGB1 (high-mobility group box 1) emerges as an important molecule of the body immune network. Accumulating data have demonstrated that HMGB1 is crucially implicated in lung diseases and acts as an independent biomarker and therapeutic target for related lung diseases. This review provides an overview of updated understanding of HMGB1 structure, release styles, receptors, and function. Furthermore, we discuss the potential role of HMGB1 in a variety of lung diseases. Further exploration of molecular mechanisms underlying the function of HMGB1 in lung diseases will provide novel preventive and therapeutic strategies for lung diseases.

The following report details the overexpression of glycation in ovarian cancer. It was submitted Oct 28, 2016;

- ***Overexpression of receptor for advanced glycation end products (RAGE) in ovarian cancer.***

Abstract

BACKGROUND:

Ovarian cancer is one of the important challenges in the field of gynecologic oncology because of some problems in understanding its etiology and pathogenesis. Receptor for advanced glycation end products (RAGE) is a multiligand trans-membranous receptor which is upregulated in some human cancers. Mechanisms of RAGE involvement in carcinogenesis of ovarian cancer are unknown.

OBJECTIVE:

This study aimed to investigate the expression of RAGE in ovarian cancers and its association with clinicopathological characteristics.

METHODS:

The RAGE expression level in ovarian cancer and corresponding noncancerous tissues were analyzed by real-time quantitative RT-PCR and immunohistochemistry techniques.

RESULTS:

Results indicated that RAGE gene was overexpressed in ovarian cancer tissue compared with adjacent noncancerous tissue (p < 0.001). A significant association between RAGE expression and tumor size (p = 0.04), depth of stromal invasion (p = 0.031), lymphovascular invasion (p = 0.041) and stage of cancer (p = 0.041) was observed. The receiver operating characteristic (ROC) analyses yielded the area under the curve (AUC) values of 0.86 for RAGE in discriminating ovarian cancer samples from non-cancer controls.

CONCLUSIONS:

In conclusion overexpression of RAGE in ovarian cancer may be a useful biomarker to predict tumor progression.

What interests me is that nothing is said about what creates these RAGEs. For thirty years they've been examining the nature of glycation but have said nothing about what is responsible for the major portion of glycation, glucose consumption in the form of sugar and grains. I guess that's not profitable.

What is profitable is finding more drugs to make people need more and more drugs. Evidenced here in this report dated Oct 23, 2014, yet nothing has been announced about this report, Did you hear about it?

- ***RAGE is essential for oncogenic KRAS-mediated hypoxic signaling in pancreatic cancer.***

Abstract

A hypoxic tumor microenvironment is characteristic of many cancer types, including one of the most lethal, pancreatic cancer. We recently demonstrated that the receptor for advanced glycation end products (RAGE) has an important role in promoting the development of pancreatic cancer and attenuating the response to chemotherapy. We now demonstrate that binding of RAGE to oncogenic KRAS facilitates hypoxia-inducible factor 1 (HIF1)α activation and promotes pancreatic tumor growth under hypoxic conditions. Hypoxia induces NF-κB-dependent and HIF1α-independent RAGE expression in pancreatic tumor cells. Moreover, the interaction between RAGE and mutant KRAS increases under hypoxia, which in turn sustains KRAS signaling pathways (RAF-MEK-ERK and PI3K-AKT), facilitating stabilization and transcriptional activity of HIF1α. Knockdown of RAGE in vitro inhibits KRAS signaling, promotes HIF1α degradation, and increases hypoxia-induced pancreatic tumor cell death. RAGE-deficient mice have impaired oncogenic KRAS-driven pancreatic tumor growth with significant down-regulation of the HIF1α signaling pathway. Our results provide a novel mechanistic link between NF-κB, KRAS, and HIF1α, three potent molecular pathways in the cellular response to hypoxia during pancreatic tumor development and suggest alternatives for preventive and therapeutic strategies.

Obviously, the continuing need to examine the damage, instead of warning about the glycating substance proves to be more lucrative than realizing the actual cure, removing the glycating substances from the diet. Removing the glycating substances involves conquering an addiction, though. That wouldn't be too bad if this addiction wasn't inflicted on us. But it was, making this addiction almost impossible to conquer.

This is evidenced by this study dated July 18, 2016, and shows the influence of HMGB1 and M2 like macrophages;

- ***Tumour hypoxia promotes melanoma growth and metastasis via High Mobility Group Box-1 and M2-like macrophages.***

Abstract

Hypoxia is a hallmark of cancer that is strongly associated with invasion, metastasis, resistance to therapy and poor clinical outcome. Tumour hypoxia affects immune responses and promotes the accumulation of macrophages in the tumor microenvironment. However, the signals linking tumor hypoxia to tumor-associated macrophage recruitment and tumor promotion are incompletely understood. Here we show that the damage-associated molecular pattern High-Mobility Group Box 1 protein (HMGB1) is released by melanoma tumor cells as a consequence of hypoxia and promotes M2-like tumor-associated macrophage accumulation and an IL-10 rich milieu within a tumor. Furthermore, we demonstrate that HMGB1 drives IL-10 production in M2-like macrophages by selectively signaling through the Receptor for Advanced Glycation End products (RAGE). Finally, we show that HMGB1 has an important role in murine B16 melanoma growth and metastasis, whereas in humans its serum concentration is significantly increased in metastatic melanoma. Collectively, our findings identify a mechanism by which hypoxia affects tumor growth and metastasis in melanoma and depict HMGB1 as a potential therapeutic target.

Stomach cancer is influenced as well by glycation as explained in this report submitted Oct 1, 2015;

- ***Combined targeting of high-mobility group box-1 and interleukin-8 to control micro metastasis potential in gastric cancer.***

Abstract

Micrometastasis is the major cause of treatment failure in gastric cancer (GC). Because epithelial-to-mesenchymal transition (EMT) is considered to develop prior to macroscopic metastasis, EMT-promoting factors may affect micrometastasis. This study aimed to evaluate the role of extracellular high-mobility group box-1 (HMGB1) in EMT and the treatment effect of combined targeting of HMGB1 and interleukin-8 (IL-8) at early-stage GC progression through interrupting EMT promotion. Extracellular HMGB1 was induced by human recombinant HMGB1 and pCMV-SPORT6-HMGB1 plasmid transfection. EMT activation was evaluated by immunoblotting, immunofluorescence and immunohistochemistry. Increased migration/invasion activities were evaluated by in vitro transwell migration/invasion assay using all histological types of human GC cell lines (N87, MKN28 SNU-1, and KATOIII), N87-xenograft BALB/c nude mice and human paired serum-tissue GC samples. HMGB1-induced soluble factors were measured by chemiluminescent immunoassay. Inhibition effects of tumor growth and EMT activation by combined targeting of HMGB1 and IL-8 were evaluated in N87-xenograft nude mice. Serum HMGB1 increases along the GC carcinogenesis and reaches maximum before macroscopic metastasis. Overexpressed extracellular HMGB1 promoted EMT activation and increased cell motility/invasiveness through ligation to the receptor for advanced glycation end products. HMGB1-induced IL-8 overexpression contributed the HMGB1-induced EMT in GC in vitro and in vivo. Blocking HMGB1 caused significant reduction of tumor growth, and the addition of human recombinant IL-8 rescues this antitumor effects. Our results imply the role of HMGB1 in EMT through IL-8 mediation, and a potential mechanism of GC micrometastasis. Our observations suggest combination strategy of HMGB1 and IL-8 as a promising diagnostic and therapeutic target to control GC micrometastasis.

More evidence of Glycation in Breast cancer is in this report from Dec 23, 2016;

- ***Accumulation of the advanced glycation end product carboxymethyl lysine in breast cancer is positively associated with estrogen receptor expression and unfavorable prognosis in estrogen receptor-negative cases.***

Abstract

Advanced glycation end products (AGEs) accumulate as a result of high concentrations of reactive aldehydes, oxidative stress, and insufficient degradation of glycated proteins. AGEs are therefore accepted biomarkers for aging, diabetes, and several degenerative diseases. Due to the Warburg effect and increased oxidative stress, cancer cells frequently accumulate significant amounts of AGEs. As the accumulation of AGEs may reflect the metabolic state and receptor signaling, we evaluated the potential prognostic and predictive value of this biomarker. We used immunohistochemistry to determine the AGE Nε-carboxymethyl-lysine (CML) in 213 mammary carcinoma samples and Western blotting to detect AGEs in cell cultures. Whereas no significant correlation between hormone receptor status and CML was observed in cell lines, CML accumulation in tumors was positively correlated with the presence of estrogen receptor alpha, the postmenopausal state, and age. A negative correlation was found for grade III carcinomas and triple-negative cases.

Again, this form of cancer can be curable if you remove the glycating factor. I have yet to find cancer that can't be cured by taking away the glycating factor, glucose. Why then is glucose still a recommended food, as in carbohydrates such as "whole grains"?

It amazes me how many studies they find to say the same thing over and over again. Yet they keep doing it, day after day after day, in an unending cycle of dependence. This report on the effects of RAGEs on esophageal and lung cancers;

- *Tissue-specific expression profiling of receptor for advanced glycation end products and its soluble forms in esophageal and lung cancer.*

Abstract

The receptor for advanced glycation end products (RAGE) interacts with several ligands and is involved in various human diseases. Several splicing forms of the RAGE gene have been characterized, and two general mechanisms are usually responsible for the generation of soluble receptors. However, variants distribution and respective roles in different tumors are not clear. We analyzed RAGE and hRAGEsec mRNA expression in esophageal and lung cancer by RT-polymerase chain reaction. The Agilent clipper 1000 Bioanalyzer using lab-on-a-chip technology was applied to size and quantify the polymerase chain reaction products. Western blotting was performed to measure total soluble RAGE protein levels. The results showed that RAGE and its splice variants increased in esophageal cancers and decreased in lung cancers. We conclude that RAGE presents as a major isoform; soluble RAGE may also play certain roles in esophageal cancer and lung cancer.

How many reports does the FDA or the USDA need to tell them that what they're recommending for everyone to eat, is doing them more harm than good, far more?

This report dated June 15, 2007, shows the effects of AGEs on chondrosarcoma, a bone cancer;

- *Endogenous secretory receptor for advanced glycation endproducts as a novel prognostic marker in chondrosarcoma.*

Abstract

BACKGROUND:

Chondrosarcoma, the second most frequent primary malignant bone tumor, is classified into 3 grades according to histologic criteria of malignancy. However, a low-grade lesion can be difficult to distinguish from a benign enchondroma, whereas some histologically low-grade lesions may carry a poor prognosis. The receptor for advanced glycation endproducts (RAGE) and its ligand, high-mobility group box-1 (HMGB1), was quantified in enchondromas and chondrosarcomas to determine whether these markers were associated with histological malignancy and prognosis.

METHODS:

Enchondromas (n = 20) and typical chondrosarcomas (n = 39) were evaluated for RAGE, endogenous secretory RAGE (esRAGE, a splice variant form), and HMGB1 protein expression by immunohistochemistry including laser confocal microscopy. The content of esRAGE in resected specimens was measured with an enzyme-linked immunosorbent assay. Associations of these molecules with histology and clinical behavior of tumors were analyzed.

RESULTS:

Expression of esRAGE and HMGB1 was observed in all specimens. The numbers of cells positive for esRAGE and HMGB1 expression were positively associated with the histologic grade. Expression of esRAGE was significantly higher in chondrosarcomas than in enchondromas ($P < .001$). Tissue esRAGE content was also significantly higher in grade 1 and 2 chondrosarcomas than enchondromas ($P = .0255$ and $P = .008$, respectively). High expression of esRAGE in grade 1 chondrosarcoma was associated with subsequent recurrence ($P = .0013$), lung metastasis ($P = .0071$), and poor survival ($P < .001$).

CONCLUSIONS:

Assessment of esRAGE expression should aid in diagnostic and prognostic determinations in chondrosarcoma.

This report dated Nov 23, 2016, shows the effects that glycation and AGEs have on ovarian cancer and prostate cancer,

1. Introduction

Reactive oxygen species (ROS), generated as consequence of oxidative metabolism, activate signal transduction pathways, which contribute to cellular homeostasis. Metabolically active cells, neutrophils, and macrophages from the immune system produce high levels of ROS.

7. The Function of HMGB Proteins and Other Redox Sensors during Oxidative Stress in Ovarian Cancer

OS has been proposed as a cause of ovarian cancer. HMGB1 is considered a biomarker for ovarian cancer and increased levels of interleukin-8 protein (IL-8) and HMGB1 correlate with poor prognosis in prostate and ovarian cancer cells.

8. Oxidative Stress in Prostate Cancer and the Function of HMGB Proteins and Other Redox Sensors

The human prostate anatomy displays a zonal architecture, corresponding to central, periurethral transition, peripheral zone, and anterior fibromuscular stroma. The majority of prostate carcinomas are derived from the peripheral zone, while benign prostatic hyperplasia arises from the transition zone.

Finally, several research lines outline the direct importance of HMGB proteins in prostate cancer and their implications in therapy. Increased HMGB2 expression, HMGB1 expression, or coexpression of RAGE and HMGB1 has been associated with prostate cancer progression and has been correlated with poor patient outcome.

10. Conclusions and Perspectives

ROS overproduction and imbalance are a primary cause of malignancy in the onset of cancer. Cells have evolved multiple strategies in response to ROS production and HMGB proteins play a major role in many molecular mechanisms participating in these responses. In the nucleus, HMGB proteins affect DNA repair, transcription, and chromosomal stability; in the cytoplasm, they determine key decisions that finally lead towards autophagy or apoptosis; as extracellular signals, they produce changes that affect the microenvironment of a tumor and attract cells from the immune system. In turn, the inflammatory onset can increase ROS production and therefore enhances the response. HMGB1 and HMGB2 are expressed at the highest levels in immune cells and, besides, they have been related to cancers, which are hormone-responsive, such as ovarian and prostate cancers. Since HMGB proteins have many different functions and are necessary for healthy cells, an improved strategy to modulate their role in cancer progression could be to act through other proteins interacting specifically with them. The identification of HMGB partners, which could be univocally associated with specific cancerous processes or with mechanism of cisplatin resistance, is a field of interest for ongoing translational cancer research. Interactive strategies are outstanding for the development of these research lines.

A search for cervical cancer and glycation returned 602 studies in the PMC index and started with this study;

Expression and Effects of High-Mobility Group Box 1 in Cervical Cancer

We investigated the significance of high- mobility group box1 (HMGB1) and T-cell-mediated immunity and prognostic value in cervical cancer... HMGB1 expression may activate Tregs or facilitate Th2 polarization to promote immune evasion of cervical cancer. Elevated HMGB1 protein in cervical carcinoma samples was associated with a high recurrence of HPV infection in univariate analysis... Data collected here demonstrated that the expression of HMGB1 in cervical lesions increased with tumor progression.

I wanted to see the relationship between glycation and bladder cancer. My search returned 616 studies, with the first one dated Feb 25, 2015;

- *Expression of tumor suppressive microRNA-34a is associated with a reduced risk of bladder cancer recurrence*

Bladder cancer is the 4th most common cancer among men in the U.S. and more than half of patients experience recurrences within 5 years after initial diagnosis.

Kidney disease isn't immune from the effects of glycation either, as expressed in this study from Oct 29, 1993;

Expression of receptors for advanced glycosylation end products on renal cell carcinoma cells in vitro.

Abstract

Proteins that have been modified by long-term expose to glucose accumulate advanced glycosylation end products (AGEs) as a function of protein age. In these studies, we have examined the interaction of AGE-protein with renal cell carcinoma cells (RCC) in vitro, using AGE-modified bovine serum albumin (AGE-BSA) as a probe. AGE-BSA showed a tendency to induce in vitro cell growth of RCC cells and promoted the production of interleukin-6 (IL-6), an in vitro autocrine growth factor. Reverse transcriptase-polymerase chain reaction analysis revealed that RCC cells used here express mRNA for a receptor for AGEs (RAGE). These results suggested that AGEs taken up through RAGE on RCC cells might play a role in promoting the growth of RCC cells.

This was discovered in the summer of 1993 or prior, yet nothing was ever announced by the FDA or the USDA that there might be a preventative diet to protect against cancer. Did you hear anything about sugar or carbohydrates causing this kind of damage? I didn't. Yet the evidence is clear as day from a study done over 20 years ago. Still, nobody announced these revelations as they were being discovered. This report submitted Dec 2012;

Functional amyloid formation by STREPTOCOCCUS MUTANS

In summary, there is a growing realization that amyloid formation is a directed, widespread, functional process that contributes to the biology of numerous micro-organisms, with particular relevance for adhesion and biofilm formation. We have now demonstrated amyloid formation by the cariogenic pathogen S. MUTANS, which is not surprising considering its biofilm niche. In addition to the contribution of amyloids to virulence by facilitating the adhesion, biofilm formation and invasion of pathogens, microbial amyloids have been postulated to contribute to systemic diseases, including Alzheimer's and Parkinson's, possibly by seeding amyloid formation in the brain.

What's behind liver cancer? Copied from **PMC** on liver cancer;

According to the database from GLOBOCAN 2012, liver cancer has the fifth highest incidence rate and is the second most life-threatening cancer in the world. There were an estimated 14.1 million new cases and 8.2 million cancer deaths worldwide in 2012, among which there were 782,500 new patients and 745,500 deaths caused by liver cancer.

HMGB1 has been demonstrated as a critical role in a number of cancers, including colorectal, breast, lung, prostate, cervical, skin, kidney, gastric, pancreatic, osteosarcoma and leukemia.

Recently, HMGB1 has been recognized as a pro-angiogenesis factor leading to the generation of vascular endothelial growth factor (VEGF) in colon cancer, while RAGE was identified as the requirement for cell angiogenesis in HCC (hepatocellular carcinoma).

Autophagy and apoptosis are recognized as both the programmed cell deaths. In HCC, the release of HMGB1 from nuclei to cytoplasm was reported as an inducer of autophagic cell death, which may be associated with ROS and/or Beclin-1.

In summary, HMGB1 plays a pivotal role in oncogenesis and progression in HCC which may be a potential target for therapies and is worthy of further study. (What's responsible for HMGB1?)

This free report appeared in PubMed 3/1/2016, it expresses the role AGEs and RAGE play in Colorectal cancer, yet it's been a year since this report and nothing's been publicized about this; (Again I ask myself why.)

Clinical significance of AGE-RAGE axis in colorectal cancer: associations with glyoxalase-I, adiponectin receptor expression, and prognosis.

Abstract

BACKGROUND:

Advanced glycation end products (AGEs) and their receptor RAGE emerge as important pathogenic contributors in colorectal carcinogenesis. However, their relationship to the detoxification enzyme Glyoxalase (GLO)-I and Adiponectin receptors (AdipoR1, AdipoR2) in colorectal carcinoma (CRC) is currently understudied. In the present study, we investigated the expression levels of the above molecules in CRC compared to adjacent non-tumoral tissue and their potential correlation with clinicopathological characteristics and patients' survival.

METHODS:

We analyzed the immunohistochemical expression of AGE, RAGE and GLO-1, AdipoR1, and AdipoR2 in 133 primary CRC cases, focusing on GLO-1 The tumor MSI status was further assessed in mucinous carcinomas. Western immunoblotting was employed for validation of immunohistochemical data in normal and tumoral tissues as well as three CRC cell lines. An independent set of 55 patients was also used to validate the results of univariate survival analysis regarding GLO-1.

RESULTS:

CRC tissue showed the higher intensity of both AGE and RAGE expression compared with normal colonic mucosa which was negative for GLO-1 in most cases (78 %). Western immunoblotting confirmed AGE, RAGE and GLO-1 overexpression in tumoral tissue. GLO-1 expression was directly related to RAGE and inversely related to AGE immunolabeling. There was a trend towards higher expression of all markers (except for RAGE) in the subgroup of mucinous carcinomas which, although of borderline significance, seemed to be more prominent for AdipoR1 and AGE. Additionally, AGE, AdipoR1, and Adipo R2 expression were related to tumor grade, whereas GLO-1 and AdipoR1 to T-category. In survival analysis, AdipoR2 and GLO-1 overexpression predicted shortened survival in the entire cohort and in early-stage cases, an effect which for GLO-1 was reproduced in the validation cohort. Moreover, GLO-1 emerged as an independent prognosticator of adverse significance in the patients' cohort.

CONCLUSIONS:

We herein provide novel evidence regarding the possible interactions between the components of the AGE-RAGE axis, GLO-1 and adiponectin receptors in CRC. AGE and AdipoR1 are possibly involved in colorectal carcinogenesis, whereas AdipoR2 and GLO-1 emerged as novel independent prognostic biomarkers of adverse significance for patients with early disease stage. Further studies are warranted to extend our observations and investigate their potential therapeutic significance.

I'll bet that you thought that esophageal cancer was the result of smoking only. My best friend lost his wife to esophageal cancer 30 years ago. This study shows that it's not just the smoke that causes this cancer. Glycation of carbs tends to promote this cancer just as much as the smoking.

Plasma miR-185 is decreased in patients with esophageal squamous cell carcinoma and might suppress tumor migration and invasion by targeting RAGE.

The receptor for advanced-glycation end products (RAGE) is upregulated in various cancers and has been associated with tumor progression, but little is known about its expression and regulation by microRNAs (miRNAs) in esophageal squamous cell carcinoma (ESCC). Here, we describe miR-185, which represses RAGE expression and investigate the biological role of miR-185 in ESCC. In this study, we found that the high level of RAGE expression in 29 pairs of paraffin-embedded ESCC tissues was correlated positively with the depth of invasion by immunohistochemistry, suggesting that RAGE was involved in ESCC. We used bioinformatics searches and luciferase reporter assays to investigate the prediction that RAGE was regulated directly by miR-185. Besides, overexpression of miR-185 in ESCC cells was accompanied by 27% (TE-11) and 49% (Eca-109) reduced RAGE expression. The effect was further confirmed in RAGE protein by immunofluorescence in both cell lines. The effects were reversed following cotransfection with miR-185 and high-level expression of the RAGE vector. Furthermore, the biological role of miR-185 in ESCC cell lines was investigated using assays of cell viability, Ki-67 staining, and cell migration and invasion, as well as in a xenograft model. We found that overexpression of miR-185 inhibited migration and invasion by ESCC cells in vitro and reduced their capacity to develop distal pulmonary metastases in vivo partly through the RAGE/heat shock protein 27 pathway. Interestingly, in clinical specimens, the level of plasma miR-185 expression was decreased significantly (P = 0.002) in patients with ESCC [0.500; 95% confidence interval (CI) 0.248-1.676] compared with healthy controls (2.410; 95% CI 0.612-5.671). The value of the area under the receiver-operating characteristic curve was 0.73 (95% CI 0.604-0.855). In conclusion, our findings shed novel light on the role of miR-185/RAGE in ESCC metastasis, and plasma miR-185 has potential as a novel diagnostic biomarker in ESCC.

Are these enough reports to prove how glycation directly influence cancer? After reading this can you see the logic in controlling cancer by controlling your carb intake? Where are the warnings from the FDA and the USDA? Don't they care about what they're recommending? Don't they understand, because of their recommendations, they send millions of Moms and Dads, sisters and brothers, husbands and wives to their slow, expensive, painful deaths?

These are free reports that are available to everyone. All you have to do is search for them at the National Library of Medicine in the National Institute of Health. There are literally 100s of thousands of reports on the effects of glycation that remain hidden in the PubMed and PMC databases except to the few who look through them. The only ones looking through this database are the drug companies looking for more ways to make money. Nobody is looking to warn anyone of the dangers of this food.

My question is why? The answer I get is, "there's no money in it". That's is why I said in my first book, it would be a shame if profits and money weren't the primary motivating factors in our society, but they are, and we have to live with it. That's why I choose not to buy into it. You have the same choice.

Chapter 10

Can Your Heart Disease be Cured or Just Treated?

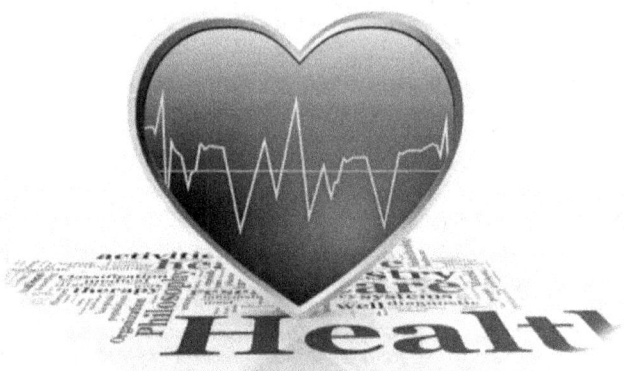

This chapter has been reserved for atherosclerosis and other heart-related diseases. Dementias and diseases of inflammation will be in the next chapter, as well with all other disorders that inflammation is responsible for.

Listed below from PubMed or PMC or the FDA are reports of studies done on the effects of glycation and its influence in any CVD or disease influenced by inflammation, which is a direct cause of glycation.

- *Advanced glycation endproducts induce apoptosis of endothelial progenitor cells by activating receptor RAGE and NADPH oxidase/JNK signaling axis.*

Elevated levels of advanced glycation endproducts (AGEs) is an important risk factor for atherosclerosis. Dysfunction of endothelial progenitor cells (EPCs), which is essential for re-endothelialization and neovascularization, is a hallmark of atherosclerosis. However, it remains unclear whether and how AGEs acts on EPCs to promote the pathogenesis of atherosclerosis. In this study, EPCs were exposed to different concentrations of AGEs. The expression of NADPH and Rac1 was measured to investigate the involvement of NADPH oxidase pathway. ROS was examined to indicate the level of oxidative stress in EPCs. Total JNK and p-JNK were determined by Western blotting. Cell apoptosis was evaluated by both TUNEL staining and flow cytometry. Cell proliferation was measured by (3)H thymidine uptake. The results showed that treatment of EPCs with AGEs increased the levels of ROS in EPCs. Mechanistically, AGEs increased the activity of NADPH oxidase and the expression of Rac1, a major component of NADPH. Importantly, treatment of EPCs with AGEs activated the JNK signaling pathway, which was closely associated with cell apoptosis and inhibition of proliferation. Our results suggest that the RAGE activation by AGEs in EPCs upregulates intracellular ROS levels, which contributes to the increased activity of NADPH oxidase and expression of Rac1, thus promoting cellular apoptosis and inhibiting proliferation. Mechanistically, AGEs binding to the receptor RAGE in EPCs is associated with hyperactivity of JNK signaling pathway, which is downstream of ROS. Our findings suggest that dysregulation of the AGEs/RAGE axis in EPCs may promote atherosclerosis and identify the NADPH/ROS/JNK signaling axis as a potential target for therapeutic intervention.

With the list growing past 17,729 studies on the effects of glycation, I think this message about the process of glycation should be wider known. This is the basis of all modern disease.

Why has it been kept hidden? Is it due to industrial concerns? What would happen to the pharmaceutical/chemical industry if you wiped 98% of all illness?

This report dictates how the modification of proteins (glycation) is involved in atherosclerosis. This is the smoking gun that carbs are dangerous foods to eat. Even though this report is from Dec 2016, it only says, again, what hundreds if not thousands of other reports dictate. They all dictate glycation is dangerous. What causes glycation should be avoided at all costs, to ensure optimal health.

- **Cellular mechanisms and consequences of glycation in atherosclerosis and obesity.**

Post-translational modification of proteins imparts diversity to protein functions. The process of glycation represents a complex set of pathways that mediate advanced glycation endproduct (AGE) formation, detoxification, intracellular disposition, extracellular release, and induction of signal transduction. These processes modulate the response to hyperglycemia, obesity, aging, inflammation, and renal failure, in which AGE formation and accumulation are facilitated. It has been shown that endogenous anti-AGE protective mechanisms are thwarted in chronic disease, thereby amplifying accumulation and detrimental cellular actions of these species. Atop these considerations, receptor for advanced glycation endproducts (RAGE)-mediated pathways downregulate expression and activity of the key anti-AGE detoxification enzyme, glyoxalase-1 (GLO1), thereby setting in motion an interminable feed-forward loop in which AGE-mediated cellular perturbation is not readily extinguished. In this review, we consider recent work in the field highlighting roles for glycation in obesity and atherosclerosis and discuss emerging strategies to block the adverse consequences of AGEs. This article is part of a Special Issue entitled: The role of post-translational protein modifications on the heart and vascular metabolism edited by Jason R.B. Dyck & Jan F.C. Glatz.

If this is the smoking gun that proves what glucose consumption does to the body in the form of atherosclerosis, how long before the FDA or the USDA will admit that this is what happens after ingesting grains? Will the Heart Association say anything about this? What about the American Diabetic Association? I wonder if this news will reach any regulatory agency. My guess is because Monsanto has something to say about it, any regulatory agency will say what Monsanto wants them to say, as they're mostly all controlled by Monsanto.

This report from Aug 1, 1989, reveals how aware we were then, that glycation as a damaging process, is caused by excess glucose in your system. One would think that 28 years would be long enough to reveal this information. Apparently, it wasn't. But now you know:

- *Nonenzymatic glycation of human blood platelet proteins.*

We studied 11 diabetic patients, all of whom had the severe atherothrombotic disease, and 11 normal controls. Overall glycation was assessed by the extent of incorporation of [3H]-NaBH4 into fructosyl lysine separated from whole platelet proteins following amino acid analysis. Fructosyl lysine represented 5.7% +/- 1.0 S.D. of the total radioactivity in the normal whole platelet samples. Increased glycation was observed in platelets from 5 of the 11 diabetics. Platelet glycation did not correlate with glycation of hemoglobin or albumin. The pattern of glycation of various platelet proteins in whole platelets, as determined by the incorporation of [3H]-NaBH4 into electrophoretically separated proteins did not display selectivity, although myosin and glycoproteins IIb and IIIa showed relatively increased levels of [3H]-NaBH4 incorporation. Artificially glycated platelet membranes exhibited glycation mainly in proteins corresponding to the electrophoretic mobility of myosin, glycoproteins IIb, and IIIa.

The previous report was published in 1989, yet have you heard anything about it? Didn't they any have an idea, at that time, what carbs were doing to the body, when ingested? I guess they needed more studies. Over 17,000 of them have been filed as of yet. Why has it taken until 2010 to learn any of this? Even today, they still are reluctant to admit such, that carbs are dangerous foods to be eating.

- *Advanced glycation end products: An emerging biomarker for adverse outcome in patients with peripheral artery disease.*

Patients with peripheral artery disease (PAD) suffer from widespread atherosclerosis. Partly due to the growing awareness of cardiovascular disease, the incidence of PAD has increased considerably during the past decade. It is anticipated that algorithms to identify high-risk patients for cardiovascular events require being updated, making use of novel biomarkers. Advanced glycation end products (AGEs) are moieties (elements) formed non-enzymatically on long-lived proteins under influence of glycemic and oxidative stress reactions. We elaborate on the formation and effects of AGEs, and the methods to measure AGEs. Several studies have been performed with AGEs in PAD. In this review, we evaluate the emerging evidence of AGEs as a clinical biomarker for patients with PAD.

Peripheral Artery disease is often the start of Atherosclerosis and all CVDs. They are a direct cause of glycation. Glycation is controllable by controlling the number of carbs you put in your mouth every time you eat.

This following study shows how your body reacts to the glucose infusion by sending out macrophages to counteract the damage presented by the glucose. The modified LDL particles are the glycated endproducts of what happens to your cholesterol with glucose in your system.

- *How do macrophages sense modify low-density lipoproteins?*

Abstract

In atherosclerosis, serum lipoproteins undergo various chemical modifications that impair their normal function. Modification of low-density lipoprotein (LDL) such as oxidation, glycation, carbamylation, glucooxidation, etc. makes LDL particles more proatherogenic. Macrophages are responsible for clearance of modified LDL to prevent cytotoxicity, tissue injury, inflammation, and metabolic disturbances. They develop an advanced sensing arsenal composed of various pattern recognition receptors (PRRs) capable of recognizing and binding foreign or altered-self targets for further inactivation and degradation. Modified LDL can be sensed and taken up by macrophages with a battery of scavenger receptors (SRs), of which SR-A1, CD36, and LOX1 play a major role. However, in atherosclerosis, lipid balance is deregulated that induces inability of macrophages to completely recycle modified LDL and leads to lipid deposition and transformation of macrophages to foam cells. SRs also mediate various pathogenic effects of modified LDL on macrophages through activation of the intracellular signaling network. Other PRRs such Toll-like receptors can also interact with modified LDL and mediate their effects independently or in cooperation with SRs.

What you should think about, is what would happen if the glucose weren't there? The cholesterol can do what it's supposed to do, feed your body.

From Dec 2016, Coronary Heart Disease and Ischemic stroke are shown to be influenced by another RAGE Gly82ser. How many more of these do they have to find before they realize that you can prevent this by keeping carbs out of the diet?

- *Association of RAGE gene Gly82Ser polymorphism with coronary artery disease and ischemic stroke: A systematic review and meta-analysis.*

Abstract

BACKGROUND:

The receptor for advanced glycosylation end products (RAGE) has been widely linked to diabetic atherosclerosis, but its effects on coronary artery disease (CAD) and ischemic stroke (IS) remain controversial. The Gly82Ser polymorphism is located in the ligand-binding V domain of RAGE, suggesting a possible influence of this variant on RAGE function. The aim of the present study is to clarify the association between the RAGE Gly82Ser polymorphism and susceptibility to CAD and IS.

CONCLUSIONS:

The current meta-analysis suggests that the RAGE Gly82Ser polymorphism is associated with an increased risk of CAD and IS, especially in the Chinese population. However, better-designed studies with larger sample sizes are needed to validate the results.

The following report submitted Sep 31, 2011, shows the influence of RAGE in VRD;

- **RAGE-dependent activation of the oncoprotein Pim1 plays a critical role in systemic vascular remodeling processes.**

Abstract

OBJECTIVE:

Vascular remodeling diseases (VRD) are mainly characterized by inflammation and vascular smooth muscle cells (VSMCs) proliferative and anti-apoptotic phenotype. Recently, the activation of the advanced glycation endproducts receptor (RAGE) has been shown to promote VSMC proliferation and resistance to apoptosis in VRD in a signal transducer and activator of transcription (STAT)3-dependent manner. Interestingly, we previously described in both cancer and VRD that the sustainability of this proliferative and antiapoptotic phenotype requires activation of the transcription factor NFAT (nuclear factor of activated T-cells). In cancer, NFAT activation is dependent on the oncoprotein provirus integration site for Moloney murine leukemia virus (Pim1), which is regulated by STAT3 and activated in VRD. Therefore, we hypothesized that RAGE/STAT3 activation in VSMC activates Pim1, promoting NFAT and thus VSMC proliferation and resistance to apoptosis. Methods/Results- In vitro, freshly isolated human carotid VSMCs exposed to RAGE activator Nε-(carboxymethyl)lysine (CML) for 48 hours had (1) activated STAT3 (increased P-STAT3/STAT3 ratio and P-STAT3 nuclear translocation); (2) increased STAT3-dependent Pim1 expression resulting in NFATc1 activation; and (3) increased Pim1/NFAT-dependent VSMC proliferation (PCNA, Ki67) and resistance to mitochondrial-dependent apoptosis (TMRM, Annexin V, TUNEL). Similarly to RAGE inhibition (small interfering RNA [siRNA]), Pim1, STAT3 and NFATc1 inhibition (siRNA) reversed these abnormalities in human carotid VSMC. Moreover, carotid artery VSMCs isolated from Pim1 knockout mice were resistant to CML-induced VSMC proliferation and resistance to apoptosis. In vivo, RAGE inhibition decreases STAT3/Pim1/NFAT activation, reversing vascular remodeling in the rat carotid artery-injured model.

CONCLUSIONS:

RAGE activation accounts for many features of VRD including VSMC proliferation and resistance to apoptosis by the activation of the STAT3/Pim1/NFAT axis. Molecules aimed to inhibit RAGE could be of a great therapeutic interest for the treatment of VRD.

Advanced glycation end products increase lipids accumulation in macrophages through upregulation of receptor of advanced glycation end products: increasing uptake, esterification and decreasing efflux of cholesterol.

BACKGROUND:

Previous reports have suggested that advanced glycation end products (AGEs) participate in the pathogenesis of diabetic macroangiopathy. Our previous study has found that AGEs can increase the lipid droplets accumulation in aortas of diabetic rats, but the current understanding of the mechanisms remains incomplete by which AGEs affect lipids accumulation in macrophages and accelerate atherosclerosis. In this study, we investigated the role of AGEs on lipids accumulation in macrophages and the possible molecular mechanisms including cholesterol influx, esterification, and efflux of macrophages.

METHODS:

THP-1 cells were incubated with PMA to differentiate to be macrophages which were treated with AGEs in the concentration of 300 μg/ml and 600 μg/ml with or without anti-RAGE (receptor for AGEs) antibody and then stimulated by oxidized-LDL (ox-LDL) or Dil-ox-LDL.

Lipids accumulation was examined by oil red staining. The cholesterol uptake, esterification, and efflux were detected respectively by fluorescence microscope, enzymatic assay kit, and fluorescence microplate. Quantitative RT-PCR and Western blot were used to measure the expression of the molecular involved in cholesterol uptake, synthesis/esterification, and efflux.

RESULTS:

AGEs increased lipids accumulation in macrophages in a concentration-dependent manner. 600 µg/ml AGEs obviously upregulated oxLDL uptake, increased levels of cholesterol ester in macrophages, and decreased the HDL-mediated cholesterol efflux by regulating the main molecular expression including CD36, Scavenger receptors (SR) A2, HMG-CoA reductase (HMGCR), ACAT1 and ATP-binding cassette transporter G1 (ABCG1). The changes above were inverted when the cells were pretreated with the anti-RAGE antibody.

CONCLUSIONS:

The current study suggests that AGEs can increase lipids accumulation in macrophages by regulating cholesterol uptake, esterification and efflux mainly through binding with RAGE, which provide a deep understanding of mechanisms how AGEs accelerating diabetic atherogenesis.

This is the proof that AGEs inhibit proper cell nutrition by preventing the flow of cholesterol into the cell. This allows accumulation of LDL particles in your blood. Usually, with a carbohydrate diet, those LDL particles are going to be ApoB particles and those are the most proliferate in all disease. Again, this is something you have full control over, as you don't have to eat this food. There are plenty of healthier alternatives.

The next study details how *glycol-AGEs* work their way into the cellular wall of your arteries creating Atherosclerosis. What you should think about, does this always happen with glucose in your system? Can you live without glucose? If you answered YES to both of those questions, you're on your way understanding how to make your body healthier.

- *Glycolaldehyde-derived advanced glycation end products (glycol-AGEs)-induced vascular smooth muscle cell dysfunction is regulated by the AGES-receptor (RAGE) axis in endothelium.*

Advanced glycation end-products (AGEs) are involved in the development of vascular smooth muscle cell (VSMC) dysfunction and the progression of atherosclerosis. However, AGEs may indirectly affect VSMCs via AGEs-induced signal transduction between monocytes and human umbilical endothelial cells (HUVECs), rather than having a direct influence. This study was designed to elucidate the signaling pathway underlying AGEs-RAGE axis influence on VSMC dysfunction using a co-culture system with monocytes, HUVECs and VSMCs. AGEs stimulated the production of reactive oxygen species and pro-inflammatory mediators such as tumor necrosis factor-α and interleukin-1β via extracellular-signal-regulated kinases phosphorylation and nuclear factor-κB activation in HUVECs. It was observed that AGEs-induced pro-inflammatory cytokines increase VSMC proliferation, inflammation and vascular remodeling in the co-culture system. This result implies that RAGE plays a role in AGEs-induced VSMC dysfunction. We suggest that the regulation of signal transduction via the AGEs-RAGE axis in the endothelium can be a therapeutic target for preventing atherosclerosis.

Do you have any idea of how to regulate the transduction of AGEs? It's simple, go keto. Will an industry that depends on your illness, tell you that? Since it's this industry that regulates the regulatory agencies, I doubt that you'll ever hear it from them. That's why it's so important to follow this advice to stay healthy, stay away from unhealthy substances. Now that you know how unhealthy glucose is, due to its glycative effects it's easier to ignore.

If you need more reports to prove how glucose directly influence heart disease, there are literally thousands of them. After reading them, it's easier see the logic in controlling your cardiovascular disease by controlling your carb intake? Where are the warnings from the FDA and the USDA? Don't they care about what they're recommending? Don't they understand because of their recommendations, they send millions of Moms and Dads, sisters, and brothers, husbands and wives to their slow, expensive, painful deaths?

These are free reports that are available to everyone. All you have to do is search for them at the National Library of Medicine in the National Institute of Health. There are literally 100s of thousands of reports on the effects of glycation that remain hidden in the PubMed and PMC databases except to the few who look through them. The only ones looking through this database are the drug companies looking for more ways to make money. Nobody is looking to warn anyone of the dangers of this food.

My question is why? The answer I get is, "there's no money in it". That's is why I said in my first book, it would be a shame if profits and money weren't the primary motivating factors in our society, but they are, and we have to live with it. That's why I choose not to buy into it. It's the same choice you have.

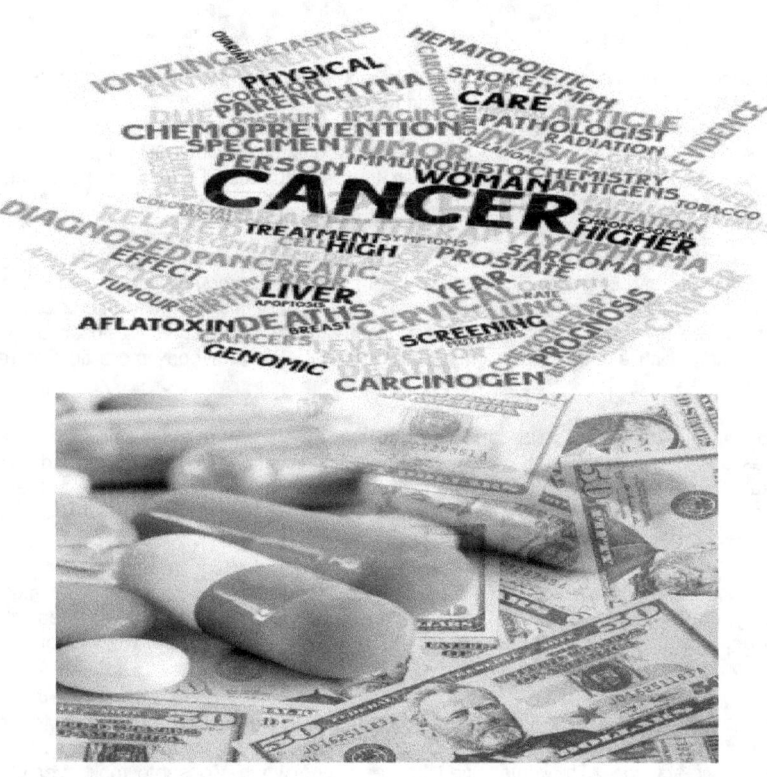

CHAPTER 11

CAN YOUR DEMENTIA, OSTEOPOROSIS, IBS/IBD, ASTHMA OR OTHER DISEASE OF INFLAMMATION BE CURED OR JUST TREATED?

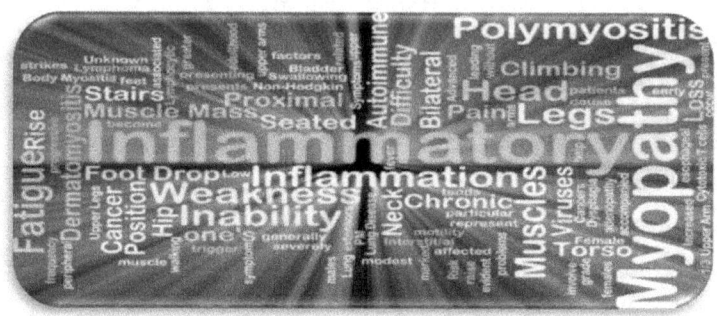

This poses an interesting question, osteoporosis, and dementia have something in common? Yes, they do. They are diseases of inflammation and inflammation is a product of glycation. It's these glycative cytokines and plaques that are responsible for all the damage that creates all diseases of inflammation. They are also responsible for IBS/IBD, Lupus, Fibromyalgia, Psoriasis, COPD, and every other disease that is influenced by inflammation, which would include most heart diseases and cancer.

Unfortunately, like arthritis, much of the damage has already been done and can't be undone. However, you can stop the decline immediately and start some recovery. Just realize that the recovery will take twice as long as it took for you to create this quagmire of disease in the first place. That only means that you must stop the glycation as soon as possible. (I suggest immediately, with a 3-day water only fast.) This will give your body more time to repair the damage.

Since the body needs proteins and cholesterol to operate and doesn't need the sugar, that leaves only one type of food to be responsible for glycation, carbs. I've learned through my research that the body can create all the glucose it needs with a process called gluconeogenesis. Gluconeogenesis is a process your body goes through whenever is needs glucose and has none readily available.

It produces this glucose with your own glycogen. That's what your body turns glucose into when you eat sugar and carbs. That is what makes me question our need to eat glucose. If your body can create what it needs, why eat it? You can live perfectly well without it because your body can make it.

Why then, were we fed the line, for 50 years that we had to make grains (the foundation of glucose in the body) the largest part of our diet? Could it be because these studies started about 60 years ago? They intensified 30 years ago when Monsanto took over GD Searle pharmaceuticals. This was also about the time when the whole grain ruse started convincing the public to consume massive amounts of this carcinogenic, atherosclerotic, inflammatory food. Do you wonder now, why all the disease exists?

When you cure a disease, you have nothing to treat. Where's the money flow in our medical industry? It flows through the treatment process. Every hospital proves this, every weight loss clinic proves this, every orthopedic clinic proves this. Actually, every clinic proves this. If a cure was found for all modern disease, what would it do to the health and medical industries? Reduce it to treating emergencies only? In another chapter of this book, I show you how reducing carb consumption will reduce emergencies as well. (That's where this really gets good.) It has something to do with its effect on your emotions.

Listed below from PubMed or PMC or the FDA are reports of studies done on the effects of glycation and its influence in osteoporosis or any disease influenced by inflammation.

Enzymes affecting your emotions are influenced by these foods affecting inflammation as well as cancer, which I've listed here. Probably the first condition to hit you will be IBS or IBD, Irritable Bowel Syndrome or Inflammatory Bowel Disease. This was just submitted this year in Feb;

- *Prevalence and Impact of Inflammatory Bowel Disease-Irritable Bowel Syndrome on Patient-reported Outcomes in CCFA Partners.*

Abstract

BACKGROUND:

Inflammatory bowel disease (IBD) patients with persistent symptoms despite no or minimal inflammation are frequently described as having an overlap of IBD and irritable bowel syndrome (IBD-IBS). Limited data are available on how IBS impacts the individual patient with IBD. In this study, we aimed to evaluate the prevalence of IBD-IBS and investigate its impact on patient-reported outcomes.

METHOD:

We performed a cross-sectional analysis of the CCFA Partners Study. Bivariate analyses and logistic regression models were used to investigate associations between IBD-IBS and various demographic, disease factors, and patient-reported outcomes including anxiety, depression, sleep disturbances, pain interference, and social satisfaction.

RESULTS:

Of the 6309 participants included, a total of 1279 (20%) reported a coexisting IBS diagnosis. The prevalence of IBD-IBS in this cohort was similar within disease subtypes. A diagnosis of IBD-IBS was associated with higher narcotic use compared with those with no IBS diagnosis for both Crohn's disease, 17% versus 11% (P < 0.001) and ulcerative colitis/indeterminate colitis, 9% versus 5% (P < 0.001). Quality of life, as measured by Short Inflammatory Bowel Disease Questionnaire (SIBDQ) was lower in patients with IBD-IBS compared with those without. IBD-IBS diagnosis was associated with anxiety, depression, fatigue, sleep disturbances, pain interference, and decreased social satisfaction.

CONCLUSIONS:

In this sample of patients with IBD, the high prevalence of concomitant IBS diagnosis was observed. IBD-IBS diagnosis was associated with increased narcotic use and adverse patient-reported outcome. Appropriate diagnosis, treatment, and counseling may help improve the functional status of IBD-IBS patients and decrease narcotic use.

My appropriate treatment for this disorder isn't a treatment. Those always lead to more treatments. I propose a cure. All the inflammation involved in these disorders can be controlled by your intake of carbs, meaning, by going keto you can avoid all inflammation. How far do you think would that go to providing you relief from your pain?

Novel Insights into the Relationship between Diabetes and Osteoporosis

Abstract

Only three decades ago adipose tissue was considered inert with little relationship to insulin resistance. Similarly, bone has long been thought purely in its structural context. In the last decade, emerging evidence has revealed important endocrine roles for both bone and adipose tissue. The interaction between these two tissues is remarkable. Bone marrow mesenchymal stem cells give rise to both osteoblasts and adipocytes. Leptin and adiponectin, two adipokines secreted by fat tissue, control energy homeostasis, but also have complex actions on the skeleton. In turn, the activities of bone cells are not limited to their bone remodeling activities, but also to modulation of adipose sensitivity and insulin secretion. This review will discuss these new insights linking bone remodeling to the control of fat metabolism and the association between diabetes mellitus and osteoporosis.

Conclusion

Chronic hyperglycemia profoundly affects multiple tissues and directly affects the frequency of complications in diabetes mellitus. Hypoinsulinemia is the primary hormonal disturbance leading to T1DM, whereas insulin resistance causing hyperglycemia is the principal event in T2DM. As discussed, bone mineral density is a relatively poor surrogate for defining bone structure during long-standing hyperglycemia. Low bone mass is often detected in T1DM although the pathogenesis is likely to be multifactorial. On the other hand, BMD can be low, normal or increased in T2DM. Yet both forms of diabetes are associated with an increased risk of fracture. In part, higher rates of fracture can be related to neuropathic, nephropathic and retinopathic changes that lead to a greater risk of falling. In addition, low body weight, hypoinsulinemia, low serum levels of IGF-I and altered gonadal steroids favor a catabolic state in the skeleton of Type I diabetics. The presence of obesity and T2DM, although associated with increased cortical bone mass, does not translate to a lower fracture risk, and paradoxically may enhance risk. Hyperglycemia can lead to degenerative changes in bone quality through advanced end product glycation, which particularly affects collagen cross-linking. Not surprisingly, one of the classic late clinical features of diabetes mellitus, i.e. vascular calcification, is associated with lower bone mass and impaired bone strength. Those two processes may be linked to reduced renal function and aberrant deposition of calcium in blood vessels rather than in the appropriate collagen matrix. Notwithstanding the potential numerous insults associated with sustained hyperglycemia, several recent developments suggest there is now a greater awareness of the skeleton as both a target of diabetic complications and a potential pathogenetic factor in the disease itself.

Could this indicate that it might be healthier to feed your kids fats and proteins instead of carbs, to help save them from broken bones? How about yourself?

The following study looked at the brains of Alzheimer's disease patients. It's dated Jan 3, 2017. They officially label Alzheimer's disease as type 3 diabetes;

- *Type 3 Diabetes Mellitus: A Novel Implication of Alzheimer Disease.*

Abstract

The brain of patients with Alzheimer disease (AD) showed the evidence of reduced expression of insulin and neuronal insulin receptors, as compared with those of age-matched controls. This event gradually and certainly leads to a breakdown of the entire insulin-signaling pathway, which manifests insulin resistance. This, in turn, affects brain metabolism and cognitive functions, which are the best-documented abnormalities in the AD. These observations led Dr. de la Monte and her colleagues to suggest that AD is actually a neuroendocrine disorder that resembles type 2 diabetes mellitus. The truth would be more complex with understanding the role of Aβ derived diffusible ligands, advanced glycation end products, and low-density lipoprotein receptor-related protein 1. However, now it's known as "brain diabetes" and is called type 3 diabetes mellitus (T3DM). This review provides an *overview of "brain diabetes" focusing on the reason why the phenomenon is called T3DM.*

Evidence of inflammation's role in myasthenia gravis, dated Jan 3, 2017; I used to have a granddaughter with myasthenia gravis, as I recall at that time, there was no known cause. I guess the cause wasn't known then. It's a nice thing to know that it is now, but who are suggesting that we remove the instigating factor from this equation, the glucose that is responsible for the glycation? It's nicer to realize that there are a growing number of us;

- *Profile of upregulated inflammatory proteins in sera of Myasthenia Gravis patients.*

Abstract

This study describes specific patterns of elevated inflammatory proteins in clinical subtypes of myasthenia gravis (MG) patients. MG is a chronic, autoimmune neuromuscular disease with antibodies most commonly targeting the acetylcholine receptors (AChRab), which causes fluctuating skeletal muscle fatigue. MG pathophysiology includes a strong component of inflammation and a large proportion of patients with early onset MG additionally present thymus hyperplasia. Due to the fluctuating nature and heterogeneity of the disease, there is a great need for objective biomarkers as well as novel potential inflammatory targets. We examined the sera of 45 MG patients (40 AChRab seropositive and 5 AChRab seronegative), investigating 92 proteins associated with inflammation. Eleven of the analysed proteins were significantly elevated compared to healthy controls, out of which the three most significant were: matrix metalloproteinase 10 (MMP-10; $p = 0.0004$), transforming growth factor alpha (TGF-α; $p = 0.0017$) and extracellular newly identified receptor for advanced glycation end-products binding protein (EN-RAGE) (also known as protein S100-A12; $p = 0.0054$). Further, levels of MMP-10, C-X-C motif ligand 1 (CXCL1) and brain-derived neurotrophic factor (BDNF) differed between early and late onset MG. These novel targets provide valuable additional insight into the systemic inflammatory response in MG.

The following report was submitted Dec 29, 2016, and explains the damage that oxidative stress, apoptosis, autophagy and inflammation play in kidney disease and they have plenty to say about it;

- *Inflammation, oxidative stress, apoptosis, and autophagy in diabetes mellitus and diabetic kidney disease: the Four Horsemen of the Apocalypse.*

Abstract

Diabetic kidney disease (DKD) can occur in approximately 30-40% of both type 1 and type 2 diabetic patients. The well-established features of DKD include increased serum glucose levels along with chronic low-grade inflammation, OxS, increased advanced glycation end products, sorbitol accumulation, increased hexosamine, and protein kinase C pathway activation. On the other hand, accumulating evidence suggests that novel pathways including apoptosis and autophagy might also play important roles in the pathogenesis and progression of DKD. In this review, the integrated mechanisms of inflammation, oxidative stress, apoptosis, and autophagy are discussed in the pathogenesis as well as the progression of DM and DKD.

This following report dated Feb 2017 shows the importance of sRAGE involved in lung infections and other inflammatory precursors to lung cancer;

- **THE SHEDDING-DERIVED SOLUBLE RECEPTOR FOR ADVANCED GLYCATION ENDPRODUCTS SUSTAINS INFLAMMATION DURING ACUTE PSEUDOMONAS AERUGINOSA LUNG INFECTION.**

Abstract

BACKGROUND:

The membrane-bound isoform of the receptor for advanced glycation end products (FL-RAGE) is primarily expressed by alveolar epithelial cells and undergoes shedding by the protease ADAM10, giving rise to soluble cleaved RAGE (cRAGE). RAGE has been associated with the pathogenesis of several acute and chronic lung disorders. Whether the proteolysis of FL-RAGE is altered by a given inflammatory stimulus is unknown. Pseudomonas aeruginosa causes nosocomial infections in hospitalized patients and is the major pathogen associated with chronic lung diseases.

CONCLUSIONS:

These data are the first to suggest that inhibition of FL-RAGE shedding, by affecting the FL-RAGE/cRAGE levels, is a novel mechanism for controlling inflammation to acute P. aeruginosa pneumonia. sRAGE in the alveolar space sustains inflammation in this setting.

Below is evidence that the destruction of glycation starts before you were ever born, thanks to your mother's glucose ingestion. This is where your addiction began. Do you think if she knew how much harm she was inflicting, she would do it again? That might depend on her addiction;

From the study report itself, dated Nov 2016;

- *AGEs induce ectopic endochondral ossification in intervertebral discs*

Abstract

Ectopic calcifications in intervertebral discs (IVDs) are known characteristics of IVD degeneration that are not commonly reported but may be implicated in structural failure and dysfunctional IVD cell metabolic responses. This study investigated the novel hypothesis that ectopic calcifications in the IVD are associated with advanced glycation end products (AGEs) via hypertrophy and osteogenic differentiation. Histological analyses of human IVDs from several degeneration stages revealed areas of ectopic calcification within the nucleus pulposus and at the cartilage endplate. These ectopic calcifications were associated with cells positive for the AGE methylglyoxal-hydroimidazolone-1 (MG-H1). MG-H1 was also co-localized with Collagen 10 (COL10) and Osteopontin (OPN) suggesting osteogenic differentiation. Bovine nucleus pulposus and cartilaginous endplate cells in cell culture demonstrated that 200 mg/mL AGEs in low-glucose media increased ectopic calcifications after 4 d in culture and significantly increased COL10 and OPN expression. The receptor for AGE (RAGE) was involved in this differentiation process since its inhibition reduced COL10 and OPN expression. We conclude that AGE accumulation is associated with endochondral ossification in IVDs and likely acts via the AGE/RAGE axis to induce hypertrophy and osteogenic differentiation in IVD cells. We postulate that this ectopic calcification may play an important role in accelerated IVD degeneration including the initiation of structural defects. Since orally administered AGE and RAGE inhibitors are available, future investigations on AGE/RAGE and endochondral ossification may be a promising direction for developing a non-invasive treatment against the progression of IVD degeneration.

This report makes me wonder, how long will it take until the FDA or the USDA to wake up and realize that what they're recommending everyone eat is actually what's making everyone sick. Then I think about who controls the FDA and the USDA, it somehow nullifies my curiosity, I know who is responsible. A multinational chemical company intent on bolstering their profits at whatever cost, regardless of what may be brought about their actions.

It's when those actions bolster the profits of another related industry that I get bothered. When I see people conned into consuming foods that make them sicker every day, I get a little upset. When I see this, I see my mother dying because she bought into this ruse herself. This makes this ruse the most dangerous con game ever to hit mankind.

The following report submitted Mar 2, 2009, details the beginning of glycation from the fundamental elements of glucose, glyoxal and methylglyoxal, and their roles in aging and disease;

- *Protein and nucleotide damage by glyoxal and methylglyoxal in physiological systems - role in aging and disease*

Glyoxal and methylglyoxal are potent glycating agents. Glycation of proteins is a complex series of parallel and sequential reactions collectively called the Maillard reaction. It occurs in all tissues and body fluids. Early stage reactions in glycation of protein by glucose lead to the formation of fructosyl-lysine (FL) and N-terminal amino acid residue-derived fructosamines. Later stage reactions form stable end-stage adducts called advanced glycation endproducts (AGEs). FL degrades slowly to form AGEs – and also glyoxal and methylglyoxal. In contrast, glyoxal and methylglyoxal react with proteins to form AGE residues directly and relatively rapidly.

Glycation by glyoxal and methylglyoxal, and the related influence of Glo1 are now emerging as playing a critical role in aging and disease processes – vascular complications associated with diabetes renal failure, Alzheimer's disease, and tumorigenesis and multidrug resistance in cancer chemotherapy. They may also have roles in pathologic anxiety, autism, obesity and other disorders.

Again, this is just one of 804 return reports from a search of Lymphoma and glycation. To think that one has nothing to do with the other is what the FDA and the USDA seem to be doing in the continued recommendations to eat the food that does the glycating. If you were to tell me that the influence of Monsanto's execs in the offices and agencies had nothing to do with these decisions to alert the public about the dangers in what they're eating, I'd have to tell you that you are completely misinformed. Can I sell you some ocean front property in Kansas?

Does this mean that you're stupid? Absolutely not. It just means that you've been duped like everyone else. It's really easy to do. All you have to do is taste the food. One taste and you're hooked. Since it doesn't kill you immediately, it's assumed safe. This assumption is what's killing America and the rest of the world. This is the most deadly assumption to make, bread is safe to eat. Bread nowadays is deadly...very deadly

When I searched glycation and asthma, it returned 45 studies showing the influence that glycation has on asthma. The first one explains how more severe asthma can be characterized by clustering of AGEs;

- *A Systemic Inflammatory Endotype of Asthma With More Severe Disease Identified by Unbiased Clustering of the Serum Cytokine Profile.*

Asthma is considered as a clinical and molecularly heterogeneous disorder. Systemic inflammation is suggested to play an important role in a group of asthma patients. We hypothesized that there is a subgroup of patients with asthma characterized by systemic inflammation. In this study, we aimed to discriminate asthma subtypes based on circulating biomarkers and to determine whether a systemic inflammatory endotype of asthma could be identified. In the present cross-sectional study, 50 patients with untreated asthma were prospectively recruited from a single academic outpatient clinic, and characterized with respect to clinical, functional, and inflammatory parameters. The expression profiles of 20 serum cytokines were assessed by anti-human cytokine antibody array. Then, hierarchical clustering analysis was performed based on the principal component analysis (PCA)-transformed data to classify the clinical groups. PCA showed that 6 independent components accounted for 80.113% of the variance, and PCA-based hierarchical clustering identified 3 endotypes. One of the endotypes was evidenced by elevated systemic inflammation markers such as leptin, vascular endothelial growth factor (VEGF), and reduced levels of soluble receptor for advanced glycation end products (sRAGE), an anti-inflammatory molecule. More female patients were included, with higher circulating neutrophil counts and more severe symptoms. In conclusion, we identified an endotype of asthma characterized by systemic inflammation and severe symptoms. Increased levels of VEGF, leptin and decreased level of sRAGE may contribute to the systemic inflammation of this asthma endotype.

With inflammation being a major influence on asthma, would it make sense to control the inflammation first and foremost?

This report from Oct 16, 2015, details how high fructose corn syrup is associated with chronic bronchitis;

- *Intake of high fructose corn syrup sweetened soft drinks is associated with prevalent chronic bronchitis in U.S. Adults, ages 20-55 y.*

High fructose corn syrup (HFCS) sweetened soft drink intake has been linked with asthma in US high-schoolers. Intake of beverages with excess free fructose (EFF), including apple juice, and HFCS sweetened fruit drinks and soft drinks, has been associated with asthma in children. One hypothesis for this association is that underlying fructose malabsorption and fructose reactivity in the GI may contribute to in situ formations of enFruAGEs. EnFruAGEs may be an overlooked source of advanced glycation end-products (AGE) that contribute to lung disease. AGE/ RAGEs are elevated in COPD lungs. EFF intake has increased in recent decades, and intakes may exceed dosages associated with adult fructose malabsorption in subsets of the population. Intestinal dysfunction has been shown to be elevated in COPD patients. The objective of this study was to investigate the association between HFCS sweetened soft drink intake and chronic bronchitis (CB), a common manifestation of COPD, in adults.

HFCS sweetened soft drink intake is correlated with chronic bronchitis in US adults aged 20-55 y, after adjusting for covariates, including smoking. Results support the hypothesis that underlying fructose malabsorption and fructose reactivity in the GI may contribute to chronic bronchitis, perhaps through in situ formations of enFruAGEs, which may contribute to lung disease. Longitudinal and biochemical research is needed to confirm and clarify the mechanisms involved.

The next report I looked at was from Nov 10, 2016, and it displays the extent this industry will go to, to simply allow this addiction to kill as many people as it possibly can, by it to continue. Its purpose is to show the benefits of Bazedoxifene, a new drug being tested for reducing apoptosis and oxidative stress when all they have to do is to recommend the cessation of the consumption of grains and sugar that leads to the glycation that is responsible for all these diseases. They're not interested in arresting it or abating it. Their sole interest is to expand its influence, to addict more and more people. This appears to be done solely to increase the profits of the pharmaceutical industry. It explains the benefits of a new drug that the industry wants to impose upon the people, probably in the guise of helping the people;

- *BAZEDOXIFENE AMELIORATES HOMOCYSTEINE-INDUCED APOPTOSIS AND ACCUMULATION OF ADVANCED GLYCATION END PRODUCTS BY REDUCING OXIDATIVE STRESS IN MC3T3-E1 CELLS.*

Abstract

Elevated plasma homocysteine (Hcy) level increases the risk of osteoporotic fracture by deteriorating bone quality. However, little is known about the effects of Hcy on osteoblast and collagen cross-links. This study aimed to investigate whether Hcy induces apoptosis of osteoblastic MC3T3-E1 cells as well as affects enzymatic and nonenzymatic collagen cross-links and to determine the effects of bazedoxifene, a selective estrogen receptor modulator, on the Hcy-induced apoptosis and deterioration of collagen cross-links in the cells. Hcy treatments (300 µM, 3 mM, and 10 mM) increased intracellular reactive oxygen species (ROS) production in a dose-dependent manner. Propidium iodide staining showed that 3 and 10 mM Hcy induced apoptosis of MC3T3-E1 cells. Moreover, the activities of caspases-8, 9, and 3 were increased by 3 mM Hcy. The detrimental effects of 3 mM Hcy on apoptosis and ROS *production were partly reversed by bazedoxifene and 17β estradiol. In addition, real-time PCR, immunostaining and Western blot showed that 300 µM Hcy decreased the expression of lysyl oxidase (Lox). Furthermore, 300 µM Hcy increased extracellular accumulation of pentosidine, an advanced glycation end product. Treatment with bazedoxifene ameliorated Hcy-induced suppression of Lox expression and increase in pentosidine accumulation. These findings suggest that high-dose Hcy induces apoptosis of osteoblasts by increasing oxidative stress, and low-dose Hcy decreases enzymatic collagen cross-links and increases pentosidine accumulation, resulting in the deterioration of bone quality. Bazedoxifene treatment effectively prevents the Hcy-induced detrimental reactions of osteoblasts. Thus, bazedoxifene may be a potential therapeutic drug for preventing Hcy-induced bone fragility.*

Even though we've had an idea of the damage of glycation and what causes it for over 30 years, This industry is still concentrating on making new drugs. Drugs always have side effects that lead to more drugs, yet this is this industry's modus operandi. They don't know how to operate otherwise. It's the ties to the grains industry that I object to and the power we've given to these industries, simply to allow the public to continue to feed their addiction. You might as well tell us to stand in front of a racing bus or semi. You're basically selling us the same thing, future time in the hospital;

- *BAZEDOXIFENE AMELIORATES HOMOCYSTEINE-INDUCED APOPTOSIS AND ACCUMULATION OF ADVANCED GLYCATION END PRODUCTS BY REDUCING OXIDATIVE STRESS IN MC3T3-E1 CELLS.*

Abstract

Elevated plasma homocysteine (Hcy) level increases the risk of osteoporotic fracture by deteriorating bone quality. However, little is known about the effects of Hcy on osteoblast and collagen cross-links. This study aimed to investigate whether Hcy induces apoptosis of osteoblastic MC3T3-E1 cells as well as affects enzymatic and nonenzymatic collagen cross-links and to determine the effects of bazedoxifene, a selective estrogen receptor modulator, on the Hcy-induced apoptosis and deterioration of collagen cross-links in the cells. Hcy treatments (300 µM, 3 mM, and 10 mM) increased intracellular reactive oxygen species (ROS) production in a dose-dependent manner. Propidium iodide staining showed that 3 and 10 mM Hcy induced apoptosis of MC3T3-E1 cells. Moreover, the activities of caspases-8, 9, and 3 were increased by 3 mM Hcy. The detrimental effects of 3 mM Hcy on apoptosis and ROS production were partly reversed by bazedoxifene and 17β estradiol. In addition, real-time PCR, immunostaining and Western blot showed that 300 µM Hcy decreased the expression of lysyl oxidase (Lox). Furthermore, 300 µM Hcy increased extracellular accumulation of pentosidine, an advanced glycation end product. Treatment with bazedoxifene ameliorated Hcy-induced suppression of Lox expression and increase in pentosidine accumulation. These findings suggest that high-dose Hcy induces apoptosis of osteoblasts by increasing oxidative stress, and low-dose Hcy decreases enzymatic collagen cross-links and increases pentosidine accumulation, resulting in the deterioration of bone quality. Bazedoxifene treatment effectively prevents the Hcy-induced detrimental reactions of osteoblasts. Thus, bazedoxifene may be a potential therapeutic drug for preventing Hcy-induced bone fragility.

This displays the true despair of this problem, an industry more intent on driving profits than healing the people they affect. Their only interest is in making more drugs to allow the continuation of an addiction that's putting more people in the hospital than any other one thing. To me, that is the definition of criminal behavior. This is a clear indication of legal extortion....and we allow it to continue, just to feed our addiction.

This next report dated Oct 18, 2016, shows the influence of Metformin on the AGE population in our blood. It turns out to be another way to get you to take more drugs, as this drug encourages increased levels of CML (another AGE).

- ***PLASMA LEVELS OF PENTOSIDINE, CARBOXYMETHYL-LYSINE, SOLUBLE RECEPTOR FOR ADVANCED GLYCATION END PRODUCTS, AND METABOLIC SYNDROME: THE METFORMIN EFFECT.***

Abstract

Metabolic syndrome (Mets) is considered one of the most important public health problems. Several and controversial studies showed that the role of advanced glycation end products (AGEs) and their receptor in the development of metabolic syndrome and therapeutic pathways is still unsolved. We have investigated whether plasma pentosidine, carboxymethyl-lysine (CML), and soluble receptor for advanced glycation end products (sRAGE) levels were increased in patients with Mets and the effect of metformin in plasma levels of pentosidine, CML, and sRAGE. 80 control subjects and 86 patients were included in this study. Pentosidine, CML, and sRAGE were measured in plasma by enzyme-linked immunosorbent assay (ELISA). Plasma pentosidine, CML, and sRAGE levels were significantly increased in patients compared to control subjects (P < 0.001, P < 0.001, and P = 0.014, resp.). Plasma levels of pentosidine were significantly decreased in patients who received metformin compared to untreated patients (P = 0.01). However, there was no significant difference between patients treated with metformin and untreated patients in plasma CML levels. Plasma levels of sRAGE were significantly increased in patients who received metformin and ACE inhibitors (P < 0.001 and P = 0.002, resp.). However, in a multiple stepwise regression analysis, pentosidine, sRAGE, and drugs treatments were not independently associated. Patients with metabolic syndrome showed increased levels of AGEs such as pentosidine and CML. Metformin treatment showed a decreased level of pentosidine but not of CML. Therapeutic pathways of AGEs development should be taken into account and further experimental and in vitro studies merit for advanced research.

The purpose of this study was to look at Metformin's effect on two different AGEs, pentosidine and CML. Again the emphasis is on finding ways to keep the glycating substances in the diet and offering treatment only, not in finding a cure. That would involve removing the glycating substances from the diet and that would hurt the grain industry. Their treatment though involves the continuation of their prescribed drug regimen. This is why they pay the prettiest reps to sell their drugs to all the doctors who prescribe them.

Dated May 2016 is this report on the role of DAMP in inflammation, cancer, and tissue repair;

- **KEY ROLE OF DAMP IN INFLAMMATION, CANCER, AND TISSUE REPAIR.**

Abstract

PURPOSE:

This review aimed to take stock of the current status of research on damage-associated molecular pattern (DAMP) protein. We discuss the Janus-faced role of DAMP molecules in inflammation, cancer, and tissue repair. The high-mobility group box (HMGB)-1 and adenosine triphosphate proteins are well-known DAMP molecules and have been primarily associated with inflammation. However, as we shall see, recent data have linked these molecules to tissue repair. HMGB1 is associated with cancer-related inflammation. It activates nuclear factor-kB, which is involved in cancer regulation via its receptor for advanced glycation end-products (RAGE), Toll-like receptors 2 and 4. Proinflammatory activity and tissue repair may lead to pharmacologic intervention, by blocking DAMP RAGE and Toll-like receptor 2 and 4 roles in inflammation and by increasing their concentration in tissue repair, respectively.

METHODS:

We conducted a MEDLINE search for articles pertaining to the various issues related to DAMP, and we discuss the most relevant articles especially (ie, not only those published in journals with a higher impact factor).

FINDINGS:

A cluster of remarkable articles on DAMP has appeared in the literature in recent years. Regarding inflammation, several strategies have been proposed to target HMGB1, from antibodies to recombinant box A, which interacts with RAGE, competing with the full molecule. In tissue repair, it was reported that the overexpression of HMGB1 or the administration of exogenous HMGB1 significantly increased the number of vessels and promoted recovery in skin-wound, ischemic injury.

IMPLICATIONS:

Due to the bivalent nature of DAMP, it is often difficult to explain the relative role of DAMP in inflammation versus its role in tissue repair. However, this point is crucial as DAMP-related treatments move into clinical practice.

Are these enough reports to prove what directly influences diabetes? After reading this can you see the logic in controlling your diabetes by controlling your carb intake? Where are the warnings from the FDA and the USDA? Don't they care about what they're recommending? Don't they understand because of their recommendations, they send millions of Moms and Dads, sisters, and brothers, husbands and wives to their slow, expensive, painful deaths?

- *Monocyte Chemotactic Protein-1, Fractalkine, and Receptor for Advanced Glycation End Products in Different Pathological Types of Lupus Nephritis and Their Value in Different Treatment Prognoses.*

BACKGROUND:

Early diagnosis is important for the outcome of lupus nephritis (LN). However, the pathological type of lupus nephritis closely related to the clinical manifestations; therefore, the treatment of lupus nephritis depends on the different pathological types.

OBJECTIVE:

To assess the level of monocyte chemotactic protein (MCP-1), fractalkine (Fkn), and receptor for advanced glycation end product (RAGE) in different pathological types of lupus nephritis and to explore the value of these biomarkers for predicting the prognosis of lupus nephritis.

METHODS:

Patients included in this study were assessed using renal biopsy. Class III and class IV were defined as the proliferative group, class V as a non-proliferative group, and class V+III and class V+IV as the mixed group. During the follow-up, 40 of 178 enrolled patients had a poor response to the standard immunosuppressant therapy. The level of markers in the different response groups was tested.

RESULTS:

The levels of urine and serum MCP-1, urine and serum fractalkine, and serum RAGE were higher in the proliferative group, and lower in the non-proliferative group, and this difference was significant. The levels of urine and serum MCP-1 and serum RAGE were lower in the poor response group, and these differences were also significant. The relationship between urine MCP-1 and urine and serum fractalkine with the systemic lupus erythematosus disease activity index was evaluated.

CONCLUSION:

The concentration of cytokines MCP-1, fractalkine, and RAGE may be correlated with different pathology type of lupus nephritis. Urine and serum MCP-1 and serum RAGE may help in predicting the prognosis prior to standard immunosuppressant therapy.

Do you have Lupus? Were you told not to eat your bagels for breakfast? If you weren't, then it's probably because someone needed you back for treatment.

This following report dated

- **HMGB1 Promotes Systemic Lupus Erythematosus by Enhancing Macrophage Inflammatory Response.**

Background/Purpose: HMGB1, which may act as a proinflammatory mediator, has been proposed to contribute to the pathogenesis of multiple chronic inflammatories and autoimmune diseases including systemic lupus erythematosus (SLE); however, the precise mechanism of HMGB1 in the pathogenic process of SLE remains obscure.

Method: The expression of HMGB1 was measured by ELISA and western blot. The ELISA was also applied to detect proinflammatory cytokines levels. Furthermore, nephritic pathology was evaluated by H&E staining of renal tissues. Results: In this study, we found that HMGB1 levels were significantly increased and correlated with SLE disease activity in both clinical patients and a murine model. Furthermore, gain- and loss-of-function analysis showed that HMGB1 exacerbated the severity of SLE. Of note, the HMGB1 levels were found to be associated with the levels of proinflammatory cytokines such as TNF-α and IL-6 in SLE patients. Further study demonstrated that increased HMGB1 expression deteriorated the severity of SLE via enhancing macrophage inflammatory response. Moreover, we found that receptor of advanced glycation end products played a critical role in HMGB1-mediated macrophage inflammatory response.

Conclusion: These findings suggested that HMGB1 might be a risk factor for SLE, and manipulation of HMGB1 signaling might provide a therapeutic strategy for SLE.

With this kind of evidence, do you think this might suggest that a ketogenic diet would be healthier?

Another study proving the role of glycation in the pathogenesis of arthritis proves once again how inflammation is the result of glycation, something you have control over:

- **The potential role of advanced glycation end products (AGEs) and soluble receptors for AGEs (sRAGE) in the pathogenesis of adult-onset Still's disease.**

BACKGROUND:

Accumulating evidence has demonstrated a pathogenic role of advanced glycation end products (AGEs) and receptors for AGEs (RAGE) in inflammation. Soluble RAGE (sRAGE), with the same ligand-binding capacity as full-length RAGE, acts as a "decoy" receptor. However, there has been scanty data regarding AGEs and sRAGE in adult-onset Still's disease (AOSD). This study aimed to investigate AGEs and sRAGE levels in AOSD patients and examine their association with clinical characteristics.

METHODS:

Using ELISA, plasma levels of AGEs and sRAGE were determined in 52 AOSD patients, 36 systemic lupus erythematosus(SLE) patients and 16 healthy controls(HC). Their associations with activity parameters and disease courses were evaluated.

RESULTS:

Significantly higher median levels of AGEs were observed in active AOSD patients (16.75 pg/ml) and active SLE patients (14.80 pg/ml) than those in HC (9.80 pg/ml, both $p < 0.001$). AGEs levels were positively correlated with activity scores ($r = 0.836$, $p < 0.001$), ferritin levels ($r = 0.372$, $p < 0.05$) and CRP levels ($r = 0.396$, $p < 0.005$) in AOSD patients. Conversely, significantly lower median levels of sRAGE were observed in active AOSD patients (632.2 pg/ml) and active SLE patients (771.6 pg/ml) compared with HC (1051.7 pg/ml, both $p < 0.001$). Plasma sRAGE levels were negatively correlated with AOSD activity scores ($r = -0.320$, $p < 0.05$). In comparison to AOSD patients with monocyclic pattern, significantly higher AGEs levels were observed in those with polycyclic or chronic articular pattern. With treatment, AGEs levels declined while sRAGE levels increased in parallel with the decrease in disease activity.

CONCLUSION:

The elevation of AGEs levels with concomitant decreased sRAGE levels in active AOSD patients, suggests their pathogenic role in AOSD.

Juvenile arthritis is shown in this study to be the product of glycation, again something you have control over by what goes into your body for food. If you or your child suffers from this, your only cure is to stop the glycation. The older you are, the less you can reverse. But if you're young enough, you may be able to reverse a majority of it.

- *The presence of high mobility group box-1 and soluble receptor for advanced glycation end-products in juvenile idiopathic arthritis and juvenile systemic lupus erythematosus.*

Background

The involvement of high mobility group box-1 (HMGB1) in various inflammatory and autoimmune diseases has been documented but clinical trials on the contribution of this pro-inflammatory alarmin in children with juvenile idiopathic arthritis (JIA) and systemic lupus erythematosus (SLE) are basically absent. To address the presence of HMGB1 and a soluble receptor for advanced glycation end products (sRAGE) in different subtypes of JIA and additionally in children with SLE, we enrolled a consecutive sample of children harvested peripheral blood as well as synovial fluids (SF) at diagnosis and correlated it with ordinary acute-phase reactants and clinical markers.

Methods

Serum and synovial fluids levels of HMGB1 and sRAGE in a total of 144 children (97 with JIA, 19 with SLE and 27 healthy controls) were determined by ELISA.

Results

The children with JIA and those with SLE were characterized by significantly higher serum levels of HMGB1 and significantly lower sRAGE levels compared to the healthy controls. A positive correlation between serum HMGB1 and ESR, CRP, α2 globulin was found while serum sRAGE levels were inversely correlated with the same inflammatory markers in children with JIA. Additionally, high level of serum HMGB1 was related to hepatosplenomegaly or serositis in systemic-onset JIA.

Conclusion

The inverse relationship of the HMGB1 and its soluble receptor RAGE in the blood and SF indicates that inflammation triggered by alarmins may play a role in the pathogenesis of JIA as well as SLE. HMGB1 may serve as an inflammatory marker and a potential target of biological therapy in these patients. Further studies need to show whether the determination of HMGB1 levels in patients with JIA can be a useful guideline for detecting disease activity.

What's important is that you stop the introduction of glucose as soon as possible to arrest the glycation. The secret to this cure is an end to all glycation. The magic of this cure is the end of the hunger cycle and pain. (I've noticed that they go together.)

These are free reports that are available to everyone. All you have to do is search for them at the National Library of Medicine in the National Institute of Health. There are literally 100s of thousands of reports on the effects of glycation that remain hidden in the PubMed and PMC databases except to the few who look through them. The only ones looking through this database are the drug companies looking for more ways to make money. Nobody is looking to warn anyone of the dangers of this food.

My question is why? The answer I get is, "there's no money in it". That's why I said in my first book, it would be a shame if profits and money weren't the primary motivating factors in our society, but they are, and we have to live with it. That's why I choose not to buy into it. It's the same choice you have.

Abstinence Is

The Only Path to

Health & Justice!

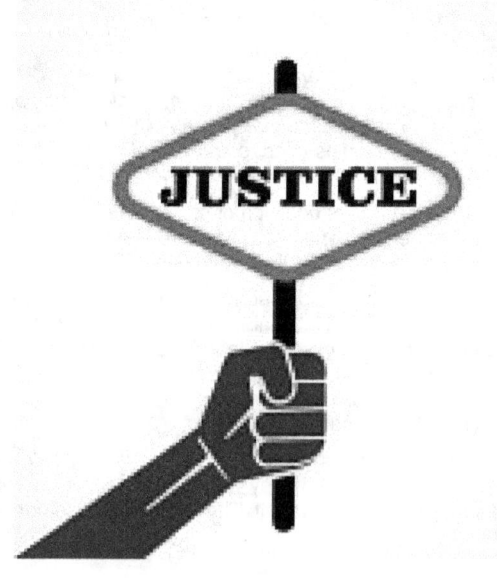

PART IV – REGULATION

WHOSE?

USDA's?

FDA's?

or

Monsanto's.

CHAPTER 12

FDA's Take on Gluten

Whose regulation, you ask? Who's not in this game. Who isn't even at first here. Only Monsanto is on any bases in this game. Monsanto controls all the bases in this game, from the FDA to the USDA to the CDC to probably the NIH, who houses and disseminates this information to the public as well. Our FDA takes the same stance as the USDA does in this Ruse, Their goal is to promote what the farmer (Monsanto) can grow the most of. This to me is what's scary, and why I won't buy into their ruse.

It would be nice if this was a problem with just the grain industry and Monsanto but it's not. It also involves the USDA and the FDA and what has influenced them to not issue warnings for this allergen and the effects it's having on the drug industry as well. The more I look at it, the more I see that it is a problem with overextending corporate entities intermingling their influence into regulatory agencies and offices to influence the agencies. Knowing the dealings that Monsanto has had in the past with competitors, regulatory agencies and offices, and their own judicial problems, it's not hard to fathom at all, the involvement they would have, in the non-disclosure of these studies. It's actually easy to see their involvement as being the same as the sugar industries', as they covored up the studies showing their food as being this dangerous. They didn't just cover up the studies condemning glucose, they initiated reports themselves that showed glucose was healthy. That is a complete falsehood from the truth of what glucose does. What glucose does is the same thing that grains do, except that grains do it worse to you than the sugar does, because of the gliadin in the gluten that's in most grains.

Gluten does the same thing as sugar. Why won't the FDA recognize that? They have all the studies that point to it. Don't they read them?

The following is an excerpt from an FDA study on Gluten as an allergen (1 of 173 studies).

THE FOOD ALLERGEN LABELING AND CONSUMER PROTECTION ACT (FALCPA) OF 2004

FALCPA is an amendment to the Federal Food, Drug, and Cosmetic Act and requires that the label of a food that contains an ingredient that is or contains protein from a "major food allergen" declare the presence of the allergen in the manner described by the law.

GLUTEN

WHY IS THERE A CONCERN ABOUT GLUTEN?

Gluten describes a group of proteins found in certain grains (wheat, barley, and rye.) It is of concern because people with celiac disease cannot tolerate it. Celiac disease (also known as celiac sprue) is a chronic digestive disease that damages the small intestine and interferes with absorption of nutrients from food. Recent findings estimate that 2 million people in the

U.S. have celiac disease or about 1 in 133 people.

WHAT DOES FALCPA REQUIRE WITH REGARD TO GLUTEN?

FALCPA requires FDA to issue a proposed rule that will define and permit the voluntary use of the term "gluten-free" on the labeling of foods by August 2006 and a final rule no later than August 2008.

WHAT HAS FDA DONE IN RESPONSE TO THE FALCPA MANDATE?

FDA held a public meeting in August 2005 to obtain expert comment and consultation from stakeholders to help FDA develop a regulation to define and permit the voluntary use on food labeling of the term "gluten-free" (Public Meeting On Gluten-Free Food Labelling). The meeting focused on food manufacturing, analytical methods, and consumer issues related to reduced levels of gluten in food.

FDA's *gluten-free definition* is that the food contains less than 20 ppm of gluten.

They consider wheat and gluten as undeclared allergens yet they refuse to acknowledge its allergenic properties to the extent that they won't require a warning label for it. Yet they know what damage it does. This is evidenced by the reports listed in chapter 4. All they require is a mention of wheat in the ingredients and nothing more. That is their warning.

Their negligence in regards to our health in this manner is unconscionable. I can only assume that they've been influenced by the other side of the industry that provides crop seed for the farmers that grow the food that the FDA approves for us to eat. The other side of this industry, owned by the same corporations, is the pharmaceutical industry. They provide us with all of the drugs that we take to fight the disease caused by the food provided their sister crop seed industry.

What I wonder is, what does the FDA consider stakeholders? Are they the corporate entities who have an interest in proliferating wheat and gluten? Since we now know that this happened with sugar, why wouldn't the same thing happen with gluten? We know that gluten breaks down into nothing more than glucose, I can see where the same situation would exist today, that existed 50 -60 years ago. In fact, I believe it's an ongoing problem that won't be resolved until the consumer does something about it.

Just like in the tobacco industry, "selling a product that is already sold for them as it's addictive", the same mantra is heard in the grain industry concerning their gluten. "How can people refuse to buy our products? They're addictive so people will want them more and more of them. The beauty of this addiction is that it feeds the other side of the same industry, the pharmaceutical industry.

I salute the FDA for monitoring products claiming to be gluten-free yet have more than a trace of gluten in them, such as the *Investigation* into General Mills for selling Cheerio's that had more than the allowed limit of 20 ppm of gluten. Yet knowing what damage gluten does to the body, I have to wonder why do they still allow it to be marketed without any warnings? The tobacco companies can't market their products without warnings. Why is the food industry allowed to? The evidence lies within the vaults of the NIH's PubMed, showing all the damage it does. Why do they ignore that evidence? I think it has to do with not enough funds or people to look over these studies. There is – after all – over 11,685 studies done on the glycation which is caused by the digestion of gluten to introduce glucose into your blood. That was the last count a couple days ago. Today I don't know how many research studies have been added. When I first checked last week, there were 11,667. This is something that is that important, yet the neither the FDA nor the USDA says anything about its dangers.

What dangers, you say? The evidence lies in the excerpts below, from 10 of their 173 studies on gluten;

"Gluten is the protein that naturally occurs in wheat, rye, barley, and crossbreeds of these grains. Most people can eat gluten, but in people with celiac disease, gluten intake gradually damages the intestines, prevents the absorption of vitamins and minerals, and can lead to other health problems. Symptoms can include diarrhea, fatigue, headaches, abdominal pain, brain fog, rashes, nausea, vomiting, and other reactions."

"People who have an allergy to wheat run the risk of serious or life-threatening allergic reaction if they eat wheat. Symptoms may include swelling, itching or irritation of mouth or throat, difficulty breathing, nasal congestion, itchy or watery eyes, rash or hives, headaches, nausea, vomiting, cramps, diarrhea, or anaphylaxis, a potentially life-threatening reaction."

What I can't understand, with this kind of disruption of bodily functions, why doesn't this require a warning like cigarettes? It's clearly killed more people.

"Unlike food allergies, clinical signs and symptoms do not appear to be reliable markers of disease activity because many individuals affected with celiac disease may be entirely asymptomatic. This tells me that a lot more people suffer from the disease than what has been diagnosed. Furthermore, although biomarkers of genetic susceptibility (e.g., presence of DQ2 and/or DQ8 HLA alleles) and gluten exposure [e.g., antibodies for gliadin (AGA), endomysial (EMA), and tissue transglutaminase (tTG)] have been defined for use in noninvasive diagnosis of individuals with celiac disease, these biomarkers have not been shown to correlate with disease severity nor to be useful in assessing daily responses to gluten exposures. Rather, evidence of intestinal mucosal inflammation is the gold standard biomarker for diagnosis of celiac disease and for assessment of disease severity. Intestinal mucosal inflammation may occur long before the development of clinical signs or a rise in antibody titers following a gluten challenge. Intestinal inflammation is assessed by intestinal biopsy, which is an invasive procedure, associated with false negatives (due to sampling error), and is impractical for frequent monitoring of disease activity or severity."   Revised Threshold Report Page 58 of 108

"Unpublished data described in Moneret-Vautrin and Kanny (2004) show that 83% of wheat allergic children reacted to less than 2 g of wheat flour while only 18% of wheat allergic adults responded at this level. Unpublished data described in Moneret Vautrin (2004) on wheat flour challenges using 32 children and 32 adults with wheat allergy, reported a LOAEL of ≤ 1.8 mg protein for allergic children (the lowest tested dose) and 52.8 mg protein for allergic adults. Scibilia et al. (2006) reported that 2 of 13 responders reacted to the lowest dose of wheat flour tested (100 mg of a mix of bread and durum flour, approximately 15 mg protein) in DBPCFCs. In total, 31% of the patients who reacted did so to challenge doses less than or equal to 240 mg of wheat protein." Approaches to Establish Thresholds for Major Food Allergens

My question is how many people eat this amount? Most people eat around 150mg of wheat products in a day, not enough to express symptoms of celiac disease, but enough to do unnoticed damage.

"The foods of concern for individuals with, or susceptible to, celiac disease are the cereal grains that contain the storage proteins prolamin and glutelin (commonly referred to as gluten in wheat), including all varieties of wheat (e.g., durum, spelt, Kamut), barley (where the storage proteins are called hordeins), rye (where the storage proteins are called secalins), and their cross-bred hybrids (such as triticale). The proportion of individuals with celiac disease that are also sensitive to the storage proteins in oats (avenins) has not been determined but is likely to be less than 1% (Kelly, 2005)."

"The clinical manifestations of celiac disease are highly variable in character and severity. The reasons for this diversity are unknown but may depend on the age and immunological status of the individual, the amount, duration, or timing of exposure to gluten, and the specific area

and extent of the gastrointestinal tract involved by disease (Dewar et al., 2004). These clinical manifestations can be divided into gastrointestinal, or "classic," and non-gastrointestinal manifestations. Gastrointestinal manifestations usually present in children 4 to 24 months old and include abdominal pain and cramping, bloating, recurrent or chronic diarrhea in association with weight loss, poor growth, nutrient deficiency, and (in rare cases) a life-threatening metabolic emergency termed celiac crisis, characterized by hypokalemia and acidosis secondary to profuse diarrhea (Farrell and Kelly, 2002; Baranwal et al., 2003). Non-gastrointestinal manifestations are more insidious and highly variable and are the common presenting signs in older children and adults. These manifestations are frequently the result of long-term nutrient malabsorption, including iron deficiency anemia, short stature, delayed puberty, infertility, and osteoporosis or osteopenia (Fasano, 2003). In children, progressive malabsorption of nutrients may lead to growth, developmental, or neurological delays (Catassi and Fasano, 2004). Extra-intestinal manifestations such as dermatitis herpetiformis, hepatitis, peripheral neuropathy, ataxia, and epilepsy have also been associated with celiac disease (Fasano and Catassi, 2001). Individuals with untreated celiac disease are also at increased risk for potentially serious medical conditions, such as other autoimmune diseases (e.g., Type I diabetes mellitus) and intestinal cancers associated with high mortality (Farrell and Kelly, 2002; Peters et al., 2003; Catassi et al., 2002). For example, individuals with celiac disease have an 80-fold greater risk of developing adenocarcinoma of the small intestine, a greater than two-fold increased risk for intestinal or extraintestinal lymphomas (Green and Jabri, 2003) and a 20-fold greater risk of developing enteropathy-associated T cell lymphoma (EATL) (Catassi et al.,"

"There is no standard protocol for gluten challenges, and challenge studies have varied greatly in amount and duration of gluten exposure. Although some studies have been designed to determine the acute effects (i.e., after 4 hours) of exposure to gluten (Sturgess et al., 1994; Ciclitiraet al., 1984), most challenges consist of an open challenge to a fixed or incremental dose of daily gluten over a minimum period of 4 weeks. Many challenge studies use a high exposure (≥ 10 g/day) to gluten, because this is believed to shorten time to disease confirmation or relapse and, therefore, to minimize discomfort to subjects (Rolles and McNeish, 1976). However, some studies have shown that low daily exposures to gluten also can elicit a disease response (Catassi et al., 1993; Laurin et al., 2002; Hamilton and McNeill, 1972)."

"At this time there is no correlative information on the efficacy of using these tests to predict or help prevent adverse effects in individuals with celiac disease."

There is now!

"Although gluten-free diets are considered the only effective treatment for individuals with celiac disease, it has been recognized that it is difficult, if not impossible, to maintain a diet that is completely devoid of gluten (Collinet al., 2004). Therefore, several attempts have been made to define gluten-free in regulatory contexts. Efforts by the Codex Alimentarius to define an international standard for "gluten-free" labeling date back to 1981. At that time, due to the lack of sensitive, specific analytical methods, a threshold value of 0.05 g nitrogen per 100 g dry matter was set for wheat starch, on the assumption that wheat protein would be the only source of nitrogen in starch (Codex Standard 118-1981). The Codex Committee on Nutrition and Foods for Special Dietary Uses is developing a revised standard. The current draft proposal would define three categories of gluten-free foods: processed foods that are naturally "gluten-free" (≤ 20 ppm of gluten), products that had been rendered "gluten-free" by processing (≤ 200 ppm), and any mixture of the two (≤ 200 ppm). The Australia New Zealand Food Agency (ANZFA) defines gluten to mean "the main protein in wheat, rye, oats, barley, triticale and spelt relevant to the medical conditions, Coeliac disease, and dermatitis herpetiform." ANZFA recognizes two classes of foods, gluten-free foods (" ...no detectable gluten") and low-gluten foods (" ...no more than 20 mg gluten per 100 gm of the food") (ANZFA Food Code Standard 1.2.8). The Canadian standard for "gluten-free" is more general, simply stating that "No person shall label, package, sell or advertise a food in a manner likely

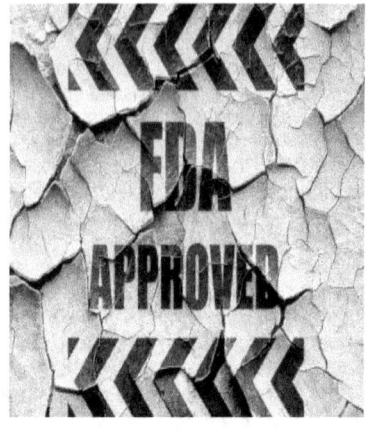

to create an impression that it is a "gluten-free" food unless the food does not contain wheat, including spelt and Kamut, or oats, barley, rye, triticale or any part thereof" (Canadian Food and Drugs Act Regulation B.24.018)." Approaches to Establish Thresholds for Major Food Allergens and for Gluten in Food. III, IV, V.

This is their admission of how difficult the food industry has made it to burb this addiction. Here's my solution; step 1, recognize the addiction, step two - vow to break it, step 3 - never touch starchy food again, ever. (Unless you want to commit suicide. This is the most painful way to do it, though.)

Now that you know what grains this involves you can get an idea of what not to eat.

"Like food allergies, celiac disease affects only a small proportion of the U.S. population (estimated at 1%, 3.1 million) (NIH, 2004). Susceptibility to celiac disease is genetically determined and is linked to the presence of the DQ2 or DQ8 HLA alleles. However, carrying these alleles does not necessarily lead to celiac disease. Both acute and chronic morbidity have been well documented for individuals with the symptomatic celiac disease. A gluten-free diet has been shown to greatly reduce the risk for cancer and overall mortality for these individuals. The potential benefit of a gluten-free diet has not been established for individuals with silent or latent celiac disease."

I submit that this is a disease of a much grander scale, than what's reported, as far too often this disease goes completely unrecognized and thus undiagnosed. I hear complaints from many carboholics about many of the disorders at the top of this list. That tells me that they each have an allergic intolerance to gluten and they don't even know it. Because of its addictive nature, they'll never know it, unless they can give it up. The above paragraphs apply to those with celiac disease, yet I contend that everyone experiences some of the above reactions to some degree. This happens even more so if you consume more of their products. I thought

I could eat this food for 58 years until I learned that I had allergies to it. Now I know that I have numerous allergic intolerances to this food. They present themselves every time I try to eat it again.

My guess is that 95% of the population is exactly the same as I am, allergic to the protein in gluten. I contend that the obesity and diabetes rates that exist today confirm this. The death rates of all the diseases caused by glycation prove it. That forces me to ask, with all the evidence available in your archives FDA, why doesn't this food require a warning?

They require other carcinogens to display warnings. Why not this one? This food is not only carcinogenic, it's atherosclerotic and inflammatory. What more could you want in a poison?

THIS IS WHAT THE FDA CLAIMS THEY'RE CONCERNED ABOUT;

"In 21 Code of Federal Regulations (CFR) part 117 (part 117), we have established our regulation entitled "Current Good Manufacturing Practice, Hazard Analysis, and Risk-Based Preventive Controls for Human Food." We published the final rule establishing part 117 in the

Federal Register of September 17, 2015 (80 FR 55908). Part 117 establishes requirements for current good manufacturing practice for human food (CGMPs), for hazard analysis and risk-based preventive controls for human food (PCHF), and related requirements."

After reviewing over half of the documents available and an examination of all the titles of the documents, I see nothing that bans the inclusion of any of these dangerous foods in our food products made for public consumption (processed foods, including bread). It seems their interest lies only in compliance with the labeling of the product. They want to make sure that a package that's sold as gluten-free has to have less than 20ppm gluten in the product.

They don't even feel that it's important enough to warn you that a product contains gluten, and they don't feel it important enough to warn you of the dangers of gluten on the package like they do with the dangers of cigarettes. They recognize the danger of tobacco, why can't they recognize the dangers of gluten and wheat? It seems that they're content with the warning you how much a product is gluten-free, but not how much gluten it has in it as if it does no harm at all. C'MON MAN. I have access to the same studies they have. They're all located at **PUBMED.COM** and they all explain the dangers this food presents. If I can learn about what this food does, they have to know. Why are they so willing to ignore it? Why are they so willing to treat this food as though there's nothing wrong with it?

The first page of studies I opened brought me to this study, the twelfth study out of 1797 studies on the list and reveals the dangers of just breathing the dust from these cereal grains. The grain induced asthma which affects those who work in the various fields in the grain industry, as stated by the **Allergy, Asthma & Immunology Research:**

"Asthma caused by an allergy to proteins from cereal grains is one of the most common types of occupational asthma (OA) and its prevalence does not seem to be declining. The main professions affected are bakers, confectioners, pastry factory workers, millers, farmers, and cereal handlers. Although wheat is the most commonly involved cereal, other grains (e.g. rye, barley, rice) also play a role. In addition, flour from other sources (e.g. soya, Lupin), pests, and several flour additives used in the baking industry to improve fermentation and elasticity of the dough, as well as to improve storage of the bread, may also give rise to IgE-mediated allergy." "This disorder has been classically considered a form of allergic asthma mediated by IgE antibodies specific to cereal flour antigens, mainly wheat, rye, and barley,"

In the tenth study on the list published, in July 2009, it's been found that the globulins in wheat can cause type1 diabetes. T1D is an autoimmune disorder that was thought to have no cause. At least, all the studies I've looked at didn't reveal this. According to *BioMed Central*;

"Taken together, the results indicate that a diverse group of globulins exists in wheat, some of which could be associated with the PATHOGENESIS of T1D in some susceptible individuals. These data expand our knowledge of specific wheat globulins and will enable further elucidation of their role in wheat biology and human health.

I have read elsewhere that it might be thought that an allergen might trigger an autoimmune response that shuts down the hormones that trigger insulin manufacture in the pancreas. It appears that this is that finding. Wheat can be responsible for type 1 diabetes. Have you seen any warnings for that? I haven't. Have any been issued? I haven't seen them. Why haven't they been issued? How many parents have fed their kids bread to find out that their children are diabetic because of this auto-immune disorder? Why is bread still considered by so many to be a necessity of life? It doesn't appear so. It appears more likely to be a destroyer of life.

We can end this. We can change our diet.

THIS IS WHAT I'M CONCERNED ABOUT;

47,397 DEATHS EVERY DAY FROM CVDS

THE ATHEROSCLEROTIC EFFECT

47,397 people died each day, worldwide, from cardiovascular disease in 2013. That breaks down to over 1800 Americans that died every day from cardiovascular disease in 2013. That's about 79 people every hour. That's 17.3 million annually, worldwide. That was up from 12.3 million (25.8%) in 1990. According to **Wikipedia**;

"CORONARY ARTERY DISEASE AND STROKE ACCOUNT FOR 80% OF CVD DEATHS IN MALES AND 75% OF CVD DEATHS IN FEMALES. MOST CARDIOVASCULAR DISEASE AFFECTS OLDER ADULTS. IN THE UNITED STATES 11% OF PEOPLE BETWEEN 20 AND 40 HAVE CVD, WHILE 37% BETWEEN 40 AND 60, 71% OF PEOPLE BETWEEN 60 AND 80, AND 85% OF PEOPLE OVER 80 HAVE CVD. THE AVERAGE AGE OF DEATH FROM CORONARY ARTERY DISEASE IN THE DEVELOPED WORLD IS AROUND 80 WHILE IT IS AROUND 68 IN THE DEVELOPING WORLD."

This rate is increasing each year by an ever-increasing rate, outpacing itself every year. This statement proves how slow this damage of glycation manifests. But it does manifest every time you eat anything that breaks down into glucose. And that includes all carbs, all sugars.

THE CARCINOGENIC EFFECT

According to the NCBI's PubMed;

A total of 1,658,370 new cancer cases and 589,430 cancer deaths are projected to occur in the United States in 2015.

1614 Americans die every day from cancer, in the US alone, due to ECC. That's 67 people every hour who die from cancer in the US alone. My mother was one of them. That's why I constructing this book. I know I'm not alone in the way I feel about the despair of cancer and number of lives it ruins. The changes that have to be made to correct this dilemma that our food industry has inflicted upon us, have to be made with a concerted effort by everyone involved. Otherwise, the health of our society will never recover.

Consumers should refrain from buying this food so that the manufacturers and growers will start growing and manufacturing something else more nutritious.

THE INFLAMMATORY EFFECT

In 2015, there were approximately 48 million people worldwide with the AD. In 2010, dementia resulted in about 486,000 deaths, according to Wikipedia. That's 19,440 Americans every year. That's 53 people every day that this disease takes and it won't stop until you stop the glycation. The only way you can stop the glycation is to take away the glucose that triggers it. This is curable. It's going to require that everyone conquer their own addiction. That means that they have to stop starting the addiction by keeping it out of all baby food.

How many people do you know who aren't affected by arthritis? I only know of a few who claim that they aren't. Arthritis is the widest spread manifestations of glycation. This is due to the fact that inflammation exists in the blood and it affects every bone and organ that your blood flows through. Because of this, the arthritis is always the first to be felt. The other manifestations usually aren't felt until it is too late. That's the manifestations of atherosclerosis and cancer and Alzheimer's disease. By the time you feel those, you're already deep into the drug cycle, and that's a cycle that ends only in death or abstinence.

Probably the first of these inflammatory manifestations to fully hit you is IBF or a condition preceding Irritable Bowel Syndrome as this is a major disorder that can be attributed directly to inflammation as evidenced by this report submitted Dec 16 last year;

BACKGROUND:

Irritable bowel syndrome (IBS) and inflammatory bowel disease (IBD) patients report similar gastrointestinal (GI) symptoms, yet comparisons of symptom severity between groups and with the general population (GP) are lacking.

The Overlap between Irritable Bowel Syndrome and Non-Celiac Gluten Sensitivity: A Clinical Dilemma

The spectrum of gluten-related disorders has widened in recent times and includes celiac disease, non-celiac gluten sensitivity, and wheat allergy. The complex of symptoms associated with these diseases, such as diarrhea, constipation or abdominal pain may overlap for the gluten-related diseases, and furthermore, they can be similar to those caused by various other intestinal diseases, such as irritable bowel syndrome (IBS). The mechanisms underlying symptom generation are diverse for all these diseases. Some patients with celiac disease may remain asymptomatic or have only mild gastrointestinal symptoms and thus may qualify for the diagnosis of IBS in the general clinical practice. Similarly, the overlap of symptoms between IBS and non-celiac gluten sensitivity (NCGS) often creates a dilemma for clinicians. While the treatment of NCGS is the exclusion of gluten from the diet, some, but not all, of the patients with IBS also improve on a gluten-free diet. Both IBS and NCGS are common in the general population and both can coexist with each other independently without necessarily sharing a common pathophysiological basis. Although the pathogenesis of NCGS is not well understood, it is likely to be heterogeneous with possible contributing factors such as low-grade intestinal inflammation, increased intestinal barrier function and changes in the intestinal microbiota. Innate immunity may also play a pivotal role. One possible inducer of innate immune response has recently been reported to be an amylase-trypsin inhibitor, a protein present in wheat endosperm and the source of flour, along with the gluten proteins.

The question I keep asking myself is why does this have to keep happening? Why hasn't the FDA warned us about the dangers of this food? They have access to all of the same reports that I do, yet they still refuse to acknowledge that this food is dangerous. *DOES THEIR INTEREST LIE ELSEWHERE? IS THERE* **corporate influence** *INVOLVED WITH THIS, LIKE THERE WAS WITH SUGAR? THIS IS SUGAR! SO WHY ARE THEY STILL COVERING IT UP?*

"The sugar industry actively took steps for years to influence public's perception of the nutritional value of their product, when they clearly knew of the dangers it posed. "Food companies have spent billions of dollars to cover up the link between sugar consumption and health problems. That's the conclusion of a new report from the Center for Science and Democracy at the Union of Concerned Scientists (UCS)."

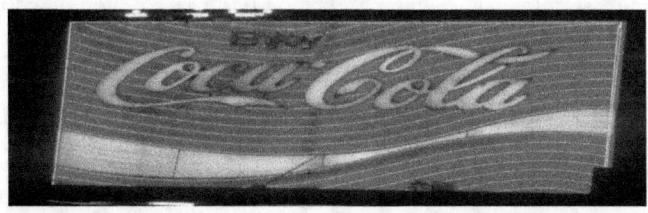

According to *The Guardian*;

"SUGAR LOBBY PAID SCIENTISTS TO BLUR SUGAR'S ROLE IN HEART DISEASE" –
REPORT

"New report highlights battle by the industry to counter sugar's negative health effects, and the cushy relationship between food companies and researchers". " Influential research that downplayed the role of sugar in heart disease in the 1960s was paid for by the sugar industry, according to a report released on Monday.

These actions are responsible for more deaths than all the world wars combined. Their actions have killed, hurt or harmed more than 500,000,000 people in the last 30 years alone. (At 17.3 million for heart disease alone, 500 million is a lowball estimate for death coming from cancer and dementia as well.) All total, the death rate for **ECC** is over 24,000,000 each year. That's over 65,753 deaths each day, simply from excessive carbohydrate consumption. (Remember carbs = sugar.)

With backing from a sugar lobby, scientists promoted dietary fat as the cause of coronary heart disease instead of sugar, according to a historical document review **published in JAMA Internal Medicine.** This was criminal, yet nothing was done about it. Though the review is nearly 50 years old, it showcases a decades-long battle by the sugar industry to persuade the public about the product's positive health effects, when it really has had none, ever. Why isn't this agency being held accountable? Maybe we should review who controls the agencies of the FDA and the USDA. (Knowing Monsanto, the EPA also.)

The findings come from documents recently found by a researcher at the University of **San Francisco**, which show that scientists at the Sugar Research Foundation (SRF), known today as the Sugar Association, paid scientists to do a 1967 literature review that overlooked the role of sugar in heart disease. Wasn't that a clear case of bribery that should have been prosecuted?

SRF set an objective for the review, funded it and reviewed drafts before it was published in the New England Journal of Medicine, which did not require conflict of interest disclosure until 1984. The three Harvard scientists who wrote the review made what would be $50,000 in today's dollars from the review. Because of this bribery, over 500,000,000 have suffered from these diseases that sugar is responsible for. From diabetes to heart disease to dementia to cancer to arthritis...(you should be familiar with the list by now).

Marion Nestle, nutrition, food studies and public health professor at New York University, said the food industry continues to influence nutrition science, **in an editorial published alongside the JAMA report;**

"TODAY, IT IS ALMOST IMPOSSIBLE TO KEEP UP WITH THE RANGE OF FOOD COMPANIES SPONSORING RESEARCH – FROM MAKERS OF THE MOST HIGHLY PROCESSED FOODS, DRINKS, AND SUPPLEMENTS TO PRODUCERS OF DAIRY FOODS, MEATS, FRUITS, AND NUTS – TYPICALLY YIELDING RESULTS FAVORABLE TO THE SPONSOR'S INTERESTS," NESTLE SAID. "FOOD COMPANY SPONSORSHIP, WHETHER OR NOT INTENTIONALLY MANIPULATIVE, UNDERMINES PUBLIC TRUST IN NUTRITION SCIENCE, CONTRIBUTES TO PUBLIC CONFUSION ABOUT WHAT TO EAT, AND COMPROMISES DIETARY GUIDELINES IN WAYS THAT ARE NOT IN THE BEST INTEREST OF PUBLIC HEALTH."

"THE CUSHY RELATIONSHIP BETWEEN FOOD COMPANIES AND RESEARCHER HAS BEEN CAPTURED IN RECENT INVESTIGATIONS BY THE ASSOCIATED PRESS AND NEW YORK TIMES. THE AP REVEALED IN JUNE THAT CANDY TRADE GROUPS WERE FUNDING RESEARCH INTO SWEETS. AND IN 2015, THE NEW YORK TIMES SHOWED HOW COCA-COLA HAS FUNDED MILLIONS IN RESEARCH TO DOWNPLAY THE LINK BETWEEN SUGARY BEVERAGES AND OBESITY."

The **Sugar** Association said in a statement that SRF *"should have exercised greater transparency" in its research, but also accused the study authors of having an "anti-sugar narrative".*

"We question this author's continued attempts to reframe historical occurrences to conveniently align with the currently trending anti-sugar narrative, particularly when the last several decades of research have concluded that sugar does not have a unique role in heart disease," the Sugar Association said. "Most concerning is the growing use of headline-baiting articles to trump quality scientific research – we're disappointed to see a journal of JAMA's stature being drawn into this trend."

The findings were based on documents found by Cristin Kearns, a postdoctoral fellow at UCSF, in library archives. The scientists and executives involved are no longer alive.

*In recent years, the link between fat and heart disease has become a more contentious topic – a 2010 review of scientific studies of fat **in the American Journal of Clinical Nutrition** found that "there is no convincing evidence that saturated fat causes heart disease". The role of sugar in heart disease is still being debated."*

Even according to **Mother Jones**;

*"The industry's tactics—similar to those used by Big Tobacco in downplaying the adverse health effects of smoking—were explored by Gary Taubes and Cristin Kearns Couzens in the 2012 Mother Jones investigation "**Big Sugar's Sweet Little Lies**." But this latest report draws on some **newly released documents** submitted as evidence in a recent federal court case involving the two biggest players in the sweetener industry: the Sugar Association and the Corn Refiners Association (the trade group for manufacturers of high fructose corn syrup)."*

When will it stop?

Until we let this industry know that we won't accept their definition of healthy food and stop buying their versions of it, you're going to be eating it until you start buying their drugs. And you'll still keep eating it. Only when it becomes unprofitable will it be eliminated.

*"Obesity and **diabetes mellitus** are often linked to cardiovascular disease, as are a history of chronic **kidney disease** and **hypercholesterolemia**. In fact, cardiovascular disease is the most life-threatening of the diabetic complications and diabetics are two- to four-fold more likely to die of cardiovascular-related causes than nondiabetics."*

According to the World Heart Association;

"Up to 90% of cardiovascular disease may be preventable if established risk factors are avoided. " Their goal is 25 by 25. "25x25, achieving a 25% relative reduction in overall mortality from cardiovascular disease, cancer, diabetes or chronic respiratory disease by 2025. In September 2011, the United Nations held a High-Level Meeting in New York on the subject of NCDs, including cardiovascular disease (CVD), cancers, diabetes and chronic respiratory diseases."

They're actively taking steps to lower the death rate of CVDs by recommending everyone to eat right, quit smoking, and exercise, all of which will lower this number one killer of people. Eating right, in my opinion, is by far the best way to combat CVDs, diabetes, obesity, hypertension, high cholesterol (which is really a problem of unbalanced cholesterol), arthritis and worst of all, dementia and Alzheimer disease.

In all of my research, I can't find anything that says to limit the use of bread and starchy carbohydrates made from grains. Yet all research I've looked at from PubMed and even the FDA show that this food does cause these disorders. Every time I look at the data, I'm forced to ask myself, why hasn't the FDA, WHA, or the ADA condemned this food? These agencies have to know what's going on, yet they refuse to act. Who is blocking this action? Why does *MYPlate.gov* still recommend them?

After researching my book ***IT'S TIME FOR A CURE,*** I've learned that this food is at the base of all of the diseases listed above, forcing me to ask, why hasn't the FDA or the WHF warned us of this food? The only reason I can come up with is that it is being protected from prosecution by the industry that provides the crop seed for the farmer as well as the drugs to combat arthritis caused by what their seed grows into.

After finding this, I don't wonder at all why the FDA isn't protecting us. It's because they're protecting Monsanto as Michael Taylor was their deputy commissioner since 2010; *Michael R. Taylor is an American lawyer. Since 2010 he has been the Deputy Commissioner for Foods at the United States Food and Drug Administration*

His past associations include 4 years with Monsanto. Do you wonder if he left with any stock options? Does he still have an interest in Monsanto's business? Their offices are loaded with people as such, corrupting the integrity of our food chain.

From Wikipedia;

Between 1996 and 2000, after briefly returning to King & Spalding, Taylor worked for Monsanto as a Vice President for Public Policy. n 1999, a lawsuit (Alliance For Bio-Integrity v. Shalala) and GAO report revealed considerable disagreement within the FDA concerning decisions about biotechnology products made during Taylor's tenure. The lawsuit and report also said that Taylor had recused himself from matters related to Monsanto's BGH and had "never sought to influence the thrust or content" of the agency's policies on Monsanto's products.

Was this following study something that he didn't want to be exposed? Or was he worried about any of the other 11,750 studies done on glycation, the end result of glucose consumption, or carb consumption?

From PubMed's study; ***Characterization of Proteins from Grain of Different Bread and Durum Wheat Genotypes****: "Wheat is unique among the edible grains because wheat flour has the protein complex called "gluten" that can be formed into the dough with the rheological properties required for the production of leavened bread. The rheological properties of gluten are needed not only for bread production, but also in the wider range of foods that can only be made from wheat, viz., noodles, pasta, pocket bread, pastries, cookies, and other products. The gluten proteins consist of monomeric gliadins and polymeric glutenins. Glutenins and gliadins are recognized as the major wheat storage proteins, constituting about 75–85% of the total* *grain proteins with a ratio of about 1:1 in common or bread wheat and they tend to be rich in asparagine, glutamine, arginine or proline but very low in nutritionally important amino acids lysine, tryptophan, and methionine."*

"Very low in nutritionally important amino acids" interests me. Amino acids are proteins. When you take away the protein, you're left with little else but carbohydrates. This fact combined with the fact that gliadins have been shown to provoke the body to release anti-gliadin antibodies, which also have been shown to have the ability to attach themselves to Purkinje cells in the cerebellum, make this food suspect, at the least.

When an anti-gliadin antibody attaches itself to a cell in the cerebellum, the brain renders that cell useless and discards it. Although many parts of your brain can grow new cells to replace discarded cells, this area of the brain can't. That means whenever an anti-gliadin antibody attaches itself to a Purkinje cell, that part of the brain never comes back. Yes, that does mean brain damage for those who release these anti-gliadin antibodies.

The question this brings up is how many of us release these antibodies? Judging from the amount of Alzheimer's disease invading the civilized world, I would say a majority of people display this form of intolerance....a rather large majority. The next question this generates is, am I one of them? Are you one of them? I found out that I am. Have you yet?

42,657 DEATHS EACH DAY WORLDWIDE FROM CARDIOVASCULAR DISEASE

Heart disease kills more people every year than any other single cause. Over 42,000 people die from this disease every day and the only reason it exists is the high amount of sugar we put into our bodies. It brings about the glycation that **ECC** is responsible for and it's this glycation that is responsible 42,000 deaths from cardiovascular disease every day. That's 1,680 Americans every day. That's 33 people for every state every day, dying from a cardiovascular disease caused by nothing other than ECC, Excessive Carbohydrate Consumption.

But that's not all it is responsible for. We have to look at Alzheimer's disease and dementia. We have to consider cancer, and we have to worry about the amount of high blood pressure and high cholesterol ECC is responsible for. All of these disorders are money producing the diseases that this industry generates, simply for the sake of profit. It's this profit that is killing everyone

13,698 DAILY DEATHS GLOBALLY FROM ALZHEIMER DISEASE

13.698 die each day, worldwide, due to Alzheimer disease. That amounts to over 500 deaths daily in the US, which means that at least 20 people in this country will die this hour alone, due to Alzheimer disease. Nothing contributes to Alzheimer disease as much as bread consumption. It's the starchy carbs that break down to glucose, and it's the glucose that glycates the cholesterol and protein that builds up the plaque and inflammation in your blood that leads to Alzheimer disease, cancer, arthritis, Atherosclerosis as well as most all other CVDs, as well as hypertension and high cholesterol.

11,232 DEATHS DAILY FROM CANCER WORLDWIDE

11,232 people die every day globally due to some form of cancer and with all the evidence available that wheat contributes to the spread of multiple forms of cancer, why hasn't the FDA made any statements about the dangers this food presents to the human body. Evidence shows these devastating effects going back to the bones of earliest cavemen that have been discovered.

I recently watched a Nova program on a 5,000-year-old iceman mummy that had been frozen in an ice flow until he was discovered in 1991. They found remnants of einkorn wheat in his upper digestive tract suggesting his last meal was bread made from the flour of einkorn wheat. His bones also showed "disease of a modern lifestyle", as they like to call it. What is this disease of a modern lifestyle? Arthritis! This is evidence of the glycation that occurred in this man from eating the carb-loaded grain from einkorn wheat. Even as difficult as it was to digest einkorn wheat at that time, due to its fibrous nature, it still did the same damage then, that it does today to everyone who continues to eat this food.

Copied from NOVA on PBS concerning a 4,000-year-old frozen mummy;

"Oeggl reconstructed the Iceman's last meal from his microscopic analysis of a tiny sample removed from the mummy's transverse colon, the part of the intestine just beyond the stomach. When the Iceman was discovered in 1991, x-rays and CAT-scans of the corpse revealed that his internal organs had shrunken so drastically in the 5,300 years in the glacier that Dr. Dieter Zur Nedden, the radiologist who examined the images, could barely distinguish them. Instead of filling the chest cavity with their billowy white form, the lungs looked like wisps of clouds.

But at the top of the colon, Zur Nedden made out a slight bulge, which the radiologist suspected was a clump of half-processed food. The progress of the food indicated that the Iceman had last eaten about eight hours before he died, possibly of hypothermia, on the Hauslabjoch pass, which cuts over the main Alpine ridge dividing Austria from Italy at 10,500 feet above sea level.

Not until several years after the discovery did the Innsbruck scientists finally cut a holo into the mummy, insert an endoscope, and snip out about .004 ounces from the colon. Dr. Werner Platzer, the University of Innsbruck anatomist then in charge of research on the corpse, gave .0016 ounces milligrams of the material to Oeggl, who had already been studying the rich botanical finds from the site.

Pollen provided a snapshot of the environment the Iceman was exposed to in the hours before his death

Oeggl's sample was barely the size of his little fingernail. Under the microscope, he quickly identified the flake-like, semi-digested material that made up the bulk of the sample as einkorn, the most important wheat of the Neolithic, the period of prehistory in which people lived in semi-permanent settlements and survived by agriculture and keeping animals. The discovery of einkorn, which does not occur naturally in Europe, in the Iceman's intestinal tract suggested that he had contact with an agricultural community. The dominance of bran in the sample led Oeggl to believe that the wheat had been finely ground into meal and made into bread, rather than eaten as a porridge, where the grains would have been eaten whole and found in larger pieces in the colon. But the bread would have been little like modern bread. In order to get bread to rise when yeast is added, the wheat grains must contain a high level of gluten, which lends the dough a durable elasticity and therefore holds the pockets of air. Einkorn has low levels of gluten, so the bread made with it was probably hard, somewhat like a cracker, and rather tough on the teeth.

Using an electron microscope Oeggl also spotted tiny particles of charcoal attached to the bran, probably remnants of the baking process on a hot rock, or next to a fire. In addition to the einkorn, the cells of at least one other plant, possibly some herb, were present in the sample, and Oeggl concluded that they, too, had been part of his meal. He also found a tiny muscle fiber and a burned bit of bone, evidence that the Iceman might also have eaten a meat. What kind of meat Oeggl cannot yet say, nor can he determine how much of the meal the sample represented. Not everything passing through the Iceman's gut had been swallowed intentionally or was even desirable. Oeggl also found the eggs of the human whipworm. Many people alive today who do not live in areas with flush toilets also carry the worm, which can cause unpleasant symptoms like stomach ache and diarrhea, or even lead to malnutrition. The scientists have no way of knowing whether the Iceman had any such complaints.

Scientists may never know what prompted the Iceman to leave the relatively hospitable valley with no water or food to speak of. The sample also contained many different varieties of pollen, whose strange and beautiful forms Oeggl saw under the electron microscope. Though some peoples are known to eat pollen, Oeggl believed that the quantity in his colon was too small to represent a meal. Instead, the pollen accidentally ended up in the man's stomach because they either had landed in food or water he ingested, or were inhaled and became trapped in HIS saliva which he then swallowed. Scientists had long wondered where the Iceman was coming from and where he was headed, but until the discovery of the pollen inside the corpse, no scientist had any convincing documentation for his last day. But the pollen provided a snapshot of the environment the Iceman was exposed to in the hours before his death.

This feature originally appeared on the site for the Nova program *ICE MUMMIES*.

Although not shown in this excerpt, the Iceman did show signs of modern day disease in his bones. it was evident mostly around his joints in the form of arthritis. This arthritis is directly due to his diet of einkorn wheat.

As it does now, it did it then. The glucose glycates the cholesterol it comes in contact with, causing arthritis. It did so then, as it does now. It just did it slower, due to the indigestibility of the einkorn wheat. But it happened, never-the-less.

The damage it did at that time was much less than what it does now. This is due to the lack of fiber it comes with, in today's strains of wheat, mostly the common bread wheat made of **Triticum aestivum,** and, spelt, rye and emmer. It also comes from more glutinous wheat like durum as well.

Even though arthritis seldom kills its victim, the damage it does doesn't go away, ever. It's stuck to you like paint on a wall and you can't scrape it off. Most of the today's wheat has more gluten protein than it's ever had in its history, making it gluier and stickier, which makes it that much more dangerous, as this is what builds up the plaque in your system and you already know what damage plaque does. This points to the fact this food which is eaten on a daily basis does so little damage incrementally to the consumer that it's never noticed until it's too late. The disease has already manifested itself and the price is now being paid for a lifetime of consumption.

Perhaps the biggest question this brings up is, with all of this information available for this many years, why hasn't the FDA warned us that this food has these capabilities to do this kind of damage to the human body. Should the public be able to make an informed decision as to whether or not to continue to eat this food? Or should the FDA continue to ignore the evidence and fail to even let the public know what this food does? The question I want to ask, was and is there outside influence in their decision to not expose this information?

THE EVIDENCE IS PILING UP. THE FDA NOR THE USDA CAN'T HIDE THEIR COMPLICITY MUCH LONGER.

Someone is trying to hide this information. They want to leave it up to an uneducated public to automatically know what these studies have shown. In whose best interest would it be to keep this information hidden? Whose business would hurt the most if bread and corn and wheat products all of a sudden became taboo? The grain industry? Monsanto? The more I look into this, the more it spells out cover-up and because this is how the FDA treats this, it creates a lot of fear in me as to how healthy the rest of our food supply is.

I contend that The FDA has to know of the damage these grains do to the body when ingested, so why do they allow these industries to continue to peddle their wares as if they're healthy? (This is the definition of inside influence.)

Food, Inc. is a 2008 American documentary film directed by filmmaker Robert Kenner. The academy award-nominated film examines corporate farming in the United States, concluding that agribusiness produces food that is unhealthy, in a way that is environmentally harmful and abusive to both animals and employees. The film is narrated by Michael Pollan and Eric Schlosser

The film received positive responses and was nominated for several awards, including the academy award and the independent spirit awards in 2009, both for best documentary feature.

The film's first segment examines the industrial production of meat (chicken, beef, and pork), calling it inhumane and economically and environmentally unsustainable. The second segment looks at the industrial production of grains and vegetables (primarily corn and soybeans), again labeling this economically and environmentally unsustainable. The film's third and final segment is about the economic and legal power, such as food labeling regulations, of the major food companies, the profits of which are based on supplying cheap but contaminated food, the heavy use of petroleum-based chemicals (largely pesticides and fertilizers), and the promotion of unhealthy food consumption habits by the American public. It shows companies like Walmart transitioning towards organic foods as that industry is booming in the recent health movement.

Monsanto, the USDA and the FDA

FOOD, INC is an eye-opening documentary that deals with the agricultural industry's influence in the USDA and the FDA, concentrating on the meatpacking industry's influence. In 2008 the Chief of Staff for the USDA was a former chief lobbyist for the beef industry. The head of the FDA was a former executive vice president for the national food processors Association. A majority of the staff at both the FDA and the USDA came from Monsanto or its subsidiaries, posing clear conflicts of interests when it comes to protecting consumers. These industries; Monsanto, Bayer, Syngenta have spread their influence throughout the offices and agencies of the USDA and the FDA and are ultimately responsible for more death and disease than all violence, which includes war and crime, as well as all automobile accidents, all other addictions, including heroin, amphetamines, and alcohol. This addiction can be blamed for every other addiction that exists, simply because of the control, this addiction has over your hormones combined with the fact that this addiction was forced upon you right after birth.

Food, Inc talks about the revolving door between Monsanto's corporate offices and the various regulatory agencies that are supposed to protect us, the consumer. Donald Rumsfeld was CEO of Searle, which was owned by Monsanto. You know of his close ties to the Bush White House, John Ashcroft (Missouri Senator) received record donations from Monsanto. According to *Food, Inc.* for 25 years our government agencies that are set up to protect us were dominated by the industry they regulate. This is how Monsanto self-regulates. They pretty much own the gov't agencies. That makes it convenient to keep control of your drugs and how much you pay for them.

Justice Clearance Thomas was a Monsanto attorney prior to being named a Supreme Court Justice, which wouldn't matter too much except for the fact that he wrote the decision the court made, that allows Monsanto to prohibit farmers (both contracted and uncontracted) from cleaning their own seeds to use for next year's planting (according to *Food, Inc)*.

Something as natural as a seed is what the Supreme Court has allowed Monsanto to patent. The consequence of this has been disastrous for the farmer. It's been far worse for the consumer. Now, Monsanto controls all the food you buy, if you're buying the carbs their crops are made into. Most all seed companies are owned by Monsanto. If a farmer wants to grow a crop, they have to buy seed for that crop from Monsanto. This is unless you're old enough to have your own seed that you've never bought. You've just kept re-using your crop from last year for this year's seed. This requires cleaning a portion of your crop to use as seed for next year's crop. This is how farmers improved their own crops. They would pick out the best section of their fields to clean for next year's crops.

This is where the problem begins for these farmers. Seed cleaners used to have thriving businesses in the Midwest. Now, few if any of them exist. This is an industry that's been put to death by Monsanto and their patented seeds. Monsanto guarantees their demise by threatening any farmers that use their services, legal action. This is to inhibit any farmer from cleaning their own seeds. (Monsanto uses the patent clause in their contracts to prosecute farmers for growing their GMO seeds when in all actuality their crops have been cross-pollinated by their neighbor's GMO crops.)

Say goodbye to homegrown in your food. It all belongs to Monsanto now. Don't forget though, they also made your Celebrex.

Crops that are grown in an open field are open to the environment. Being open to the environment leaves them open to cross-pollination. This cross-pollination happens when neighboring field's GMO crops and portions of a non-GMO field get contaminated with GMO cross-pollination. Monsanto makes their farmers sign a "no clean" contract, saying that they can't clean a portion of their seed to save for planting next year. If caught doing so, they're open for prosecution. However, the farmer growing his own seed that's been contaminated by GMO cross-pollination is now open to prosecution by Monsanto, your food provider.

This puts your food if you're eating carbs, completely under the control of the same company that controls the drug industry that treats you for the conditions their foods give you. This is the glucose ruse, the ultimate carb haul, the emanate destroyer of health and life. This may be the superlative of corporate chicanery, your health risked, all for the sake of profit, and what drives profit? The ~~desire~~ hunger for security drives the desire for profit. It's the same hunger as that for food. It a hunger for security, it's an impulse to stay alive and hopefully make life easier to ensure a longer life.

It would be OK if you had a choice in the matter. But you didn't. (Would you choose an addiction, if you had a choice?) This one has been forced upon you just like it was me and if I could break the cycle, with all the issues I have, you can too.

These industries and agencies are directly responsible for over 950,000 deaths each and every year. That total continues to climb and it will continue until everyone decides, like me, that it's time for a cure.

Decisions have been made in the past that clearly benefited industry while presenting clear dangers to humans. By allowing contaminated food with worthless nutritional values or food contaminated by bacteria to sneak into our food supply, as well as by polluting our rivers and lakes in the process, with contaminated groundwater from runoff from chemical fertilizers, pesticides and herbicides, Monsanto has probably contributed more to the damage of mankind than any other one entity. This is the primary reason this is unsustainable and has to be changed.

It all starts with the grain industry, along with our insatiable appetites for high starch and sugary foods (which is all forced upon us by this industry) the corn producers, the wheat growers, and the crop seed companies owned by Monsanto, Novartis, Syngenta, Bayer *ET AL*. Because their food requires treatment with medications that this industry controls, they have full control over what happens inside your body when you bend to their will and buy their products.

The Iowa Corn Fed Beef Controversy

The grain industry in Iowa promoted *"Iowa Corn Fed Beef"*, to sell more corn, their largest industry. This had multiple, unforeseen consequences that not only damaged our food supply, but it polluted our resources more than what could have ever been foreseen.

The increase in industrial beef production that this promotion has generated has damaged the quality of the beef as well as damage the environment with the pesticides and herbicides needed for growing the corn to use as feed for the cattle. This has acted as a double whammy for our environment.

The huge cattle farms act as methane farms contributing more to global warming than much of anything else in the environment. On top of that, the chemicals sprayed on the fields of corn that's to be used for feed ultimately put these chemicals into our food supply as well as washing off the crops to contaminate groundwater and runoff into the streams and rivers polluting drinking water. This led to multiple outbreaks of cancer in downstream communities.

The cattle eat these glyphosate herbicide infected grains, (mostly soy and corn) which infects the meat which you eat. This is basically putting this enzyme changing chemicals in your body. Can you see how the ingestion of enzyme changing chemicals could have an impact on your health? This is just a taste (no pun intended) of what this industry is putting our society through. How safe would you consider your food is from these chemicals?

A lot of this feed corn that's been genetically modified to accept the Roundup weedkiller that's been sprayed on it, finds its way through the food supply into your processed foods, to make ingredients for foods that you commonly eat. I'll bet you didn't know you were buying cancer when you bought those corn chips last time, did you? How about that power bar or soy milk? If you're not reading labels on the food you're buying, how do you know you're not subjecting your body to this damage?

Or how about when you bought that formula or medicine for your baby? The #1 or #2 ingredient in many Similac infant formulas and Pedialyte, is corn syrup and corn syrup solids right behind water. Often the second or third ingredient is soy protein. Arguably the 2 heaviest sprayed crops in our food supply are soybeans and corn, ensuring your baby's diet is herbicide laden. Do you think that could cause some future need for further medication for your baby, in the future? And don't forget, drug use always leads to more and more drug use, especially when the drug is basically sugar. The only thing that can stop it is to either, quit the carbs and go keto, or die prematurely of any disease of your body's choice.

Because of our propensity to feed our addiction to sugar (which includes all grains), the products that this industry has devised to get us to eat more of their junk food, are putting everyone who is suckered into this cycle, in the hospital with serious disorders. You should know the range of disorders this incurs by now, from arthritis to cancer to hypertension to

CVDs, anything involving inflammation including all dementia. The scale is staggering. The toll is staggering.

This is clearly a case where self-policing doesn't work. It's taking its toll on Americans, currently at a rate of 196 of us every hour, because it isn't working. From all ECC caused forms of death, this glucose addiction is costing our country 959,993 premature deaths, every year that could have been prevented by a simple change of diet. That's 2,630 mothers and fathers every day or 109 family members every hour. Evidence can be seen in the number of heart disease deaths, cancer deaths, Alzheimer's deaths, and this doesn't mention all the pain, discomfort, and drug abuse that comes along with the disease. All of this is due to the pain and discomfort the disease inflicts.

When I consider how close I was to suicide because of my pain and seeing no way out of it, I have to consider many suicides as being caused by carbohydrates now. If carbs weren't at the root of my pain, I definitely wouldn't have been as close to suicide as I was, for I would not have had as much pain. That and the fact that sugar does mess with your emotions by messing with your hormones makes it much easier to see how suicide could be considered caused by ECC. Depression is another manifestation of glucose addiction, I know, I was there. It's become clear to me that if you don't die of old age, and I mean really old age, (as in 100 years old or older) your death is going to be a result of your addiction.

Although this is nice for the profits of Monsanto, Syngenta and Bayer who also make drugs that treat the diseases their foods cause; it's leading our country down a path of destruction that we'll never recover from if you keep eating the food they keep pushing you to eat. They are counting on the addiction that they've inflicted upon the American people as well as the world to pad their profits and boost the influence, both commercially and politically.

This industry's desire to make certain that sugar gets into as much baby food as they can pack it into, to make sure that every baby who eats it becomes addicted to it, making them lifetime _USERS_ of their poison. This unwilling addiction to sugar, by the public at large, has brought this industry to a level of evil that's never been seen in any industry. This industry is so intent on keeping us addicted to its lure, simply to increase their profits, that they are now responsible for over 65,753 deaths, worldwide daily. Yes, I said 65,753 deaths daily. If this doesn't bother you, then you have no conscience. Yes, this is something to be appalled about and appalled I am and you should be too. This is simply more proof that it's time for a cure.

It was recently revealed that the sugar industry took steps to cover up the reports of damage that their food offered, so why wouldn't it make sense that this closely related industry, the grain industry, would take those same steps to cover up the same information about what their foods provided? Was this another case of the industry policing itself and its watchdog, as well? Does this make a valid argument for the self-policing of corporate entities like this, instead of government regulations? This is the epitome of corporate propaganda generated to bolster profits by building their influence in the regulatory departments that are responsible for our health. This is my worst dream come true, someone else controlling my health by controlling my food.

For the sake of profit, this industry has poisoned not only us the consumer, but the space we have to live in as well, as they've contaminated our environment and condemned our society to a cycle of dependence that can only end with a premature death. There is an alternative. You can always join me and go keto. It'll not only save your life, it will extend it.

Our health is at stake here and we've allowed the USDA and the FDA to escape judgment. That in my estimation is borderline criminal. 2,893 deaths nationally, each day from CVDs, cancer, and Alzheimer disease combined. All three of these disorders are directly due to _ECC, EXCESSIVE CARBOHYDRATE CONSUMPTION_, which can be controlled. That's enough people to wipe out 4 towns, the same size I grew up in. That's unconscionable and we let it happen. Shame on us, for allowing this ruse to continue.

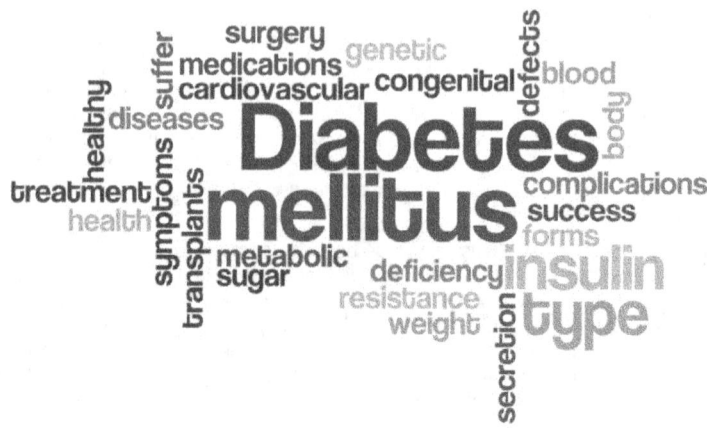

We have direct control of these disorders. We don't have to let this continue, but we do, simply to feed our addiction. We have a societal addiction to glucose. Because it's not just sugar, it's what breaks down into glucose, and that includes not only sugar but all carbohydrates that break down to their most basic molecule, glucose. It's our addiction to this glucose that clouds our judgment, masks our emotions, and controls our desires by gumming up the neurons in our brains every time we eat this food. This is exactly what makes it addictive and hands total control over to the glucose, every time you eat it Yes, we do have full control over this, and you can stop it. We have to stop the celebration of our individual addiction, to stop the addiction on a societal level. We need to un-brainwash ourselves and learn to see pain every time we see bread, pasta, cereal, and sugar because that's all it brings.

You have the power to stop this, and by stopping it,

it gives you far more POWER than what you ever could have imagined you would have.

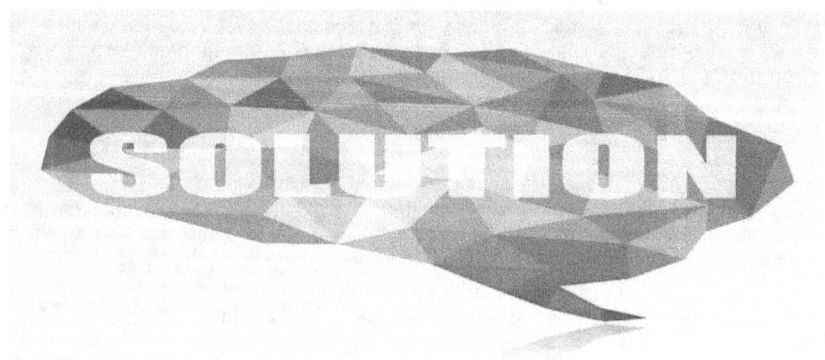

CHAPTER 13

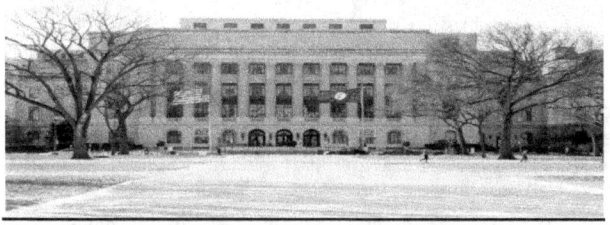

USDA'S INVOLVEMENT

With the same commingling of execs and offices of the USDA and Monsanto, as between the FDA and Monsanto, Monsanto has set itself up to be producer and regulator in full control over all of the food that we are forced to put on our tables. That is if you're forced to eat at a restaurant or buy food at a grocery store. If you're one of those people, your food is more than likely, a product of Monsanto. It's also a product of Monsanto's chemicals, chiefly their herbicide Roundup, a glyphosate herbicide that inhibits how enzymes work in the environment as well as your body.

That wouldn't be so bad if Monsanto didn't force all farmers to grow their crop seed each and every year. That gives them full control over every muffin you sink your teeth into, even those bran muffins, the ones that are supposed to be so healthy.

What Monsanto knows that they're not telling the USDA, is that the corn, wheat, and soybeans that their farmers grow for us are at the root of most all glycation that occurs in the body. What they're afraid of the USDA knowing, is that this glycation is at the root of all modern diseases, from atherosclerosis to hypertension, from arthritis to IBS or irritable bowel syndrome, to dementia including Alzheimer's disease and Parkinson's disease. All of these diseases and disorders are treated by the drug industry that Monsanto owned as well. That's what's scary…very scary. The company that's responsible for your food is the same company that treats you for the ailments their food brings. To me that's criminal. Now, Bayer wants to buy out Monsanto. What do you think that will do to your food supply? Bayer is a German company, you know.

Monsanto doesn't want either the USDA or the FDA to be too aware of what their food does, yet all of the studies mentioned above are available through PubMed. If I have access to these studies, I know they do as well. What don't I know is what do they refuse to look at them? They only have to look at a few. I found two or three damning studies on the first page of search returns for the term, glycation. Glycation has a nasty tendency to muck up everything in the body that blood effects. Monsanto doesn't want the USDA or the FDA to realize this. Their practice of striving for total control over our food source drives the profits of their crop seed companies, (of which they're dozens). Having that control over our food gives them control over our drug use, as it's their food that makes us sick. That makes us require their medications to treat the disease their food gives those who eat it.

They've tried denying that their food is as dangerous as it is by publishing their own research reports showing different results that "prove" their food is healthy when it's not. It's obvious that they don't want this information known by either the USDA or the FDA.

Fortunately for Monsanto, they already have they own retired execs running the FDA and the USDA. Apparently, it's not in their best interest to make this information known to the public. I'm sure they fear the consequences of their actions, for producing a food this dangerous. I would be if I were them.

With all the agencies the USDA has control over, it's no wonder that they can't see that the food they recommend we eat, has had more studies done on the glycation of it than any other food. We've learned that glycation is the real poisoning of America, and with glycation being involved in every modern disease known to man (simply because of the glycation is caused), glycation is something that our food industry should be working to stem as it's this glycation that's at the root of all "modern" diseases.

FYI fact: There were 50,000 food safety inspections in 1972. That was reduced to just over 9,000 in 2008. There aren't fewer consumers. Is it due to a lack of funding or a lack of willingness on the USDA's and FDA's desire to control these pandemics

If there were only 9000 in 2008, reduced from 50,000 in 1972, when the threat level was much lower, the FDA is only succeeding at failing us on an unprecedented basis. I'm sure this is due to funding cutbacks from the government but I'm also sure it involves something related to departmental offices being run by corporate management brought in from corporations they're supposed to regulate, proving once again that money talks and (unfortunately) the bottom line is what wins here and the bottom line is greed. If the USDA and the FDA can allow a food this dangerous through its monitoring, I'm afraid to even think about what else has snuck through? The beef industry has already displayed their contempt for regulation through the mass production of beef that their industry is responsible for, especially in the last 30 years. (Including that beef that's imported from Paraguay, the most GMO soy loaded feed made for feedlots.) That's a whole other story about how this industry is ruining the lives of our South American neighbors by poisoning their crops and the lives of their farmers. This is just so you can have cheap beef.

According to their Website, USDA.gov their agencies and offices include the following (I'm listing all of them so you'll know the enormity of this agency). It has to be enormous, 19 agencies and 17 offices, all designed to protect you. Your health is at stake and a majority of this Departments' agencies and offices are failing to keep your food safe for consumption.

AGENCIES:

AGRICULTURAL MARKETING SERVICE (AMS)

AMS facilitates the strategic marketing of agricultural products in domestic and international markets while ensuring fair trading practices and promoting a competitive and efficient marketplace. AMS constantly works to develop new marketing services to increase customer satisfaction. It's responsible for developing quality grade standards for agricultural commodities, administering marketing regulatory programs, marketing agreements and orders, and making food purchases for USDA food assistance programs.

Program and Service Highlights:

Agricultural Transportation

Country of Origin Labeling

Farmers Market

Farmers Market Promotion Program

Federal-State Marketing Improvement Program

Food Purchases

Grade Standards

Local Food Marketing

Market News Reports

National Organic Program

I have to wonder if they check the quality and safety of the grain they're approving for consumption, whether it's for livestock feed or human consumption. Are they aware that what they're approving is contaminated? I'm curious as to how they grade this substandard grain that's putting so many people in the hospital? Evidently they not detecting the Roundup that's it's laden with.

AGRICULTURAL RESEARCH SERVICE (ARS)

ARS is USDA's principal in-house research agency. ARS leads America towards a better future through agricultural research and information.

(ARS) works to ensure that Americans have reliable, adequate supplies of high-quality food and other agricultural products. ARS accomplishes its goals through scientific discoveries that help solve problems in crop and livestock production and protection, human nutrition, and the interaction of agriculture and the environment.

Programs and service highlights:

National Research

International Research

Research Partnerships and Technology

Research Locations

National Agricultural Library

The question I'd like to ask this department is how much research do you pay attention to when you recommend what food to eat. Does your research cover the effects of grains after they've been consumed? They claim to be interested in nutrition. Are they? Or are they interested in their own bottom line with their stock options with Monsanto?

Animal and Plant Health Inspection Service (APHIS)

APHIS provides leadership in ensuring the health and care of animals and plants. The agency improves agricultural productivity and competitiveness and contributes to the national economy and the public health.

(APHIS) is responsible for protecting and promoting U.S. agricultural health, administering the Animal Welfare Act, and carrying out wildlife damage management activities.

Programs and service highlights:

Cattle Disease Information

Plant Health Import Permits

Plant Export Certificates and Forms

Animal Health Permits

Animal and Animal Product Export Information

Wood Packaging Material

- **Animal Welfare Act (AWA) Licensing and Registration**

CENTER FOR NUTRITION POLICY AND PROMOTION (CNPP)

CNPP works to improve the health and well-being of Americans by developing and promoting dietary guidance that links scientific research to the nutrition needs of consumers.

(CNPP) works to improve the health and well-being of Americans by developing and promoting dietary guidance that links scientific research to the nutrition needs of consumers.

Programs and service highlights:

ChooseMyPlate

MyPlate Blast Off Game and Information for Children

SuperTracker and Other Tools

Dietary Guidelines for Americans

Healthy Eating Index

Nutrition Insights

These are the offices that are supposed to ensure that the food you eat on a daily basis, no matter where it comes from or where you buy it (grocery store or restaurant), is going to keep you healthy. Have you ever considered the value of their work or the quality of the food they approve for your table? With the high rates of Atherosclerosis, cancer, inflammatory diseases and dementia, it appears that they are failing on a massive scale.

(Unless you were looking at it from a corporate point of view where this is an investors dream, this is a consumer's nightmare.) Regardless of how unscrupulous this is, it's going to continue to happen as long as this agency recommends the consumption of these foods.

Myplate.gov, which is administered by the CNPP, has replaced the food pyramid for our dietary guidelines. Myplate.gov is now our dietary guidelines and it still insists that grains remain a part of our diet. I've asked them about this and have received one reply from someone who didn't even know what glycation is or what it is responsible for. I'm still waiting for my reply for that and another email I've not so recently sent them.

Economic Research Service (ERS)

ERS is USDA's principal social science research agency. Each year, ERS communicates research results and socioeconomic indicators via briefings, analyses for policymakers and their staffs, market analysis updates, and major reports. (ERS) provides economic research and information to inform public and private decision making on economic and policy issues related to agriculture, food, natural resources, and rural America. Through a broad range of products, ERS research provides not only facts, but also expert economic analysis of many critical issues facing farmers, agribusiness, consumers, and policymakers. ERS expertise helps these stakeholders conduct business, formulate policy, or just learn about agriculture, food, natural resources, and rural America.

Programs and service highlights:

Food and Nutrition Assistance

Food Safety

Farm Sector Income & Finances

Food Markets and Prices

Natural Resources and Environment

Agricultural Markets and Trade

Rural Communities and Development

Farm and Commodity Policy

Agricultural R&D and Productivity

Amber Waves Magazine

State Fact Sheets

Commodity Outlook Reports

These are the offices regulate the safety of our food. I wonder if they are aware of the dangers of grains in the food supply. One would think that they are, but with 109 people dying every hour, I have to wonder.

Farm Service Agency (FSA)

The Farm Service Agency implements agricultural policy, administers credit and loan programs, and manages conservation, commodity, disaster and farm marketing programs through a national network of offices. (FSA) administers farm commodity, crop insurance, credit, environmental, conservation, and emergency assistance programs for farmers and ranchers.

Programs and service highlights:

Farm Loan Programs

Disaster Assistance

Price Support

Conservation Programs

Daily Market Prices

Commodity Procurement

This is the agency that watches over the farmer and their needs and concerns. Their interest doesn't concern the safety of the food we eat or how nutritious it is. They're simply concerned about the farmer's ability to grow it. They offer the assistance programs that help fund the industry.

Food and Nutrition Service (FNS)

FNS increases food security and reduces hunger in partnership with cooperating organizations by providing children and low-income people access to food, a healthy diet, and nutrition education in a manner that supports American agriculture and inspires public confidence. (FNS) administers the food and nutrition assistance programs in the U.S. Department of Agriculture. FNS provides children and needy families with better access to food and a more healthful diet through its programs and nutrition education efforts.

Programs and service highlights:

Women, Infant, and Children (WIC) Program

Supplemental Nutrition Assistance Program

School Meals

Food Distribution Programs

Disaster Assistance

Child and Adult Care Food Program

Summer Food Service Program

Farmers Markets Nutrition Programs

Nutrition Education

This is the agency that makes sure the disadvantaged have an adequate food supply. One of their major concerns is to distribute the grains that are used in our food supply to those who don't have the ability to purchase their own. This ensures that everyone who lives in this disadvantaged lifestyle doesn't get the proper nutrition they need to sustain a healthy living and in turn, makes them dependant on the pharmaceutical industry for their future health. Don't forget that pharmaceuticals only lead to more and ultimately more pharmaceuticals. This is the never-ending cycle of dependence that this industry wants to keep the public in. This cycle is at the government expense though, and that means that we, the taxpayer get to foot the bill.

It's too bad that they don't realize to conquer hunger you must first conquer the hunger cycle. If the USDA read any of the reports in the PubMed or PMC archives, they'd know that it's the grains and sugar in the diet that create hunger cycle more than anything else. If you were on a ketogenic diet, you could see the logic in this statement, to stop hunger you have to stop the hunger cycle.

This is where their logic is flawed; they think that feeding hungry people grains to fill their bellies will take care of the hunger. It won't, it will only make them hungrier; it's the law of carbohydrate consumption, it a continuous hunger cycle that you're really condemning them to. You're also condemning them to a lifetime of medication need.

Food Safety and Inspection Service (FSIS)

FSIS enhances public health and well-being by protecting the public from foodborne illness and ensuring that the nation's meat, poultry, and egg products are safe, wholesome, and correctly packaged. (FSIS) is the public health agency in the U.S. Department of Agriculture responsible for ensuring that the nation's commercial supply of meat, poultry, and egg products is safe, wholesome, and correctly labeled and packaged, as required by the Federal Meat Inspection Act, the Poultry Products Inspection Act, and the Egg Products Inspection Act.

Program and Service Highlights;

Food Safety Education

Science

Regulations and Policies

Food Recalls

Food Defense and Emergency Response

Fact Sheets

Ask Karen

If this agency had anything to do with the production of sugar and grains, I'd be in contact with them. But they don't.

It appears that this following agency ensures that the poison we grow in the US makes its way around the world to infect as many people as possible.

Foreign Agricultural Service (FAS)

FAS works to improve foreign market access for U.S. products. This USDA agency operates programs designed to build new markets and improve the competitive position of U.S. agriculture in the global marketplace. (FAS) is responsible for collecting, analyzing, and disseminating information about global supply and demand, trade trends, and market opportunities. FAS seeks improved market access for U.S. products; administers export financing and market development programs; provides export services; carries out food aid and market-related technical assistance programs; and provides linkages to world resources and international organizations.

Program and Service Highlights;

Trade News

Trade Policy

Commodity Information

Country Information

Export Programs

Food Aid Programs

Attache Reports

Export Sales Reports

North American Free Trade Agreement (NAFTA) Information

*The **U.S.-Central America-Dominican Republic Free Trade Agreement (CAFTA-DR)***

This may be done to ensure the viability of the pharmaceutical industry, as all of those grains foods can only lead to more pharmaceutical needs. If you can spread this problem around the world, what do you think that would do for your profit margin if you're a pharmaceutical company? (Evidently, Monsanto, thinks the same way.) Maybe that's why we shouldn't allow anyone with corporate ties in any way, to work in any of our regulatory agencies. That would mean that government employees couldn't own any corporate stock. I wonder how many do today. Do you think that could constitute any conflicts of interest?

Forest Service (FS)

FS sustains the health, diversity, and productivity of the Nation's forests and grasslands to meet the needs of present and future generations. (FS) administers programs for applying sound conservation and utilization practices to natural resources of the national forests and national grasslands, for promoting these practices on all forest lands through cooperation with states and private landowners, and for carrying out extensive forest and range research.

Program and Service Highlights;

Fire Information

Maps and Brochures

Passes and Permits

Forest Inventory and Analysis

Forest Health Protection

Recreational Activities

Research & Development

This agency protects undeveloped land and has no control over what goes on your table. It's the following agency that I have issues with as they inspect the grain that's responsible for all this damage.

Grain Inspection, Packers and Stockyards Administration (GIPSA)

GIPSA facilitates the marketing of livestock, poultry, meat, cereals, oilseeds, and related agricultural products. It also promotes fair and competitive trading practices for the overall benefit of consumers and American agriculture. GIPSA ensures open and competitive markets for livestock, poultry, and meat by investigating and monitoring industry trade practices.

Programs and service highlights;

Federal Grain Inspection and Weighing Services

International Service Programs

Regulated Entities under the Packers and Stockyards Act

Packers and Stockyards Program (P&SP) Enforcement Actions

Federal Grain Inspection Service (FGIS) Providers

FGIS Handbooks and Publications

FGIS Forms

P&SP Forms

Directives and Notices

GIPSA Violation Hotline

Official U.S. Standards for Grain

Contact GIPSA

I doubt this agency even knows what they're approving when they approve this grain for consumption. If they did, they wouldn't allow this to slip right past their noses without smelling anything rotten?

NATIONAL AGRICULTURAL LIBRARY (NAL)

NAL ensures and enhances access to agricultural information for a better quality of life. (NAL) provides technical information on agricultural research and related subjects to scientists, educators and farmers using computer databases; coordinates and are the primary resource for a national network of state land-grant university and field libraries and serves as the U.S. center for the international agriculture information system.

Program and Service Highlights;

Agricultural Online Access (AGRICOLA)

Agriculture Network Information Center (AgNIC)

Alternative Farming Systems Information Center (AFSIC)

Animal Welfare Information Center (AWIC)

Digital Desktop (DigiTop) for Employees

Food and Nutrition Information Center (FNIC)

Food Safety Research Information Office

Healthy Meals Resource System

National Invasive Species Information Center (NISIC)

Nutrition.gov

Rural Information Center

SNAP-Ed Connection (formerly Food Stamp Nutrition Connection)

Water Quality Information Center

WIC Works Resource System

One would think with all the departments in this agency, at least one would understand the dangers of grains. It may not be a problem of whether or not anyone knows about it, it may be a problem of anybody caring enough to do anything about it.

National Agricultural Statistics Service (NASS)

NASS serves the basic agricultural and rural data needs of the country by providing objective, important and accurate statistical information and services to farmers, ranchers, agribusinesses and public officials. This data is vital to monitoring the ever-changing agricultural sector and carrying out farm policy. (NASS) is responsible for conducting monthly and annual surveys and preparing official USDA data and estimates of production, supply, prices, and other information necessary to maintain orderly agricultural operations. NASS also conducts the census of agriculture which is currently conducted every 5 years.

Program and Service Highlights

Today's Reports

Quick Stats - Query Database by Commodity, State, and Year

Census of Agriculture

Crop Weather by State

Agricultural Charts and Maps

Agricultural Statistics by Year

Statistics by Subject

Calendar of NASS Reports

I wonder if any of their statistics show the impact that this food has had on our society as a whole, in the way it's influenced the health and medical industries with the boom of business it's created for the pharmaceutical industry. Does the government understand that the more they support the industrial GMO farming, in this case, the more it's costing them having to treat people for the disorders that this industry is imposing upon those who buy into it? How many people do you know that didn't have their toast or bagel this morning? How many of those do you think will go without a sandwich at lunch?

This is not a small problem. It exists everywhere. This is the result of politically engineering your food supply by the industry that supplies it. This is the result of self-policing. Our problem is, it's created a land of sugar junkies clamoring for their next hit, wherever they can find it. (It'll probably be the next drive through.) You unwittingly buy right into this with every Big Mac you buy. That comfort you're buying now leads only to huge amounts of discomfort in the very near future. I'll start with headaches and stomach aches. It'll end with your body's choice of disease starting with atherosclerosis and Alzheimer's, and end with cancer or cardiovascular disease. This is a cycle that must change.

I add my name to the list of many trying to get the FDA and the USDA to act on this concern. Spearheading this list were Dr. William Davis and Dr. David Perlmutter in 2010 and 2012, with their books *Wheat Belly* and *Grain Brain*. They are still trying to right this wrong. After being on both sides of this argument and experiencing all the pain that the other side has to offer, I know for a fact that the only avenue out of this dilemma, is to go to a paleo or ketogenic diet. I just wish the FDA and the USDA could understand this.

National Institute of Food and Agriculture (NIFA)

NIFA's unique mission is to advance knowledge for agriculture, the environment, human health and well-being, and communities by supporting research, education, and extension programs in the Land-Grant University System and other partner organizations. NIFA doesn't perform actual research, education, and extension but rather helps fund it at the state and local level and provides program leadership in these areas. (NIFA) is an agency within the U.S. Department of Agriculture (USDA), part of the executive branch of the Federal Government. Congress created NIFA through the Food, Conservation, and Energy Act of 2008. NIFA replaced the former Cooperative State Research, Education, and Extension Service (CSREES), which had been in existence since 1994.

I clicked on the *research* Link to find that they're pretty proud of their involvement in

peanut research, claiming that; *North Carolina A&T research makes peanuts safer to* *eat.*

Maybe if they were to stop and realize that peanuts, like all legumes, are grains, they would understand that like grains, peanuts ultimately break down to glucose. They're just not cereal grains, so they inflict the harm slower, but they still have the capacity to inflict harm. Because they're harder to digest and do have more fiber than the starchy cereal grains, they impact the glycemic load much less, which is what keeps the blood glucose more even over time. Any doctor will tell you that will make you healthier. The problem is, healthier, in this case, is still unhealthy.

I submit that it's not peanuts that create the allergic reaction, It's the glucose. Like celiac disease with wheat, peanut allergies operate the same way because they ultimately break down to glucose and then to methylglyoxal, the most glycating substance the body creates from carbs. I contend that it's this substance that causes the allergic reaction. (If it weren't for glucose, the *lac operon* in your genome could recognize all lactose that you consume, but because of this lac operon, your gut bacteria can't recognize the lactose because it sees the glucose. It rejects the lactose making people allergic to lactose, when in all actuality; it's the glucose that's creating the problem.) Where is the warning for glucose? And where's the warning fructose as well for that matter? It glycates, almost as much, as glucose.

NATURAL RESOURCES CONSERVATION SERVICE (NRCS)

NRCS provides leadership in a partnership effort to help people conserve, maintain and improve our natural resources and environment. (NRCS) is the primary federal agency that works with private landowners to help them conserve, maintain and improve their natural resources. The Agency emphasizes voluntary, science-based conservation; technical assistance; partnerships; incentive-based programs; and cooperative problem-solving at the community level.

This is the agency responsible for the treatment of our environment including the lands and waters that create it. I found that their concern is mostly with conservation and soil health. My concern is in the growing of nonessential grains and feeding them to an unsuspecting society. I included this agency only because it is a small part of this whole complex algorithm. I haven't checked on their relationship with the EPA is though. I'm sure that they would be happy not having to check toxin levels in the soil with the loss of spraying Roundup. I can only imagine the headaches this herbicide has given them (those not owned by Monsanto).

RISK MANAGEMENT AGENCY (RMA)

RMA helps to ensure that farmers have the financial tools necessary to manage their agricultural risks. RMA provides coverage through the Federal Crop Insurance Corporation which promotes national welfare by improving the economic stability of agriculture. (RMA) promotes, supports, and regulates sound risk management solutions to preserve and strengthen the economic stability of America's agricultural producers by providing crop insurance to American producers, developing and the premium rate, administering premium and expense subsidy, approving and supporting products, and reinsuring companies.

It's a shame crop insurance doesn't cover the damage the crops do to the consumer. Where's that kind of crop insurance? In a keto diet!

RURAL DEVELOPMENT (RD)

RD helps rural areas to develop and grow by offering Federal assistance that improves quality of life. RD targets communities in need and then empowers them with financial and technical resources. USDA Rural Development is committed to the future of rural communities. Our role is to increase rural residents' economic opportunities and improve their quality of life. Rural Development forges partnerships with rural communities, funding projects that bring housing, community facilities, utilities and other services. We also provide technical assistance and financial backing for rural businesses and cooperatives to create quality jobs in rural areas. Rural Development promotes the President's National Energy Policy and ultimately the nation's energy security by engaging the entrepreneurial spirit of rural America in the development of renewable energy and energy efficiency improvements. Rural Development works with low-income individuals, State, local and Indian tribal governments, as well as private and nonprofit organizations and user-owned cooperatives.

Program and Service Highlights

Business Programs

Community Development Programs

Cooperative Programs

Housing and Community Facilities Programs

Renewable Energy and Energy Efficiency Improvements Program

Rural Utilities Service

Water and Waste Disposal Loan and Grant Program

This agency's concern is the viability of rural communities, probably in an attempt not to allow rural towns to become ghost towns, which is already beginning to happen where industrial farming is taking place. With the new industrial farming that's done today, fewer farmers are living in rural areas to support these rural communities. This is industrial farming according to the Monsanto creed. I shouldn't need to ask you why this is allowed to happen. What will I ask is, what would happen if the grain industry transformed into a healthier industry? It would have to be one that didn't involve polluting the environment with herbicides and pesticides and creating food that is responsible for all modern disease imposed upon modern man. It would have to include a withdrawal from industrial farming, A lack of the need for all the grain we consume would curtail this problem immensely. We need to bring back the small farmer.

DEPARTMENTAL MANAGEMENT (DM)

DM provides central administrative management support to Department officials and coordinates administrative programs and services. Departmental Management is USDA's central administrative management organization. Departmental Management provides budget and fiscal management, human resource, procurement and information technology support to mission areas so that they can serve customers more effectively and efficiently. Departmental Management manages the Headquarters Complex and provides direct customer service to Washington, D.C. employees.

Program and Service Highlights

Be Prepared - USDA Employee Information Center

Sustainable Operations - USDA Sustainability Efforts

Office of Small and Disadvantaged Business Utilization

TARGET Center

USDA Vendor Outreach Program

Judicial Decisions

Contract Appeal Decisions

Alternative Fuel Vehicle (AFV) Program

Workplace Violence Prevention

If this department's job is to coordinate interdepartmental management and cooperation, is it their responsibility to disseminate the information from the reports in PubMed, PMC, and the

FDA with their agency that recommends what should be in our diet? Have they educated the people at MyPlate.gov about the warnings that have been coming from PubMed and PMC about the dangers of what they're recommending everyone to consume on a regular basis? Whole grains are still recommended in every agency and association that has a diet recommendation. Even Myplate.gov and the American Dietary Association and, believe it or not, the American Diabetic Association still recommend whole grains should be a part of a healthy diet. What health grains bring is, by far, counterbalanced by the harm they inflict.

National Appeals Division (NAD)

NAD conducts impartial administrative appeal hearings of adverse program decisions made by USDA and reviews of determinations issued by NAD hearing officers when requested by a party to the appeal. (NAD) is responsible for all administrative appeals arising from program activities of the Farm Service Agency, Risk Management Agency, Natural Resources Conservation Service, Rural Business-Cooperative Development Service, Rural Housing Service, and the Rural Utilities Service.

Program and Service Highlights

Appeal Process

E-Guide to Filing an Appeal

How to Make a FOIA Request

Statutes and Regulations

Search for Decisions

The appeal that I'd like to file would be to appeal the decision to approve grains for human consumption. They're inadequate as animal feed due to all the herbicides and pesticides in them, yet they still recommend them as human food. This is unconscionable.

OFFICES

Office of Advocacy and Outreach (OAO)

The Office of Advocacy and Outreach (OAO) was established by the 2008 Farm bill to improve access to USDA programs and to improve the viability and profitability of small farms and ranches; beginning farmers and ranchers and socially disadvantaged farmers or ranchers. OAO develops and implements plans to coordinate outreach activities and services provided by the Department through working collaboratively with the field base agencies and continually assessing the effectiveness of its outreach programs.

Improving the viability and profitability of small and beginning farmers and ranchers Improving access to USDA programs for historically underserved communities Improving agricultural opportunities for farm workers

Closing the professional achievement gap by providing opportunities to talented and diverse young people to support the agricultural industry in the 21st century

If it's this department's responsibility to ensure the small farmer's growth, why are they allowing Monsanto to take over all farming in the USA? A healthy food supply cannot be supplied by a monopoly as big as Monsanto. Are they familiar with the contracts Monsanto requires their contracted farmers to sign? Are they familiar with to movement Monsanto is making to control 100% or our food supply? Are they aware of the holdings of the Monsanto execs in the drug industry that used to be owned by Monsanto? I'm sure their breakup did not leave anybody without stock options.

Office of the Assistant Secretary for Civil Rights (OASCR)

OASCR's mission is to facilitate the fair and equitable treatment of USDA customers and employees while ensuring the delivery and enforcement of civil rights programs and activities. ASCR ensures compliance with applicable laws, regulations, and policies for USDA customers and employees regardless of race, color, national origin, sex (including gender identity and expression), religion, age, disability, sexual orientation, marital or familial status, political beliefs, parental status, protected genetic information, or because all or part of an individual's income is derived from any public assistance program. (Not all bases apply to all programs.)

OFFICE OF BUDGET AND PROGRAM ANALYSIS (OBPA)

OBPA provides centralized coordination and direction for the Department's budget, legislative and regulatory functions. It also provides analysis and evaluation to support the implementation of critical policies. OBPA administers the Department's budgetary functions and develops and presents budget-related matters to Congress, the news media, and the public.

Office of the Assistant Secretary for Civil Rights ensures compliance with applicable laws, regulations, and policies for USDA customers and employees regardless of race, color, national origin, sex (including gender identity and expression), religion, age, disability, sexual orientation, marital or familial status, political beliefs, parental status, protected genetic information, or because all or part of an individual's income is derived from any public assistance program. (Not all bases apply to all programs.)

Program and Service Highlights

Program Discrimination Complaints

Office of the Assistant Secretary for Civil Rights

Early Resolution and Conciliation

If this department is interested in civil rights, then I have a complaint about them right now. My rights have been violated, by this food being imposed upon me, by making sure it's in my baby food, and anything I want to drink (except for plain water), and everything I want to eat. I didn't ask for this but it causes a lot of discomfort for me and everyone else who eats it. All of our rights were violated in serving this food to us without our consent or approval.

Office of the Chief Economist (OCE)

OCE advises the Secretary on the economic situation in agricultural markets and the economic implications of policies and programs affecting American agriculture and rural communities. OCE serves as the focal point for economic intelligence and analysis related to agricultural markets and for risk assessment and cost-benefit analysis related to Departmental regulations affecting food and agriculture. (OCE) advises the Secretary on the economic implications of policies and programs affecting the U.S. food and fiber system and rural areas as well as coordinates, reviews, and approves the Department's commodity and farm sector forecasts.

Program and Service Highlights

World Agricultural Outlook Board (WAOB)

Office of Risk Assessment and Cost-Benefit Analysis

Climate Change Program Office

Sustainable Development

Agricultural Labor Affairs

Office of Energy Policy and New Uses

Weather and Climate

Office of Environmental Markets

If this office is to oversee the offices affecting the food and fiber system, what's happened to the regulation regarding the use of pesticides and herbicides on crops? Is there none?

Office of the Chief Financial Officer (OCFO)

OCFO shapes an environment for USDA officials eliciting the high-quality financial performance needed to make and implement effective policy, management, stewardship, and program decisions. (OCFO) provides financial leadership for USDA, which administers $100 billion of loans as well as significant guarantees and insurance in support of America's farmers and ranchers.

Program and Service Highlights

USDA Budget

USDA Performance and Accountability Report

USDA Strategic Plan

National Finance Center (NFC)

Employee Personal Page

Financial Management Modernization Initiative (FMMI)

I wonder how many loans they've given that have benefited the industrial farming side of this equation. Are they helping to promote this huge industrial farming that's detrimental not only to the environment but to our food supply? How can that be to our benefit?

Office of the Chief Information Officer (OCIO

OCIO has the primary responsibility for the supervision and coordination of the design, acquisition, maintenance, use, and disposal of information technology by USDA agencies. OCIO's strategically acquires and uses information technology resources to improve the quality, timeliness, and cost-effectiveness of USDA services.

Program and Service Highlights

Directives

Enterprise Architecture

Enterprise IT Solutions

Enterprise Network Services

Forms Management

Governance and Strategic Investment (GSI)

Information Collection

IT Capital Planning & Investment Control

IT Security

Quality of Information Guidelines

Records Management

Section 508

This is the IT dept of the USDA. My question for this dept, does their information collection include reports from PubMed and PMC for educational purposes for recommending diets through Myplate.gov?

Office of the Chief Scientist (OCS)

OCS provides scientific leadership to the Department by ensuring that research supported by and scientific advice provided to the Department and its stakeholders is held to the highest standards of intellectual rigor and scientific integrity. It also identifies and prioritizes Department-wide agricultural research, education, and extension needs. (OCS) was established in accordance with the Food, Conservation, and Energy Act of 2008 to provide strategic coordination of the science that informs the Department's and the Federal government's decisions, policies and regulations that impact all aspects of U.S. food and agriculture and related landscapes and communities.

OCS advises USDA's Chief Scientist and the Secretary of Agriculture in the following areas of science:

Agricultural Systems and Technology

Animal Health and Production, and Animal Products

Plant Health and Production, and Plant Products

Renewable Energy, Natural Resources, and Environment

Food Safety, Nutrition, and Health

Agricultural Economics and Rural Communities

Our work supports larger goals of scientific prioritization and coordination across the entire Department through which federal agencies provide Senior Advisors to serve in a detailed capacity within OCS. We identify, prioritize and evaluate Department-wide agricultural research, education, and extension needs. In addition, the Office of the Chief Scientist regularly convenes a **USDA Science Council** to further facilitate cross-Departmental scientific coordination and collaboration.

That is directly from their website. To me that says that they ensure information gets from one department to another department, yet they seemed to have missed the reports from PubMed and PMC pointing to the damage grains do, especially wheat.

From a PDF document on nutrition, Executive Summary: National Nutrition Research Roadmap (2016-2021) I found this paragraph;

"For Q3T1 (Assessing Dietary Exposures), ARS scientists recognize there is a strong need for biomarkers of intake, nutrient status, and health, and are working in multiple areas related to this. For example, ARS scientists are studying the association of vitamin K with reduced cardiovascular disease and the amounts and types of dietary fatty acids that influence immunity and inflammation. There is also a need for the development of more objective measures of food intake and physical activity. To that end, scientists are testing electronic capture devices that require no input from the user and can download to databases. I can tell them right now, that fatty acids are very important for immune functions. I've found those studies in my research. If that's what I found, I'm sure that's what they'll find. I also found that all inflammation that exists is because of glucose in the blood. I wonder how long it will be until they realize that all inflammation is influenced by one thing more than anything else? I can tell them with full confidence that glucose influences inflammation more than anything else. I know because I limit my inflammation by limiting my carb intake and nothing else has worked as well. I can also tell them through experience that exercise and dietary reduction of starches, (which they still recommend being 25% of the diet) will go further than any vitamin. I wonder how long it will take this chief scientist to realize that glycation is at the root of all inflammation and that glucose is at the root of all glycation. It doesn't take any kind of a scientist to see that if you removed the glucose from the equation, the product of the equation couldn't exist. The product in this equation is all the diseases created by inflammation."

Office of Communications (OC)

OC is USDA's central source of public information. The office provides centralized information services using the latest, most effective and efficient technology and standards for communication. It also provides the leadership, coordination, expertise, and counsel needed to develop the strategies, products, and services that are used to describe USDA initiatives, programs, and functions to the public. (OC) provides leadership, expertise, counsel, and coordination for the development of communications strategies which are vital to the overall formulation, awareness, and acceptance of USDA programs and policies, and serves as the principal USDA contact point for the dissemination of consistent, timely information.

Program and Service Highlights

Creative Media and Broadcast Center

Brand, Events, Exhibits, and Editorial Review

Digital Communications

Photography Services

Printing Services

Radio News

The dissemination of consistent, timely information, is what this office's responsibility is, yet I've not heard anything from them about the information from over 11,750 studies recording the dangers of glycation, which is the result of glucose interference with your body's normal processes. With studies showing this glycation going back over 30 years (about as old as GMO seeds), why hasn't any of this *"timely information"* been *disseminated* for *30 years*? Is this due to the Monsanto influence? If any agency is not fulfilling their responsibilities to keep the public safe from their own food, it's this one. They have access to the same studies that I and thousands of others do, yet they still choose to ignore them. They still choose to recommend that this poisonous food be a part of your diet. Why?

Office of Congressional Relations (OCR)

OCR serves as the USDA's liaison with Congress. OCR works closely with members and staffs of various House and Senate Committees to communicate the USDA's legislative agenda and budget proposals. (OCR) serves as the Department's liaison with Members of Congress and their staffs. OCR works closely with members and staffs of various House and Senate Committees including the House Agriculture Committee and the Senate Committee on Agriculture, Nutrition, and Forestry to communicate USDA's legislative agenda and budget proposals. Within OCR is the Office of External and Intergovernmental Affairs (EIA) which serves as the liaison to elected and appointed officials of State, county, local, and Tribal governments. The office also serves as a liaison to USDA stakeholders.

My question to this office, have your alerted Congress of the dangers of these grains and the consequences they bring to the human physiology when consumed? Are you afraid of laws being passed that might outlaw some of this insanity? The insanity that I refer to is the insanity of buying into this glucose ruse, orchestrated by one of the most unscrupulous companies to ever conduct business. Is this the office responsible for keeping this information hidden from our lawmakers' eyes? Is this the office that should be held accountable for our current state of public health? The state of our current public health is obese and diabetic, leading to carcinogenic and atherosclerotic, all because of the inflammatory nature of glycation.

If I can learn this myself and I have a good deal of brain damage inhibiting my learning ability, why can't this office learn this to alert our Congress of this problem? The problem exists only for the consumer, as it's a boom for Monsanto and its industries. Why would they want to control this? For them, this is good business. This is what attracts stockholders.

Office of Ethics (OE)

The Office of Ethics (OE) is the centralized office responsible for coordinating and implementing USDA's Ethics program throughout the Department. OE provides ethics services to employees at all levels of USDA concerning advice and training about compliance with ethics laws and regulations, including the conflict of interest and impartiality rules, as well as the rules governing political activity by Federal employees.

A visit to this office's site brought me to a page that showed me;

THE STOCK ACT

On April 4, 2012, the President signed the Stop Trading on Congressional Knowledge Act or STOCK Act (S. 2038), which amended the Ethics in Government Act of 1978 (5 U.S.C. App. § 101 et seq.) The Act has several different provisions, some of which are effective immediately, some which become effective 90 days after enactment, some which become effective on August 31, 2012, and some which do not become effective until 18 months after enactment. The following compendium of ethics laws, regulations and guidelines govern Executive Branch employees' conduct, including USDA employees. The Department promulgated its own supplemental ethics regulation (5 CFR Part 8301) in 2006 to augment the Office of Government Ethics' Standards of Ethical Conduct. The Department's ethics regulation and other selected ethics laws and regulations are accessible from this page for ready reference (click on "General Ethics Laws and Regulations" below).

Overviews

Ethics Issuances

General Ethics Laws and Regulations

USDA Supplemental Ethics Regulations

Financial Disclosure

Fundraising & the CFC

Gifts

Holiday Guidance for Federal Personnel

Letters of Support, Recommendation, Collaboration, etc.

Lobbying

Non-Federal Organizations

Outside Employment

Political Activity

Post Employment and Seeking Employment

Procurement Integrity

Special Government Employees (SGEs)

STOCK Act

Travel & Non-Federal Assistance

I wonder what their ethic regulations say about recommending poisonous food to remain in our diet when there is proof of this food's glycative effects in over 10,000 studies in PubMed and PMC. What do their ethics say about falsifying information disseminated to the public? They still claim that whole grains are safe to eat.

Office of Environmental Markets (OEM)

OEM supports the development of emerging markets for carbon, water quality, wetlands, and *biodiversity. (OEM) provides leadership in the development of emerging markets for carbon, water quality, wetlands, and biodiversity. OEM is building national environmental market infrastructure, supporting regional market innovation, and fostering collaboration around market-based conservation within USDA and across the federal government.*

I wonder if this environmental market infrastructure includes more fields of these killing field grains? If so, they may want to re-assess their goals, if they want to protect the public and the environment.

- ### *Office of the Executive Secretariat (OES)*

OES ensures that all Department officials are included in the correspondence drafting and policy-making process through a managed clearance and control system. Keeping policy officials informed of executive documents enhances the Secretary's ability to review sound and thought out policy recommendations before making final decisions. (OES) ensures that all Department officials are included in the correspondence drafting and policy-making process through a managed clearance and control system. Keeping policy officials informed of executive documents enhances the Secretary's ability to review sound and thought out policy recommendations before making final decisions. Did this office miss the memo on glycation; its causes and effects? Do they need another one? Is it their responsibility that so few know about this? Are these the people we should hold accountable?

Faith-Based and Neighborhood Partnerships (FBNP)

USDA has a long history of working with faith-based and community organizations to help those in need, by providing federal assistance through domestic nutrition assistance programs, international food aid, rural development opportunities, and natural resource conservation.

This is the office that coordinates churches food banks to assist the needy. Every church I've been to has had one, and they all give out plenty of bread, the deadliest of foods that we can give anyone. This condemns these poor unsuspecting souls to lives of poor health and continued medication. Our food supply is inundated with this vile product, only because it's the primary bringer of people to medication, medication for pain.

Office of the Inspector General (OIG)

OIG investigates allegations of crime against the Department's program and promotes the economy and efficiency of its operations. (OGC) is an independent legal agency that provides legal advice and services to the Secretary of Agriculture and to all other officials and agencies of the Department with respect to all USDA programs and activities.

There were 50,000 food safety inspections in 1972. That was reduced to just over 9,000 in 2008. If there were only 9000 in 2008, reduced from 50,000 in 1972, when the threat level was much lower, the FDA is only succeeding at failing us on an unprecedented basis. I'm sure this is due to funding cutbacks from the government and lack of interest to protect the consumer, due to industrial control. It's related to departmental offices being run by corporate management brought in from corporations they're supposed to regulate, proving once again (unfortunately) the bottom line is what wins here and the bottom line is greed. (Yes I do consider this criminal. How many Moms, Dads, sisters and brothers, husbands and wives have they taken?)

If the USDA and the FDA can allow a food this dangerous through its monitoring, I'm afraid to even think about what else has snuck through? The beef industry has already displayed their contempt for regulation through the mass production of beef that their industry is responsible for, especially in the last 30 years.

Office of the General Counsel (OGC)

The Office of the General Counsel (OGC) is an independent legal agency that provides legal advice and services to the Secretary of Agriculture and to all other officials and agencies of the Department with respect to all USDA programs and activities.

I wonder how many lawsuits this agency is going to have to fight for advising the public to eat food that's as dangerous as whole grains. Myplate.gov still has them at 25% of our diet. Why?

Office of Tribal Relations (OTR)

The Office of Tribal Relations is located in the Office of the Secretary and is responsible for government-to-government relations between USDA and tribal governments.

I can only empathize with this office as they have to see that this garbage is provided to tribal governments as well as the public in general.

I listed all of their offices and agencies for a reason. I wanted to show you the vastness of this department. It's huge. It has to be huge to protect our food supply. As big as it is, it's not doing that. It's not doing its job. It's been hijacked by the industry that it's supposed to control. The proof lies in the extent of which disease exists today.

With all of these agencies and offices, I'm sure it's quite difficult to keep all this information straight for the public to fully understand what this agency is allowing to "fall through the cracks", as in allowing grains and sugar to be recommended food for everyone to eat, sometimes even those who have celiac disease. What this agency doesn't understand is that everyone has an intolerance to the gluten that comes in grains. It's estimated that 95% of the population have some sort of intolerance to the gliadin and gluten found in most cereal grains, especially wheat, barley, and rye.

I've already contacted the ***CENTER FOR NUTRITION POLICY AND PROMOTION0 (CNPP)*** to ask them why they still recommend including grains in the diet. They've come to their senses when it comes to sugar, why can't they, with grains, they're just as deadly as sugar, if not more so? The agency above is responsible for recommending our diet at **My Plate** and I've already asked them why they still recommend a food that can cause as much damage is this food does. I'm waiting for their reply.

There is absolutely no reason for these foods to still be recommended except for the fact that to decrease the consumption of this food would irreparably harm Monsanto and the farming industry that they control. And they control a huge portion of it.

The infiltration of their old execs and lobbyists into the offices of the FDA and the USDA is evidence indicating their complicity in the matter. With their old personnel working the offices and agencies of the USDA and the FDA, they've cleared a pathway to their full control over what goes on your table. This in return gives them control over the meds you'll be buying from them in the near future.

I noticed that there is no agency or office to review and disseminate the information in these research studies showing the damaging effects of the food they're recommending for us to eat. There's supposed to be one, but there isn't.

How do they make recommendations on what foods are good for you to eat, when you're ignoring all the studies that say otherwise? They rely on Monsanto to tell them what's healthy and what isn't. Is that a source you would trust? I hope so because you trust them with every bagel you put in your mouth.

This is an agency that recommends you eat what the farmer can grow the most of and not what's necessarily healthy for you to eat. This makes the farm industry more important than you!

PART V

A NEW TOMORROW

CHAPTER 14

FASTING AND THE KETOGENIC DIET

As far back as 500BC, physicians have used fasting as a means to find the way back to health by a simple and inexpensive manner in which one could actually heal themselves from virtually any of the modern diseases that have plagued man since the dawn of civilization. For me, it's easy to see the correlation of the emergence of modern diseases with the gradual increase of consumption of einkorn wheat, the precursor to our modern strains of wheat. From Emmer (one of the first domesticated strains) and Durum Semolina which is little higher in gluten (yet it's still considered a weak wheat as the wheat doesn't rise as well as it holds the dough together to hold the pasta shape.) Winter Red, spelt and other bread wheat or common wheat that are higher in gluten have been used for bread for thousands of years because they rise better.

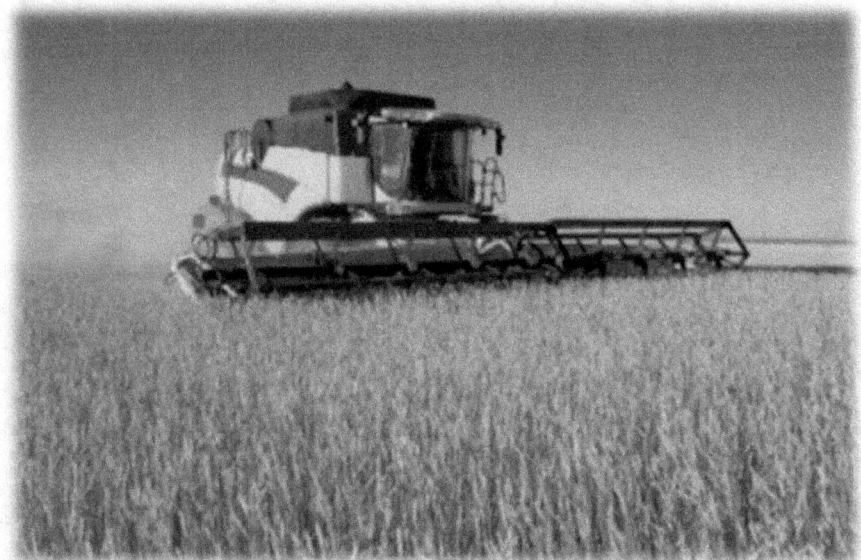

Today's forms of highly modified wheat act nothing like the strains from thousands of years ago as today's highly domesticated strains of wheat cannot survive in the wild. That's according to Wikipedia and that's due to their inability to disperse their seeds. Monsanto has made certain of that through their genetic modifying to create ender seeds that won't get pollinated so a farmer has no seed for next year's crop forcing them to buy GMO seed from Monsanto. (GMO by itself is not dangerous. It's what the modifying allows the farmer to do that makes it dangerous and that's to spray it with Roundup. Their seed is genetically modified to handle applications of the glyphosate herbicide.) This is the wheat that Monsanto is forcing their farmers to grow for your cereal, bread, and snacks. The same glyphosate exists in the cornfields as well, contaminating every corn chip that you eat. (When was the last time you ate Mexican food?)

But we're talking about wheat right now which was originally cultivated in the Fertile Crescent 10,000 years ago, approximately the same time that modern disease started showing up in the bones of the remains of the people. This is a clear indication of the glycation that wheat was responsible for, even then, even as slow as the einkorn wheat is to digest (which slows the progression of glycation). The glycation existed then as it does now, only it took it much longer to manifest. Today, it manifests itself immediately (as soon as it touches your tongue) and this is due to the fast dissolving gluten flour that's used for bread and pastries as well as pasta and cereal. It glycates more now as the grain has changed immensely in the last 10,000 years. As this food increased in prevalence in our diet, the rates of disease increased, as it's these grains that have always generated disease. They generate it so slowly that it's never noticed until it's too late or you stop eating it. This is the value of fasting and why fasting is so important to the health of anyone on this type of carbohydrate diet.

This is why fasting has always cured disease. 98% of all disease is a direct result of our diet. With that being said, it's easy to see why removing everything damaging from our diet is going to heal the damage caused by keeping those foods in the diet. Fasting produces such good results it's been the subject of over 20,000 studies on PMC in the NLM at the NIH. (PMC has reported from across the world. PubMed has 590 reports from studies done in the US alone.) It's that important, yet what has your doctor shared with you about this life-saving course of intervention? Your doctor comes into your appointed meeting with his/her prescription tablet in hand ready to prescribe pharmaceuticals. (Now it's a laptop that affords them more latitude in their diagnosis. I sometimes see a primary care physician who still carries a prescription pad with him everywhere he goes, but then he has drug reps going in and out of his office all the time, so to speak.) Their whole intent is to prescribe drugs for your ailments, which are more than likely caused by the ingestion of grain foods. Prescribing drugs is the way they're trained to treat patients, not with recommendations for diet. (Monsanto wouldn't allow that to take place as they have far more control over your life than what you could ever believe.)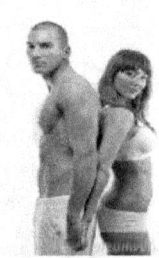

That's exactly why fasting is so healthy. It removes the worst of the toxins in our bodies that are built up from the diets of bread, wheat, and grain-based products, and doesn't put more toxins back in with the prescribed drugs. Those grain products also happen to be the most addictive, which is what makes them the hardest to give up. The addictive nature of sugar, at its worst, is displayed in this manner (when it drives pharmaceuticals). When one fasts, they give up the sugars that are doing all the glycating and it's this glycation that is at the root of all disease and this is why going without food is so healthy.

It also sets your body up for future health by resetting the hormonal structure in your body. This is mostly the result of your hormones transitioning to a starvation mode of survival, where the Ghrelin your stomach releases, sends this growth hormone throughout your body allowing it to do its magic in repairing damage and extending cell life where cell death took place before. (This is directly due to the carbohydrate influence in the diet, creating glycation.) It's the elimination of glycation that initially brings back a resemblance of health but that's not what brings future health. It's the breaking of an addiction. This addiction is built into our society so much, It starts in our prenatal body and continues through the first year of life and then on. (This is due to the prevalence of sugar and high fructose corn syrup in baby foods, formula, and infant medicines.) The prenatal effect starts with mama's diet before you're born, if your mother ate carbs, you got them before you were born. But that only explains why you're dependent. It doesn't explain how to break the dependence. That's with fasting and the keto diet, or ketogenic diet (the diet our ancestors were on, ever since our existence). The keto diet involves fasting as part of the diet, making it much easier to maintain. (There's no hunger.) Fasting does that by sending your body into ketosis.

According to Wikipedia; *in the early 20th century around 1911; Bernarr Macfadden, an American exponent of physical culture, popularized the use of fasting to restore health. His disciple, the osteopathic physician Hugh Conklin, of Battle Creek, Michigan, began to treat his epilepsy patients by recommending fasting. Conklin conjectured that epileptic seizures were caused when a toxin, secreted from the Peyer's patches in the intestines, was discharged into the bloodstream. Conklin's fasting therapy was adopted by neurologists in mainstream practice. In 1916, a Dr. McMurray wrote to the New York Medical Journal claiming to have successfully treated epilepsy patients with a fast, followed by a starch-and sugar-free diet, since 1912. In 1921, prominent endocrinologist H. Rawle Geyelin reported his experiences to the American Medical Association convention. He had seen Conklin's success first-hand and had attempted to reproduce the results in 36 of his own patients. He achieved similar results despite only having studied the patients for a short time. He reported that three water-soluble compounds, β-hydroxybutyrate, acetoacetate and acetone (known collectively as ketone bodies), were produced by the liver in otherwise healthy people when they were starved or if they consumed a very low-carbohydrate, high-fat diet.*

With fasting being able to eliminate so many disorders, a path was sought to bring this form of healing to the mainstream by creating a diet to encourage fasting. Thus the ketogenic diet was born in 1921 through the efforts of Russel Wilder. According to Wikipedia, Russel Wilder, at the Mayo Clinic, built on this research and coined the term ketogenic diet to describe a diet that produced a high level of ketone bodies in the blood (ketonemia) through an excess of fat and lack of carbohydrate.

Fasting is the quickest manner in which to allow your body to go into ketosis, yet it may not be the easiest. Although on second thought, being the quickest way may make it the easiest. I went through two weeks of withdrawal because I couldn't give up all the foods I loved to eat all at once, to allow my body to go into ketosis in a few days. I could have avoided 10 days of want by fasting and only want something to eat for a few days, as what happens when you fast for a minimum of 3 days. A longer fast is more beneficial but the three days allows your body to respond by going into ketosis which is a fat burning mode. It's this fat burning mode that forces your body to make its own glucose, which is a much cleaner glucose than you get from the sugar you eat, as it's a clean glucose made from your own glycogen or fat storage. Getting into ketosis quicker could allow you to start your fat burning diet, but continuing some carbs will only make the withdrawal more difficult as it may drop your body back out of ketosis. This was my problem and why my transition took so long. (Thankfully, they'll be no next time.)

Ketosis refers to acids in the body that are derived and used while in a state of low glucose in the blood. Because my body has been in a state of ketosis for the last 3 years, I feel qualified to speak about this lifestyle. I call it a lifestyle because it really is. It's a lifestyle completely different from the lifestyle of a carboholic. Carboholics require food every other hour or so, it's the law of glucose consumption, appetite follows glucose levels in the blood. It's that simple, blood sugar levels rise and satiety sets in, releasing hormones controlling feel-good emotions influencing behavior. But, that usually happens when the blood sugars fall again after a couple hours releasing hormones of hunger, need and want. These hormones are completely different than the satiety hormones and have a much different effect on the body, sometimes unrecognizable behavioral effects.

This is where carboholics do not have the advantage that ketonemiacs have. Ketonemiacs (those who have allowed their bodies to go into a state of ketosis) aren't controlled by their hormones, so they don't have to follow any hunger cycle. They're in full control of their hormones. This also means that they're in more control of their emotions because of that. I know that it doesn't sound like it's that big of a deal, but it's more important than you could ever imagine. First, let's look at the state of ketosis, as explained in Wikipedia;

*"KETOSIS is a metabolic state in which most of the body's energy supply comes from **ketone bodies** in the blood, in contrast to a state of **glycolysis** in which **blood glucose** provides most of the energy. Ketosis is similar to a condition called KETOACIDOSIS, in that both cause a side effect known to laypeople as ACETONE BREATH."*

*"Longer-term ketosis may result from **fasting** or staying on a low-carbohydrate diet, and deliberately induced ketosis serves as a medical intervention for various conditions, such as intractable epilepsy, and the various types of diabetes. In glycolysis, higher levels of insulin promote storage of body fat and block the release of fat from adipose tissues, while in ketosis, fat reserves are readily released and consumed. For this reason, ketosis is sometimes referred to as the body's "fat burning" mode."*

Even bodybuilders have recognized ketonemia or ketosis as being the most beneficial state to keep their body in as it's in this state where they produce more growth hormones because of the amount of Ghrelin their stomachs release to enable them to grow their muscles bigger without the carbs.

The state of ketosis is often confused with a state of ketoacidosis, which has nothing to do with being in a state of nutritional ketosis. Ketoacidosis is a state of extreme ketosis that can

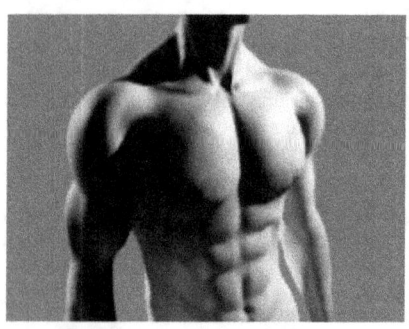

only happen to type 1 diabetics because their pancreas is incapable of secreting enough insulin to handle the amount of glucose in their system. Because of this the liver of type 1 diabetics secretes more ketones than what the body needs to operate. What if the glucose never made it into the system?

Although I appreciate ketosis as being a "fat burning mode", it's the other benefits that I appreciate more. Benefits like less pain, no headaches, no stomachaches, far more energy than what I've ever had, ability to get more work done, as I don't have to stop all the time to eat

and although I do eat at my desk, I'm usually at my desk 16-18 hours out of the day, except on therapy days. I like to take 3 hours, 3 days a week for therapy. My therapy is exercise. My brain needs it, but my body benefits. Again Wikipedia says on the subject of ketosis;

*"Ketosis is deliberately induced by use of a **ketogenic diet** as a medical intervention in cases of intractable **epilepsy**. Other uses of **low-carbohydrate diets** remain controversial. Induced ketosis or low-carbohydrate diet terms have very wide interpretation. Therefore, Stephen S. Phinney and Jeff S. Volek coined the term "nutritional ketosis" to avoid the confusion.*

*"Ketoacidosis is a metabolic state associated with high concentrations of **ketone bodies**, formed by the breakdown of fatty acids and the **deamination** of **amino acids**. Ketoacidosis is most common in untreated **type 1 diabetes mellitus** when the liver breaks down **fat** and proteins in response to a perceived need for a **respiratory substrate**. Prolonged alcoholism may lead to alcoholic ketoacidosis."*

*"In **diabetic ketoacidosis**, a high concentration of ketone bodies is usually accompanied by **insulin** deficiency, **hyperglycemia**, and **dehydration**. Particularly in type 1 diabetics the lack of insulin in the bloodstream prevents **glucose** absorption, thereby inhibiting the production of **oxaloacetate** (a crucial precursor to the β-oxidation of fatty acids) through reduced levels of **pyruvate** (a byproduct of **glycolysis**), and can cause unchecked ketone*

*body production (through fatty acid metabolism) potentially leading to dangerous glucose and ketone levels in the blood. Hyperglycemia results in glucose overloading the **kidneys** and **spilling into the urine** (transport maximum for glucose is exceeded). Dehydration results following the osmotic movement of water into **urine**. (Osmotic diuresis), exacerbates the **acidosis**."*

I bring this up to make the point that nutritional ketosis is not ketoacidosis. It's far from it. According to Wikipedia again, *"Normal **serum reference ranges** for ketone bodies are 0.5– 3.0 mg/dL, equivalent to 0.05–0.29 mmol/L." In ketosis, the levels range from 3 – 6 mg/dL. Ketoacidosis requires a level of 15 – 25 mg/dL, more the three times needed for ketosis, making it virtually impossible for anyone to into ketoacidosis if you're not a type 1 diabetic. Type 1 diabetics are required to make sure their bodies don't produce many ketones because of the risk of ketoacidosis".*

According to PMC's report on Calorie Restriction (CR) or fasting, submitted; July 2010; *Nevertheless, ongoing research continues to draw a complete picture of CR at the molecular level, which may ultimately allow for the development of therapeutics that might be able to confer at least some of the health benefits of this dietary regimen.*

Ketosis, being based on fasting, makes it the optimal diet for anybody to be on. Remaining in a state of ketosis has allowed my body to regain that which was lost 31 years ago in the car accident that left me severely disabled because of a severe closed head injury, (it was the two strokes that were the most devastating.)

It's become evident to me since I've been carb free and in a state of ketonemia or ketosis, how much our society is addicted to this drug, sugar, that does little more than to lead those who eat it to further drug use. Our food industrial complex sees to that by their advertising. I'm convinced it's because they're associated with the pharmaceutical industry. They used to be merged into one corporation that controlled the seed supply for the farmers as well as the chemicals to spray on the crops and the pharmaceuticals that treated to pain and discomfort brought on by the products made by the grains grown by those crops, made with the seed Monsanto sold to the farmer, and sprayed multiple times with glyphosate herbicide. (Yeah that was a mouthful, yet it wasn't the worst of it.) Two weeks before harvest, the crop gets desiccated to ensure a complete harvest. This may be great for the farmer and Monsanto, but it ensures more than that. It ensures that it gets into your diet and into your body.

The unfortunate result of this love affair with those snack and comfort foods is what this diet brings, at its cost of this pleasure. The price to be paid is in the discomfort that this food brings to all those who eat it, regardless of how much they eat. The food industry (Monsanto in particular) has a fortune invested in maintaining your appetite for this deadly food. They've built an industry just to treat diabetes, with all the glucose meters and pumps out there, just so addicts can get their next fix. The trouble this industry goes to just to keep their addicts happy and addicted is unsurpassed in any field.

I know now what I didn't 4 years ago when I was an addict. The amount an addict consumes at each sitting dictates how much damage it's going to do, but it's going to do damage. There is no way to avoid it. That's the way our digestion and metabolism works. That's why this addiction is by far, the worst addiction our society has to deal with. This addiction leads to every other addiction that we're actively fighting, including alcoholism, heroin and tobacco and even gambling. Yes, even gambling is driven by the glucose addiction, as gambling is driven by the hunger cycle which is one of the biggest underlying influences of a carbohydrate diet. Hunger in this diet drives absolutely everything, even breathing, and because of that, eventually drugs.

This is a cycle that I don't need. As a matter of fact, it's the last thing I need. (You don't need it either.)The biggest reason I refuse to take any of these drugs anymore is that all of them carry side effects, some major, some minor. Whether the side effects are major or minor, I don't want to experience any of them, anymore. I've had my fill of side effects, especially the ones that make my health worse, which is where most of these side effects should be classified. That only invites more treatment, which in turn invites more of my money into the pockets of the pharmaceutical industry. This is a cycle that I can't afford to be part of anymore.

After living for twenty years needing to take massive amounts of opioids for my chronic severe pain, diuretics for my high blood pressure, anti-depressants for the pain, and living with the side effects of not only the opioids, but every other drug they had me on, all twelve of them, I got fed up with it. I wasn't going to take it anymore as I just couldn't afford it. And I was only up to twelve medications. I have a friend who's on this diet, who's lowered his needs to thirteen daily medications from twenty-three. How many meds do you take every day? How many would you like to do without, if your health would allow? This is where fasting needs to replace ~~doping~~ dosing. A change in diet will go much further than any drug and the cure lasts longer than any treatment.

I prefer to live by the theory that if the meds aren't needed in the first place, my health is going to be that much better. That is why I removed everything from my diet that I could that's responsible for these horrendous diseases, which require the need for these medications. By fasting, one can reach this healing state much quicker than I did, just by cutting out my bread. Where it took me two weeks to get into full ketosis, by fasting I could have jump-started the state by starving my body, then go on from there with my ketogenic diet to keep my body in this healing state.

This is the advantage of fasting, it not only starts the healing from the beginning by putting your body in a starvation mode, it allows you to stay in that mode for the rest of your life. That one little option in itself is what's going to extend your life beyond 100 years. I can see where ultimately man will be able to extend its lifespan to over 150 years old. !00 years from now, when all mankind is on a ketogenic or paleo diet again, I can see the oldest people in the world living into their 180's, doubling today's average lifespan.

This can be easily obtained simply by allowing our bodies to heal themselves and not keep depending on drugs for the perception of healing, which ultimately brings nothing but more drug use, which ultimately is what ruins the liver and kidneys leading to all the cancers and disorders of the hepatic and renal systems. This drug dependence is driven by another dependence that we've all been born into.

I hope that you're beginning to see how our drug addictions are driven by one thread that drives all modern diseases along with it. That one thread is what ties 100% of all cancers, 98% of all heart diseases, and 99.9 % of all dementia, all arthritis, all headaches, and almost all stomach aches together is one substance that can be removed from the diet without any severe side effects.

I shouldn't need to tell you what that substance is by now. You should know. You eat it every day and you live with the effects of its addiction every day. Pain always comes with addiction. (That's what makes breaking the addiction so rewarding, limiting the pain cycle. Oh, what sweet bliss! Ending a cycle well worth ending.)

The idea then is to limit to minuscule amounts, the foods that make up these addictive substances. You should know by now what these foods are, you eat them every morning, either in your coffee as creamer, in the toast you have, or the cereal you consume. You have it every lunch with your sandwich or burrito and with every dinner with your rolls.

I have known several families that would just put a plate of bread on the table every evening. This is the display of addiction, a full out need to satisfy the taste buds by dumping more and more sugar in the body, usually in the form of the starchy carbs of bread. I've also noticed that in those houses that served bread there was always beer cans in the garbage indicating another addiction.

If you remove this one addiction from our society, you remove all addictions, as this addiction to sugar and carbs is the foundation of all other addictions as they are all based on a hunger cycle which is the result of an addiction to sugar. Do you think, that might make it the root of all evil? Maybe we should ask John Barleycorn.

I hope that you can see now that it's this addiction to sugar and carbs that are enriching the pharmaceutical industry, and that both industries are driven by the same people who have and keep a major influence in the offices of the agencies that are supposed to regulate this industry, the FDA, the USDA, the CDC and the EPA. With that kind of influence, there's only one way to fight it and that's to not buy into it.

To not buy into it does require a diet of grain abstinence, though. That requires breaking the addiction and moving to as much of a ketogenic diet, as possible. The easiest manner to do this is to do a strict three day, water only fast. The longer you can do it the better, but it must be at least 3 days with absolutely no food. That's why it's important to check with your doctor first. It's the consumption of the grain industry's products that are driving the pharmaceutical industry's profits today and will drive it tomorrow, next year, and for the next 500 and beyond. If we don't put an end to this now, our society is doomed to suffer the consequences of a carbohydrate addiction that no one is responsible for, for the rest of time.

The greed of the grain industry combined with the ambition of the pharmaceutical industry has made us all carboholic slaves to the desires of these industries. It's these industries that are rewarding from the most, from this arrangement. For me, it's scary, how much power we've given these industries, simply because we listen to their advertising. We've also let them take over the regulating agency that's supposed to control this industry. Because our health depends on it, we can't allow Monsanto to dictate how there are going to poison our food, so they can bolster the profits of the pharmaceutical industry. Not knowing what you put in your body can cost you your life. It is costing you your life if you eat carbs. Those who listen to the advertising and are influenced by it, fall prey to that influence and become their slaves for life or until they quit consuming the grains. There's very little different than that of alcoholism except that it's pretty much forced upon us, in our baby food. Mamas, feed your babies on your own milk if you want them to be healthy.

I know what you're thinking right now, what are all the foods involved in this addiction? The list is enormous and that's why this is such a dangerous addiction. This industry has virtually forced us to celebrate this addiction. It involves every one of our holidays, with the holiday season being the worst. Every celebration involves some form of sugar. From the Sugar Bowl to the Tostido's Fiesta Bowl, our celebration is never-ending. Just after the "holiday season" comes Valentine's Day barely a month later. Then, comes Easter and spring break. Are you beginning to understand why this addiction is our worst? With all the celebrating we need to keep this addiction, how do you change tradition without changing the world? The quickest way that I know is to organize an international health weekend, for 3 days, where everyone goes keto to heal their diseases and give their bodies a chance to go into ketosis, the ever healing state of metabolism.

The best advantage of this diet is the amount of control it gives you over your own emotions. You may think that you control your emotions right now, but I can tell you with full confidence, if you're on a carb diet, you have no control over your emotions. They're completely controlled by what you eat because what you eat controls your hunger cycle and it's your hunger cycle that drives every other cycle your body goes through.

Since your hunger cycle is controlled by your hormones (mostly leptin and Ghrelin), it's these hormones that are controlling your emotions. You know this every time you crave that bagel or biscotti. Once you bite into it, your saliva starts digesting that instantly gratifying food to give you that *aww* feeling, that instantly hits your brain, even before you can swallow it. This is your first sign of addiction and dependence that only gives you the perception that you have control of your own emotions. It's this cycle that is in full control of your emotions. As much as you try to control them, too often they have a tendency to slip out of your control and back into theirs.

Anyone who can't control their emotions entirely by themselves is a slave to their own hormones. This makes every carboholic a slave to their emotions and therefore a slave to these industries. This displays the dependence of the hunger cycle and the carb diet that drives that hunger cycle. You may not classify these as emotions, but I submit that they actually are. Satiety is defined as the state of being satisfied. If that is not an emotion, as it expresses feelings of calmness and security, I don't know what is. Hunger, on the other hand, is defined as a strong desire. Is not that an emotion? These emotions are controlled by both leptin and ghrelin, which ultimately are controlled by the grain industry, more than anything else. This is the ruse I refuse to take part in. I can't afford this trap anymore. The only way out for our society is to break the hold of this industry, to let them know that we're not going to stand for this kind of abuse. To go ketogenic in your diet is the best way you can get yourself to everlasting health.

With emotions being controlled by our hormonal balance like this, it's easy to see how carbs could influence that balance. For this to not have an effect on our behavior is beyond comprehension. It has to. When you combine the drive of an addiction (which is what we're talking about) with the advertisements promoting that addiction, how can it not have an effect on our health and ultimately our society? That is why I make the statement that this cycle has to change. If it doesn't cease, our health as a society will never get better. There's never been a better time for a cure, and that cure is a ketogenic diet, not only for each and everybody to be as healthy as possible, but also to regain the health of our whole society. Can you imagine a world where everyone not only controls their own emotions but they're in control of their emotions? (That includes reactions.)

Let's go back to addiction, though, for you may still not consider this an addiction. I understand few caught in an addiction can recognize that addiction when they're feeding it because the addiction has ways of hiding itself. You can ask anyone who has to have at least one beer a day. They're not addicted to their beer, as far as they're concerned, yet they have to have it. And often they don't even drink more than just one. But they still have to have that one. That is what makes it an addiction.

The body can and does live much better without beer, so it's not a substance the body requires to survive. Yet the beer drinker needs that daily beer to satisfy their addiction. To go without, many times creates more problems because of the work your hormones are doing on your emotions and worse yet your actions, by controlling how receptors work in your brain. That makes it a natural thing that you need to do, and not an addiction, to appease that desire to drink the beer. This is how addiction works and it happens to carboholics too. I know I am a carboholic. The desire for sweets is still with me. It's the last refuge of my addiction. It's something that I get to fight for the rest of my life.

The fact of the matter is, if you were fed baby food, you've been fed sugar, simply to get you to swallow it. This addicted you to glucose immediately. Actually, you've been sold the idea that sugar and carbs were healthy foods to eat. The fault was found with every other type of nutrition except grains, until recent history. For more than 60 years, we've been told to eat grains. Thirty years ago, they said whole grains are healthy. They still say "whole grains are healthy", yet according to all the studies I've seen out of the hundreds I've looked at, nothing about this food is safe to ingest, leaving me to wonder, why do they still recommend it? Then I look at who controls the FDA, the USDA and what interest they have in their industrial farming, and it becomes pretty clear whose influence this is, controlling what we eat.

This simple little act of feeding your baby formula laced with sugars to get you to eat it has addicted you to a lifetime of dependence. It addicted me. Even though I broke the addiction, I'm still affected by what control it did have over me. That's exactly why I'm pleading with you, don't let it control you. I can virtually guarantee that you won't like the end results. Whether they come sooner or later, they always come. (They're as dependable as the tide.)

When I think about this, my first response is to get angry, for I never asked for this, nor could I ever wish it upon anyone else. Yet, there is an industry that is committed to not only continuing this cycle, they're goal is to increase its scope and they're doing it on an exponential basis. You can see this in all the advertising. It's affecting you. You can see that in the rates of cancer deaths, CVD deaths, dementia deaths, etc, etc.

This is your grain industry pushing this celebration of this addiction and you're buying into it every time you feed your carb diet, by buying all your snacks, pasta, cereal, soft drinks, and beer, just for starters. I'd go on with the rest but space limits that list in this book. You can find it in both my first and second books, *It's Time for a Cure* and *Time for the Ultimate Cure*. Your best guide is to use the glycemic index as your guide for what foods that are safe to eat or not. It's the general consensus that you should keep your foods lower than 50 on the glycemic index.

My contention is to keep carbs out of your diet completely and let your body make its own glucose. The reason you want to keep your blood glucose low is to avoid the hunger cycle. The hunger cycle is emotionally the worst manifestation of a carb diet. As it controls your emotions, it controls your actions and reactions. This is an undeniable truth. You know it as well as I do. You feel it every time you taste that divine taste when you bite into it, MMM how good it is.

This is where you need to ask yourself, what is it you crave most? If what you crave has any carbohydrate in it, then that's your first indication that you're addicted. What kind of carb you crave, quite often tells how bad your addiction is. One wouldn't think that a hamburger could be a sign of addiction, when actually when you think about the taste you crave, it's a combination of everything including the bun, which happens to be the addictive ingredient in the hamburger. Everything else in the hamburger is healthy. It's just the gluten in the bun that's so addictive. I wouldn't doubt that they use extra high gluten bread dough for the buns used for these sandwiches, as it's more addictive, due to the high gluten content. I know they use high gluten bread dough for making pizza dough because it needs to rise, and the more the gluten the better it rises. That makes it taste better, but it also makes it more addictive. That's why when you're at one of these restaurants, most everyone there is overweight. They're there because they crave that high gluten bread dough. You get it in both pizzas and fast food hamburgers. This is how they make you repeat customers.

If you think my assessment is wrong, just try eating your favorite hamburger between two slices of lettuce. The taste is completely different. Most fast food restaurants offer low carb sandwiches but few order them. The only ones that I know of who order them are those who suffer from celiac disease and I believe that all of us suffer somewhat from celiac disease. I think that there are only a very few that can get through life without showing or suffering the effects of a carb diet....especially an excessive carb diet as in the case with most people worldwide today.

The reason you crave the taste of a hamburger is that of the high gluten bread dough the buns are made from because it's that bun that raises your blood glucose as soon as it hits your tongue. Therein lies the addictive nature of glucose, the constant tug on your hunger cycle. It's caused by the foods you eat if you're on a carb diet. When you stop to think about it, you know it, as well as I.

You just need to do something about it, as I did, three years ago, and then again one year ago when I went complete keto. It took me three years to go completely keto. You can do it in one month if you've got the guts to do a thirty day fast. I didn't and I may have suffered because of it. I guess I was still persuaded to eat the carbs even after I gave up the bread. If I had to do it over again, I'd fast, to go keto. The adjustment is a lot quicker.

What do you think they're advertising when they show you those commercials for pizza and their soft drinks, fruit drinks, cereals, bread, pasta, pastries, candy, etc, etc? They selling you that mmm feeling of dependence and addiction. It's that feeling you get as soon as your favorite food hits your tongue and makes you go "ooh, I needed that". That's the same feeling a junkie feels when he gets his latest fix.

That is precisely why this food can't sustain us in space and that's why the keto diet is so important. For our species to travel into space, we'll have to do away with the hunger cycle altogether.

SPACE TRAVEL WILL REQUIRE A KETOGENIC DIET

RATHER THAN A CARBOHYDRATE DIET.

To me, this is simple, yet almost impossible to see when you're stuck in the addiction that's responsible for the reason. Again, it's a matter of how the food is digested. Carbs ultimately create glycation. Fats and proteins don't. It's that simple. That and the fact that this food creates a hunger cycle that can't be controlled without ending their consumption. One needs to compare the value of the food, in respects to the number of calories per gram of nutrition. Carbs have 4 calories whereas fat has 9, per gram of nutrition. This is important to remember as it's the calories that are important to have.

Your body requires calories to survive, so it's important to know where you're getting your calories from? Are you getting more calories from less food or do you need to eat more food to get an adequate amount of calories? Carb diets require more food per calorie, plus they're the highest calorie count of any diet. Because carbs incite hunger, they require massive amounts of calories to sustain, due to leptin resistance. This hunger cycle is a cycle that should be avoided at all costs, as it's the cycle that's at the root of all evil cycles as well. This cycle will prove to be an unsustainable cycle in space, as it does little more than to create disease in the body. Instead of using your hormones to heal the body, you're using your hormones to damage the body.

This is because the body is producing insulin and using it to turn the glucose into fat. While creating insulin, the body has little reason to create glucagon, the opposite of insulin. It's the glucagon that helps create your growth hormones. The glucagon is generated during times of hunger and fasting. Ghrelin influences how much glucagon your body makes by how much insulin you use. This is the nature of leptin resistance and explains why it's important to make yourself ghrelin resistant.

That makes the type of food you eat important, very import. Is the food you eat the most "high octane" or is it low octane "dirty fuel"? Is it clean burning fat or is it dirty burning fat? If it's fat from carbs, it's going to be dirty at best. That's if you're lucky enough for it not to be polluted with glyphosate. But then, by the time we're ready to travel that far into the stars, hopefully, we'll be past the glucose ruse and the glyphosate scourge that's the evil part of it.

If Love wins out and we're able to travel to the stars with everybody on a ketogenic diet, our world will truly be a different one then. It'll no longer be a world that's a slave to the hunger cycle and all the evil that can bring. Instead, it will be a world that can see past fear and anger. It'll be a world free of suspicion and fear. I will be an all-inclusive world, with one exception, the corporate evil that exists today because of the hunger cycle will be replaced by cycles of benevolence and charity, with more intent to help than profit. Corporations in the future will break free of the hunger cycle of profit and loss and learn that true profit can only be long-term in which the benefits are available for all mankind and not just a few stockholders.

(You have to break free from the addiction to see this.)

But to explain more succinctly why we can't eat carbs in space;

1. We'd have to grow them. Where are we going to get the water to grow them? I know there are some polar ice caps on Mars, but I don't think that's going to be enough for 100's of years until we get the technology to transport the water to where we can use it to harvest crops. Those crops though, are going to inflict the same harm that they've been inflicting for 10,000 years, and that's through the glycation they create. That's going to require medication to fight the pain created by the glycation. That is a senseless proposition.

2. The hunger cycle requires feeding every 3-4 hours or at least 3 times a day, not including snacks.

3. Without a hunger cycle, there are no snacks. There's only one meal per day (if you want that one).

4. There's much less waste from the digestion process. lessening the need for sanitation supplies. This is because there's only one meal, and it's a small one, just a little protein, and a little fat.

5. We'd have to take medication for all the problems carbs do to the body. That digestion can't be changed in less than a couple thousand years, our DNA won't let it. We'll be required to address everything in space that we address right here on earth, in regards to what sugar does to the body. That influence must be removed, from any diet of a space traveler.

6. A ketogenic diet gives the body a repairing diet that will be much more advantageous where medical treatment will be limited, at best. The sensible diet to be on is one that doesn't generate any glycation or hunger, yet generates growth hormones, instead. A diet that promotes brain growth instead of brain disease will go a lot further for our species' travels in space. This is why I can only recommend our species as a whole to go on a ketogenic diet.

7. A diet of carbs will come with a diet with glyphosate in it. Glyphosate is toxic. It's carcinogenic, atherosclerotic and extremely inflammatory. This is unsustainable off of this planet, without the resources that will be needed to treat all the pain that will be created by this glyphosated, carbohydrate diet.

8. Carbohydrates will not be available without the glyphosate sprayed on them, for at least 50 if not 100 years from now. The earth may not heal from the glyphosate contamination for 500 years, if then.

9. The carb diet creates fear cycles as a result of the hunger cycle. Combine that with the brain disease the carbs create and that's a recipe for disaster. That's the maker of every phobia and mental disorder you can think of.

The food industry is using your emotions to control your behavior. That's because they can. They already control your hormones and it's your hormones that control your emotions. Is it any wonder that so many are addicted? Our food industry has done their absolute best to sell you their goods, and that means playing to your emotions in order to sell you that great taste that's going to bring you oh so much discomfort, pain, and disease.

If you had known that this could and would happen to any one of your kids, you'd do everything in your power to change it. You have the power to change it, every time you go to the store. Read the label of everything you buy. If it contains wheat, corn, soy or grains at all, don't buy it. If you do, you'll be buying into a lifetime of pain and discomfort for your family. Choose something else to feed your family. You'll be much further ahead in the long run. The money it will save you in pharmaceuticals is nothing short of astounding. In my estimation, this is criminal behavior. It's criminal behavior being done on an industrial level. Monsanto has politically engineered their control of the FDA and USDA to ensure their compliance in their dominance of our food supply.

Corporate does this on purpose. They do this because they know that we are addicted to our rate of consumption. They also know that with their lobbying power, they can get away with virtually anything. It's the same situation as that of the military-industrial complex. They support congressmen and senators in every state and district, securing their interests, with this influence. Monsanto has even gone to the extent of contracting every farmer that they can, even to the point of suing farmers, just to corner the market. The last corporations that got away with this kind of behavior were busted up by Teddy Roosevelt in the late 19th century. No industry in our history has had more influence on our health, either as an individual or as a society than this grain and sugar industry has with its addictive food. It's created a multi-trillion dollar medical and pharmaceutical industry. The thing that scares them the most is the ketogenic diet as it's the only diet that can save you and the world, from their clutches.

We've allowed these corporations to addict us worse than we've been, anytime in the history of man, and that's something for which we should be ashamed. I would be but I didn't set up the Supreme Court to allow Monsanto to patent life in patenting GMO seeds. I didn't even ask them to play with my food supply, yet this toying around with the health of all of their consumers that insist on continuing this charade, bothers me. This may end up being the bane of mankind, as it is a very deadly path for our food industry to be taking. It's one that I consider corporate terrorism.

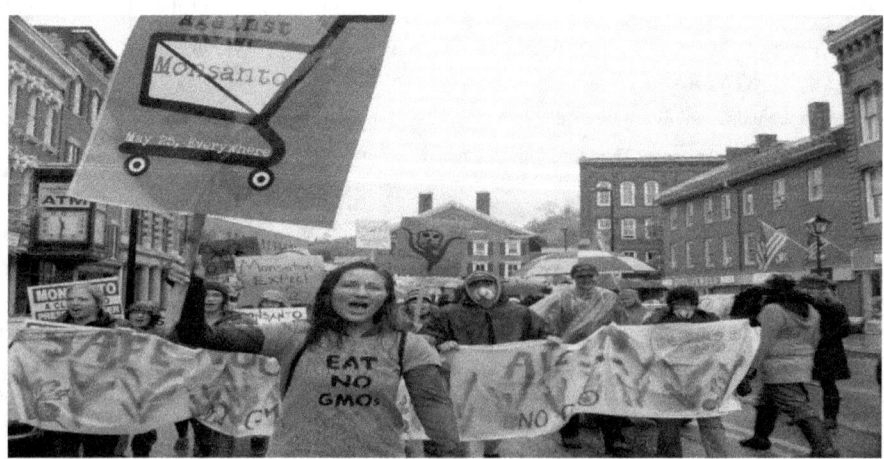

Chapter 15

WHY I STAY IN KETOSIS

Ketosis refers to acids in the body that are derived and used while in a state of low glucose in the blood. Because my body has been in a state of ketosis for the last 3 years, I feel qualified to speak about this lifestyle. I call it a lifestyle because it really is. It's a lifestyle completely different from the lifestyle of a carboholic. It's a lifestyle that's not subject to the hunger cycle.

Carboholics require food every other hour or so, it's the law of carb consumption, appetite follows glucose levels in the blood. It's that simple, blood sugar levels rise and satiety sets in, releasing hormones controlling feel-good emotions influencing behavior, sometimes unrecognizable behavior. But, that usually happens when the blood sugars fall again after a couple hours releasing hormones of hunger, need and want. These hormones are completely different than the satiety hormones and have many different effects on the body. I submit that it's this change in the hormonal influence that drives most behavior on the planet.

In my estimation, this change in our hormones is what drives a major portion of our abhorrent behavior today. This is what drives terrorism, by driving anger by driving the hunger cycle. It's my contention that if this hunger cycle can be controlled, you can control all anger and terrorism.

In this chapter, I'm going to explain the advantages of not being controlled by the hunger cycle because I believe that it's this hunger cycle that lies behind all despicable behavior. Breaking this hunger cycle puts you back in control of your own emotions and in doing so, puts you back in control of your own behavior.

According to PubMed, on the subject of ketosis;

"Hunger and satiety are two important mechanisms involved in body weight regulation. Even though humans can regulate food intake by will, there are systems within the central nervous system (CNS) that regulate food intake and energy expenditure. This complex network, whose control center is spread over different brain areas, receives information from adipose tissue, the gastrointestinal tract (GIT), and from blood and peripheral sensory receptors. The actions of the brain's hunger/satiety centers are influenced by nutrients, hormones and other signaling molecules. Ketone bodies are the major source of energy in the periods of fasting and/or carbohydrate shortage and might play a role in food intake control."

They go on to say; *"Glucose also exerts a hormonal-like action on neurons; electrophysiological recordings demonstrated, for example, that hypoglycemia activates growth hormone-releasing hormone (GHRH) neurons, suggesting a mechanistic link between low blood glucose levels and growth hormone release (Stanley et al., **2013**)."*

This is where carboholics cannot have the advantages that being in a state of nutritional ketosis has. Those who chose to live in a state of ketosis) aren't controlled by their hormones, so they don't have to follow any hunger cycle. They're in full control of their hormones. With hormones being the primary driver of appetite (Leptin & Ghrelin), they influence your appetite more than anything and are able to alter your ability to discern whether you need to eat or not. It's called leptin resistance and we'll get deeper into that later.

This also means that these hormones are in control of your emotions, because of that. I know that it doesn't sound like it's that big of a deal, but it's more important than you ever could imagine. As explained in **Why the addiction is so hard to break**, it has to do with how your hormones control your actions without you realizing it.

First, let's look at the state of ketosis, as explained in Wikipedia;

"Ketosis /kɪ'toʊsɪs/ is a metabolic state in which most of the body's energy supply comes from ketone bodies in the blood, in contrast to a state of glycolysis in which blood glucose provides most of the energy. Ketosis is similar to a condition called ketoacidosis, in that both cause a side effect known to laypeople as acetone breath. Longer-term ketosis may result from fasting or staying on a low-carbohydrate diet, and deliberately induced ketosis serves as a medical intervention for various conditions, such as intractable epilepsy, and the various types of diabetes. In glycolysis, higher levels of insulin promote storage of body fat and block the release of fat from adipose tissues, while in ketosis, fat reserves are readily released and consumed. For this reason, ketosis is sometimes referred to as the body's "fat burning" mode."

This biggest problem with a state of ketosis is that it is often confused with ketoacidosis, which has nothing to do with being in a state of nutritional ketosis. Ketoacidosis is a state of extreme ketosis that can only happen to type 1 diabetics because their pancreas is incapable of secreting enough insulin to handle even a small amount of glucose in the system. Because of this the liver of type 1 diabetics secretes more ketones than what the body needs to operate. Again Wikipedia says;

"Ketosis is deliberately induced by use of a KETOGENIC DIET as a medical intervention in cases of intractable epilepsy. Other uses of LOW-CARBOHYDRATE DIETS remain controversial. Induced ketosis or low-carbohydrate diet terms have very wide interpretation. Therefore, Stephen S. Phinney and Jeff S. Volek coined the term "nutritional ketosis" to avoid the confusion."

The worst mistake one can make about ketosis is to confuse it with Ketosis-Onset Diabetes or Ketosis-Prone Diabetes. These are conditions of extreme diabetes in which the body can't supply enough insulin for the amount of glucose in the body. It's explained in this report from Apr 23, 2013;

Ketosis-Onset Diabetes and Ketosis-Prone Diabetes: Same or Not?

Ketosis-prone diabetes (KPD) is defined as a widespread, emerging, heterogeneous syndrome characterized by patients who present with DKA or unprovoked ketosis but do not necessarily have the typical phenotype of autoimmune type 1 diabetes

While ketosis-onset diabetes patients present with ketosis or ketoacidosis without known diabetes, some investigators defined ketosis-onset diabetes as diabetes with the presence of diabetic ketosis and in the absence of glutamic acid decarboxylase (GAD) and tyrosine phosphatase (IA-2) autoantibodies.

Both of those conditions are manifestations of Diabetic Ketoacidosis (DKA). These conditions have little if anything to do with nutritional ketosis.

Although I appreciate nutritional ketosis as being a "fat burning mode", it's the other benefits that I appreciate more. I get to live with benefits like less pain, no headaches, no stomach aches, far more energy than what I've ever had, and the ability to get far more work done as I don't have to stop all the time, to eat. My efficiency in the last 6 – 12 months has been nothing short of phenomenal and although I do eat at my desk, I'm usually at my desk 16-18 hours out of the day, except on therapy days. I take 3 hours, 3 days a week for therapy. My therapy is exercise. My brain needs it, but my body benefits.

"KETOACIDOSIS IS A METABOLIC STATE ASSOCIATED WITH HIGH CONCENTRATIONS

OF KETONE BODIES, FORMED BY THE BREAKDOWN OF FATTY ACIDS AND THE DEAMINATION OF AMINO ACIDS. KETOACIDOSIS IS MOST COMMON IN UNTREATED TYPE 1 DIABETES MELLITUS, WHEN THE LIVER BREAKS DOWN FAT AND PROTEINS IN RESPONSE TO A PERCEIVED NEED FOR RESPIRATORY SUBSTRATE. PROLONGED ALCOHOLISM MAY LEAD TO ALCOHOLIC KETOACIDOSIS. IN DIABETIC KETOACIDOSIS, A HIGH CONCENTRATION OF KETONE BODIES IS USUALLY ACCOMPANIED BY INSULIN DEFICIENCY, HYPERGLYCEMIA, AND DEHYDRATION. PARTICULARLY IN TYPE 1 DIABETICS THE LACK OF INSULIN IN THE BLOODSTREAM PREVENTS GLUCOSE ABSORPTION, THEREBY INHIBITING THE PRODUCTION OF OXALOACETATE (A CRUCIAL PRECURSOR TO THE B-OXIDATION OF FATTY ACIDS) THROUGH REDUCED LEVELS OF PYRUVATE (A BYPRODUCT OF GLYCOLYSIS), AND CAN CAUSE UNCHECKED KETONE BODY PRODUCTION (THROUGH FATTY ACID METABOLISM) POTENTIALLY LEADING TO DANGEROUS GLUCOSE AND KETONE LEVELS IN THE BLOOD. HYPERGLYCEMIA RESULTS IN GLUCOSE OVERLOADING THE KIDNEYS AND SPILLING INTO THE URINE (TRANSPORT MAXIMUM FOR GLUCOSE IS EXCEEDED). DEHYDRATION RESULTS, FOLLOWING THE OSMOTIC MOVEMENT OF WATER INTO URINE. (OSMOTIC DIURESIS), EXACERBATES THE ACIDOSIS."

I bring this up to make the point that nutritional ketosis is not ketoacidosis. It's far from it. According to Wikipedia again, *"NORMAL serum reference ranges FOR KETONE BODIES ARE 0.5–3.0 MG/DL, EQUIVALENT TO 0.05–0.29 MMOL/L."*

In ketosis, the levels range from 3 – 6 mg/dL. Ketoacidosis requires a level of 15 – 25 mg/dL, more than three times the levels needed for ketosis, making it virtually impossible for anyone to go into ketoacidosis if you're not a type 1 diabetic. Actually, ketoacidosis happens when the body is overloaded with carbs and can't produce enough insulin to convert the glucose and turns to ketones in a panic. This condition requires an overload of sugar to produce the reaction. That is the last thing a diabetic wants to do. Nutritional ketosis has been instrumental in treating type2 diabetes and it's a growing sentiment that the state of ketosis and a ketogenic diet, is a cure for diabetes, even type1.

Remaining in a state of ketosis and not depending on sugar, on the other hand, has allowed my body to regain that which was lost 32 years ago in a car accident that left me severely disabled because of a severe closed head injury, (It was the two strokes that were the most devastating.)

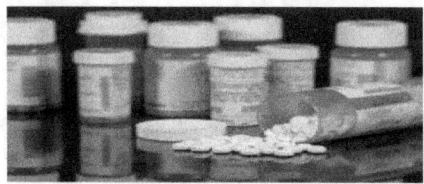

DRUGS THAT I WON'T NEED ANYMORE

Probably the first and foremost reason I choose to remain on this diet is explained by my lack of need for any of these diabetes medications. I just can't afford them or the side effects that they carry with them;

insulin, exenatide, liraglutide, pramlintide, Biguanides, metformin

Phenformin- Phenformin (DBI) was used from the 1960s through 1980s but was withdrawn due to lactic acidosis risk.

Buformin - also was withdrawn due to lactic acidosis risk.

Thiazolidinediones;

Rosiglitazone - (Avandia): the European Medicines Agency recommended in September 2010 that it be suspended from the EU market due to elevated cardiovascular risks.

Pioglitazone

Troglitazone - (Rezulin): used in 1990s, withdrawn due to hepatitis and liver damage risk

Peptide analogs; Secretagogues;

First-generation agents; tolbutamide, acetohexamide, tolazamide, chlorpropamide

Second-generation agents; glipizide, glyburide or glibenclamide, glimepiride, gliclazide, gliquidone, Meglitinides, repaglinide, nateglinide, Alpha-glucosidase inhibitors, miglitol, acarbose, voglibose.

Injectable Amylin analogs

Amylin, pramlintide, SGLT-2 inhibitors

Common generic names for many of these medicines are from Wikipedia; Many anti-diabetes drugs are available as generics. These include:[35]

Sulfonylureas- glimepiride, glipizide, glyburide

Biguanides- metformin

Thiazolidinediones(TZD) - pioglitazone, Actos generic

Alpha-glucosidase inhibitors- Acarbose

Meglitinides- nateglinide

Combination of sulfonylureas plus metformin - known by generic names of the two drugs

The above medications are used for diabetes alone. This small list is quite possibly the smallest list that one will need to choose from with a continued diet of carbohydrates. Larger lists exist for heart disease, cancer, high blood pressure, high cholesterol, arthritis, and dementia. That only covers the prescription medication. For OCD medication, you have to consider NSAIDs, the most used pain relievers, all carrying more side effects to create more need for further medication. And don't forget Tylenol. How many problems does that drug have with liver toxicity? It's been responsible for a few deaths.

Then we have to look at the Antacids and all the stomach medicine that's on the shelf. There are plenty of them and I can honestly tell you right now that 90% of these medications are not necessary unless you're on a carbohydrate diet. I haven't used any of these medications in 3 years since I gave up the bread and carbs. I used to have two or three volumes of drug catalogs full of pharmaceuticals that are needed to treat all of the diseases that are caused by the consumption of grains, from diabetes to dementia to heart disease and cancer. My first post lists all of those.

I refuse to take any of these drugs anymore because all of them carry side effects, some major, some minor. Whether the side effects are major or minor, I don't want to experience any of them. I've had my fill of side effects, especially the ones that make my health worse, which is where most of these side effects should be classified. After living for twenty years need to take massive amounts of opioids for my chronic severe pain, diuretics for my high blood pressure, anti-depressants for the pain, and living with the side effects of not only the opioids but every other drug they had me on, all twelve of them. I'm fed up with it. I'm not going to take it anymore. And I was only up to twelve medications. I have a friend who's on this diet, who's lowered his needs to thirteen daily medications from twenty-three. How many meds do you take every day?

I prefer the theory that if the meds aren't needed in the first place, my health is going to be that much better. That is why I removed everything from my diet that I could, that is responsible for these horrendous diseases, requiring the need for these medications. The one thread I found that ties 90% of all cancers (even lung cancer), 90% of all heart diseases, and 99.9 % of all dementia, all arthritis, all headaches, and almost all stomach aches together is one substance that can be removed from the diet without any severe side effects. I shouldn't need to tell you what that substance is by now. You should know. You eat it every day. You live with the effects of addiction. Pain always comes with addiction.

You eat it every morning, either in your coffee as creamer, in the toast you have, or the cereal you consume. You have it every lunch with your sandwich or burrito and with every dinner with your rolls. I have known several families that would just put a plate of bread on the table every evening. This is the display of addiction, a full out need to satisfy the taste buds by dumping more and more sugar in the body, usually in the form of starchy carbs.

The sad part of this whole argument is that I've only covered drugs for diabetes so far. I haven't even touched on drugs for heart disease, cancer, arthritis, high blood pressure, high cholesterol (probably the most dangerous), chronic pain, hyperlipidemia, obesity, etc, etc. How many side effects do think all these drugs can cause? How many more avenues can this create to develop new drugs to spring upon a mindless public clamoring for the newest drug of relief for their pain?

All of this consumption of the grain industry's products is what's driving the pharmaceutical industry today, tomorrow, next year, and will continue to drive it for the next 500 years and beyond. If we don't put an end to this now, our society is doomed to suffer the consequences of their carbohydrate addiction, a diet they're not responsible for. The greed of the grain industry combined with the ambition of the pharmaceutical industry has made us all carboholic slaves to the desires these industries. Just like the alcoholic is a slave to the liquor industry, the carboholic's masters are the grain and pharmaceutical industries. For me, it's scary how much power we've given these industries, simply because we listen to their advertising. Those who take their message to heart, and are influenced by it, fall prey to that influence and become their slaves for life or until they quit consuming the grains. It's an addiction that differs little from that of alcoholism. (Fortunately, the withdrawal symptoms aren't as bad.)

Anyone who can't control their emotions entirely by themselves is a slave to their own emotions. All addicts who recognize their addiction knows this to be true. Every addict follows their emotions before following anything else. That's because it's only their emotions that will feed the addiction. Common sense won't. It's the hormones, though that control your emotions.

Every carboholic is a slave to their hormones and hence a slave to their emotions and therefore a slave to these industries. The emotions I'm speaking about here are hunger and satiety. You may not classify these emotions, but I submit that they actually are. Satiety is defined as the state of being satisfied. If that is not an emotion, as it expresses feelings of calmness and security, I don't know what is. Hunger, on the other hand, is defined as a strong desire. Is not that an emotion? These emotions are controlled by both leptin and Ghrelin, which in turn are controlled by the grain industry, more than anything else. I refuse to take part in this trap anymore.

With emotions being controlled by our hormonal balance like this, how could the influence of anything that modifies that balance, not has an effect on our behavior? It has to. When you combine the drive of an addiction (which is what we're talking about) with the advertisements promoting that addiction, how can it not have an effect on our health and ultimately our society? That is why I make the statement that this cycle has to change. If it doesn't cease, our health as a society will never get better.

Let's go back to addiction, though, for I'm sure you don't consider this an addiction. I understand few caught in an addiction can recognize that addiction when they're feeding it because the addiction has ways of hiding it. You can ask anyone who has to have at least one beer a day. They're not addicted to their beer, as far as they're concerned, yet they have to have it. And often they don't even drink more than just one. But they still have to have that one. That is what makes it an addiction. The body can and does live much better without beer, so it's not a substance the body requires to survive. Yet the beer drinker needs that daily beer to satisfy their addiction. To go without, many times causes more problems because of the work your hormones are doing on your emotions and worse yet your actions by controlling how receptors work in your brain. That makes it a natural thing that you need to do, and not an addiction, to appease that desire to drink the beer. This is how addiction works and it happens to carboholics too. I know I am a carboholic. The desire for sweets is still with me. It's the last refuge of my addiction. It's something that I get to fight for the rest of my life.

When I think about this I get angry, for I never asked for this nor could I ever wish for it, or wish it upon anyone else. Yet, there is an industry that is committed to not only continuing this pattern, they're goal is to increase its scope. You can see this in all the advertising.

What do you think they're advertising promotes when they show you feel good commercials for their soft drinks, fruit drinks, cereals, bread, pasta, pastries, candy, etc, etc? They're using your emotions to control your behavior. That's because they can. They already control your hormones and it's your hormones that control your emotions. Is it any wonder that so many are addicted? This is the cycle of addiction that I avoid by being on my keto diet. I also avoid the cycle of hunger that everyone one carb diet has to deal with. This may be the best-unexpected benefit of a keto diet. No more cycles of pain and hunger. No more, do cycles of anger and contentment bother me nor do any cycles of fear, hate, and rage, thanks to my keto diet.

This industry has taken my right to chose simply by addicting me more, to a substance that has far deadlier consequences than it has ever had in the past. In my estimation, this is criminal behavior. It's criminal behavior being done on an industrial level. That is why I posted yesterday's post on our celebration of addiction. They do this because they know that we are addicted to our rate of consumption of their wares. They also know that with their lobbying power, they can get away with virtually anything. It's kind of the same situation as that of the military-industrial complex. They support congressmen and senators in every state and district, securing their interests, with this influence. There are very few districts or states that don't support farming, yet we allow this abuse to happen, for which we should be ashamed.

Because Monsanto is a corporation, the Supreme Court has determined that they deserve the same rights as an individual even though they don't have same moral values that most individuals have. Those who do criminal deeds we put in jail, but it's hard to put a corporation in jail for its criminal deeds.

We've made it legal for them to sell us their food contaminated with their glyphosate herbicides, regardless of how much cancer it causes. If this isn't criminal behavior, I don't know what is. That may be due to the fact that one of our Supreme Court Justices used to be an attorney for Monsanto in the late 70's. Clarance Thomas may go down in history as the Justice who did more to contribute to the ill health of-of America than any other Justice.

This is just a small iota of Monsanto's drive for profit. Justice Thomas wrote the decision that allowed Monsanto to patent something as simple as a seed. I wonder if his severance package left him with any stock options when he left Monsanto? This is what allows Monsanto to force farmers to grow their GMO seed, whether they want to or not. This is the evil of industrial farming, engineered Monsanto style.

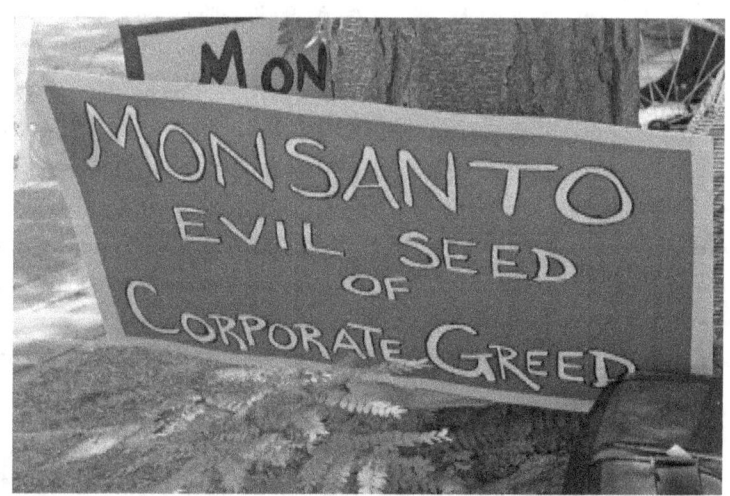

IT IS YOUR CHOICE AS YOU WILL SEE

EAT THEIR FOOD FOR YOUR MISERY

OR DO AS I DO TO BREAK THE BOARD

CHOOSE THE ONLY WAY TO MOVE FORWARD

AND END THEIR NEVERENDING CYCLE OF PAIN

SIMPLY BY ENDING YOUR APPETITE FOR GRAIN

CHAPTER 16

UNDERSTANDING THE REAL REASON WHY WE FIGHT

I can still remember it today. It was the absolute best feeling that I've ever had. I can remember exactly how I thought, what time of day it was, the room we were in. My memory of this special event is locked in my mind, forever. I thought this is so good, how can anyone fall out of love after this. I remember uttering that same feeling and hearing, "I wouldn't know. I love you too." I said again, but this time with more conviction, "I love you so much...I don't know how I could ever stop loving you."

That was the day we lost our cherries. I saw the spot on the sheets after we finished and asked her what it was, not knowing. When I did realize what it was, I felt ashamed for not knowing, then I fell deeper in love. She and I had shared something physically sacred that you experience only once in your life. When I realized what she had given up to secure my love, I relinquished my love to her without reservation or hesitation. I knew at that moment that she was my soul mate. I couldn't imagine being with anyone else or anything coming between us. I also couldn't realize what would eventually drive a wedge between us, to drive us apart.

Looking back on it now, I know exactly what it was that drove us apart. It was my pride. She was smarter than I and due to that fact, I had trouble acknowledging her superior intellect. I wasn't used to not always being "right". Because she was smarter than I, she had this habit of being right more often than I and that was tough for me to accept. I wish now that I could have worked a little harder at understanding. I've never stopped loving her and never will. She is still my soul mate, except she's with someone else because of my behavior.

Looking back on our relationship, it was rocky. I think I know why that was. I think it was because of our carbohydrate diet and the hunger cycles it put us through. I didn't know it at that time, but the hunger was the driving force behind every other cycle I went through. I was raised on bread, mostly because my mother loved it and she loved it immensely. At that time, in the fifties, bread wasn't the nasty stuff that it is now. Then it was the staff of life. Now, it's the staff of death. As I was raised on bread, I had a more active hunger cycle and because of this hunger cycle, I found myself in more trouble than most other kids my age and I was always in trouble of some sort, usually due to the fact that I couldn't control my emotions. Emotions are always the first to go on a hunger cycle. This is due to the fact that they're controlled by your hormones which are controlled by your diet. This was something it took me 60 years to learn. I wish now that I knew then what I know now, but I couldn't. I was locked into an addiction that kept me from seeing any danger signs except that I needed to make some changes.

There was an industry intent on not allowing us to know. That same industry had intentions of using our love of bread for their benefit, seeing an opportunity to make money out of an addiction that we grew into. We've had this affliction all of our lives. We were born into it as it starts before we're born, due to the consumption of it by our mothers who couldn't break away from it. That's because they're born into it. We're all born into it. It's the nature of how this grain has shaped our civilization.

It's shaped our civilization through its hunger cycle which has also forced us to reap the reward of that cycle. Like all cycles, it has its ups and downs and this is what condemns us to the karma we've created through our hunger cycles. When we're hungry, we act with less forethought and concern for long-term consequences of our actions. This doesn't allow us to see all of those manifestations, prior to our committing them. We only see the ones we want to see and this is where we get into trouble. Because of our clouded judgment, we not open to all possibilities or consequences of those possibilities and this is why our karma comes back to bite us. Too often that karma comes back in the form of terrorism when our hasty decisions are international and affect other people and nationalities. This turns the war on terrorism into a war on sugar and grains, our real nemeses.

Due to the fact that this grain has shaped our history so much, it's influenced the usurping of more territory than any other one reason. Capturing land that grew this important food meant that the conqueror could control the people that this grain fed. That meant security for the owner of such land. It was the wealth that brought this security that drove this kind of behavior, but it was the underlying hunger that drove the desire for security. This is a natural reaction to the hormonal imbalance that the hunger cycle brings with it everywhere it goes. This is due to the influence that sugar and glucose have on those hormones. They're devastating, to say the least, and they keep your hormones from being under your own control. Because of that, your hormones are under the control of what you're eating. Your diet of carbohydrates makes certain of this.

In my opinion, it's also what leads to all abhorrent behavior that in my eyes is evil. Because this behavior is driven by fear and since fear is what drives all evil, it's my opinion that this food can be considered a driver of evil. It didn't use to be like that, but it is now, especially with glyphosate that's been dumped, on these crops. Tons of the enzyme inhibiting weed killer is changing our hormonal balance to the point where it's not safe to eat bread anymore. Nor is it safe to eat corn, oats or any grain, for that matter, even sugar. They all get desiccated before harvest and this is where the danger is, in the desiccating of the crop for a complete harvest. This one action alone ensures that wo got enough glyphosate into our diets to ensure our compliance into the glucose ruse of a never-ending drug cycle that can only end in a premature death.

All grains (including sugar) are soaked in so much glyphosate that they can't help but rearrange your hormones and ultimately, health. This is why so many people are dying today from all modern disease that exists. This glyphosate actually ramps up the glycation that's responsible for these diseases and disorders and the general public isn't aware of this. They don't know what's really behind these pandemics of obesity and diabetes, cardiovascular and heart diseases as well as all cancers and dementias. They just know that what tastes good and unfortunately, that just happens to be the same thing that does all the damage. All this damage is due to the glycation that this food instigates and the fact that the glycation has been magnified by the glyphosate that it's been drenched in. This is a recipe for disaster for the health of the public. It's also a recipe for profit for;

1. the seed companies that provide the GMO seed,
2. the chemical industry that provides the glyphosate herbicide
3. pharmaceutical industries that treat you for your pain.

This profit comes from your pockets and your health. Is your addiction worth it? So, what can you do, to stay away from this glycating sugar in your diet? Nothing except to give it up...forever. This is the only way you can be free of its addiction, as it has addicted us unwittingly. It did this as soon as we were able to eat it. When one compares the ancient civilizations and their aggressive nature, the most aggressive civilizations were the ones under the influence of wheat and grains more than anything else. These crops became staples in our diet, where they used to only be eaten small amounts as it took a long time to gather it up, in order to eat it.

The Celtic empire that never had a territory, shows this clearly. The Celts were a tall people.

this is due to the protein in the wheat, amylopectin. It enabled the people who ate this einkorn wheat to grow taller and more muscular. What it did underneath the surface was completely hidden until just recently when AGEs were discovered and the real destruction of this kind of diet presented itself. That's in the glycation that these grains create.

The domestication of the grain into crops to feed the masses gave this food, power over the masses and landowners power to control that power. Landowners knew this and that's why they invaded fertile lands first. It was this land that could provide them with enough food to feed their armies. This was the perfect food to feed an army, as you could more easily control this army by controlling their hunger. Powerful warlords knew that whoever controlled the food, controlled the people.

What they didn't know, it was their own hunger that influenced this behavior and that it was the influence of their diets that influenced their hunger. That's something I didn't know until just recently. It took removing them from my diet to fully understand it, but it's plain as day, now that I'm outside of the addiction. One can seldom see an addiction when they're stuck in it and this is the inherent danger in this grain. It's always been addictive, ever since we've been eating it. It always will be and since we've eaten this food all of our lives, as we ate it when we're infants, that addicts us unwittingly and forever, unless we're aware of it wiles, its dangers, and it's addictive nature.

Any substance that affects your hormones like sugar and grains do, is going to be addictive. Alcohol proves this. So does heroin and every other drug. But then so does gambling and all risk-taking, for that fact, because it's driven by a cycle of greed, which is driven by the hunger cycle. This is why a contend that all terrorism is driven by a hunger cycle which is driven by sugar and carbs. This is also why I contend that all wars were and are ultimately driven by a hunger cycle because a power grab is a manifestation of a hunger cycle. It's the idea of security that drives someone to gain more power. It's this idea of security that's prompted by the hunger cycle. Who wants to go hungry?

Because I've broken my hunger cycle by breaking my addiction, I can see this clearly, right now. You could easier understand this concept if you can break your hunger cycle also.

THE BEST WAY TO FIGHT HUNGER FIGHTS TERRORISM AS WELL

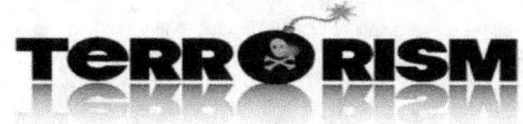

You know better than I do that hunger pervades our society. Everybody experiences hunger every day. Some people experience hunger all day all night long. At least it's thought so. Actually, those who go without food don't often experience hunger except for the ones who haven't broken the cycle of hunger. This is a cycle that controls hunger a few hours at a time at a time. This is also an addiction. This is your addiction to glucose. It works by playing with your hormones every time your blood glucose levels change. When you eat carbs your glucose levels are altered, it's this alteration of your blood glucose levels that alter the reaction of your hormones. It's those changes in your hormones that affect your behavior and makes you act in the manner you do. It's those changes in hormones that also affect your hunger cycles. I call it the *Glucose Ruse*. It's only deadly to those who buy into it. I won't because I won't pay for terrorism.

This is simple. At least, to me, it's simple. Actually, this may be the easiest and simplest cure for hunger that exists today. If you think it's time for a cure for hunger, I've got the solution for the world; to best fight hunger, you need to stop the hunger cycle. You need to do this not by feeding starving people bags of flour and corn to eat, but by giving them education about nutrition and diet to get them off of the flour and corn diet. That is what makes them hungry and dependent on the grains for their diet. They will remain dependent until they either quit eating the grains or die. The death part always comes prematurely, always. This is the addiction part of the cycle.

Since you can live better without carbs (I'm proving that), your body does not need them. That is the definition of addiction, the body requiring something it doesn't need and manifesting discomfort when it's not available for the affected to use. This is the same as what an alcoholic goes through when they can't get a drink. It's what cigarette smokers feel when they need a smoke. It's a need that has to be satisfied, but it can only be satisfied in your mind, where your hormones affect your emotions. They affect your emotions in your mind, more than anywhere else. This is your instruction center for the body, for what happens in the body and how you react to whatever stimuli affect the body.

How Sugar Creates Terrorism

Your emotions should remain in your control, not in the control of what you eat. When you allow that to happen, you're allowing the industry that controls what you eat, to control how you feel and what you do, by controlling your emotions. This is a cycle. It's a cycle of dependence. It's a cycle of dependence on the grain industry. Not the beef industry or dairy industry, simply the grain industry and its manufacturers and processors. It's this industry that's responsible for all glycation that occurs in your blood. It's this industry that's responsible for your hunger cycles and that put's responsibility on them for your changes in emotions and behavior. It can also give them some responsibility for the terrorism that exists in the world today as it's controlled by the amount of anger and hate that's expressed which in turn is controlled by what controls the hate and anger and that's a glucose diet. It's this diet, that's responsible for your emotional changes. by changing your hormones. This diet creates this hunger cycle that all who are living on it can expect to live with. Hunger is the cost of a diet of carbohydrates. It's that simple.

It's not only a cycle of hunger, it's a cycle of addiction. Every addict has to feed their addiction. When you feel hungry, what do you hunger for? What is the first thing you want to eat or drink? That tells you where your addiction lies. I know what you're thinking right now, how can hunger to eat be an addiction? That's the first question I'm asked, whenever I call this an addiction.

This is how addictions work, they force your body to want something that it really doesn't need. It creates discomfort in the body until that need is met. When that need is met, comfort takes place and damage internally begins. While your emotions are being controlled by your glucose infusion and making you feel comfortable, the glucose from the sugar and carbs is busy, very busy glycating whatever cholesterol or protein the glucose can find. Even though it's not the glycation the creates the hunger, (the hunger comes from hormone imbalance, but then, so does the pain, discomfort, irritability and general malaise that these grains bring), the glycation is now a more clarified manifestation of the real damage that takes place, every time this substance is eaten. (Thanks to Dr. Davis, Dr. Perlmutter, Dr. Volek, PubMed, and PMC.)

Those grains not only increase hunger, but they're the prime agents behind all modern diseases caused by the creation of glycation in the blood. That's exactly what these foods do. How they do it, right now, isn't important. What's important is that these foods, in the manner in which they are digested, not only create the glycation but they create hunger as well. It's this hunger they create that makes them addictive and dangerous to the point of deadly.

It has to do with the fluctuation of your hormones due to your diet of grains. Once grains are ground, they lose their fiber. This is important because it's the fiber that slows down the breakdown of the sugars in the grains that influence your blood glucose. The slower those sugars are introduced into your system, the slower they raise your blood glucose. Most diabetics know this, as it's the quick rise in blood glucose that is responsible for the glycation and the release of hormones that actually work to increase your hunger.

Leptin which is supposed to keep you from being hungry is actually increased to the point where it does little good for your body anymore. There's so much of it in your body that you don't recognize what you've already eaten and this is what's dangerous. It's this leptin resistance that makes you hungry.

This is what drives the hunger cycle and most all restaurants know this. (This is why they give you bread as soon as they seat you.) This is what makes everyone hungry. My theory is to eliminate this cycle, and to do that, means changing the equation, the equation of digestion. The best way to change that equation is to changes the factors of the equation, in this case, one factor. All you have to do to cure hunger and glycation is to remove that which creates hunger and glycation, carbohydrates from the equation and thus the diet. The solution is that simple. Maybe not easy, but simple.

When one considers the fact that the primary driver of hunger is a carbohydrate diet, it's easy to see that the solution for hunger is to eliminate the cycle of hunger by changing the diet. Taking carbohydrates out of the diet removes the hunger factor and thus the hunger cycle. Anyone doubting this can go on the diet that I've been on for three years and they'll know this to be true. Three years on the diet that I've been on will not only convince anyone of this concept, it will also improve their health in unimaginable ways. The last time I got hungry was 3 yrs 3 months ago. That was when I broke my addiction to glucose. Others who are on this diet will tell you the same thing, they don't get hungry and the reason they don't get hungry is that they don't have the glucose going through their systems to create the hunger cycle.

Because this is an addiction, those who still eat carbs, can't see it. You have to break the addiction to know this. That's the way it is with any addiction, you can't see it while you're in it. Yet, almost everyone knows that sugar is addictive. I think because nobody wants to equate that sugar with carbs, they don't want to fully grasp that the carbs they were told they need, is sugar. Carbs, something you were told you had to have, breaks down to the exact same thing as sugar, and that's glucose, and glucose glycates and makes you hungry.

Yet, they're still telling everyone to eat whole grains, as though they're healthy. It's always been spoken of in that manner because it justified our need for it. That, my friends, is the definition of dependency and I think you know what that deals with when the dependency deals with a substance. This dependency has infiltrated the agencies that are supposed to regulate it, yet they're blind to it as well. They're blind to it electively as they're instructed to by the industry that's orchestrated this whole ruse. That's the industry that's put their people in place, to afford them this control, Monsanto.

Well here's your news flash; sugar including carbs is addictive. That means that carbs are just an addictive food to eat as that of sugar. It's also deadly, deadlier than alcohol, deadlier than heroin, deadlier than cigarettes and drug addiction. Sugar addiction or ECC, (Excessive Carbohydrate Consumption) is responsible for more deaths than all world wars and terrorism combined. ECC is the deadliest addiction a person or society can have. Its toll on our society is massive, as it's responsible for over 2000 deaths every day in the US alone. That number jumps to over 50,000 worldwide (daily). The grief it creates is incalculable.

I can guarantee a manifestation of disease-causing AGEs to anyone who consumes a diet of grains. How much they consume will dictate how much glycation they get to deal with, but they will deal with it, guaranteed. The manner in which you cure the glycation will also cure the hunger. What it does to wipe out the hunger cycle (and it does it altogether), it also does to the glycation cycle. That is how you cure hunger.

That is also how you conquer and cure all modern diseases. You can do it in one fell swoop. This is exciting. To me, the cure for hunger is the same cure for all the modern diseases that are responsible for over 2000 deaths every day. If you cure one, you cure the other. That will go miles to cure the problem of hunger around the world. We need to stop supplying the world with our killing field grains. It's the hunger that proves the addictive nature of carbs. Once you break the addiction, you lose the hunger cycle and without a cycle to create your hunger, the hunger can't exist. Hunger is then cured. You just have to solve the problem of too many people going without nutritious food and being subjected to a diet of non-nutritious food, which includes the category of grains.

It's the cycle of hunger that's responsible not only for growth, but also for all harm done in the name of growth or progress, as well as advancement, or security, or improvement. Those are all desires driven by the cycle of hunger. It's this cycle of hunger that drives these emotions. Deep down inside, you know this to be true. After you eat, when your blood sugars are at their highest, you are at one of your most relaxed attitudes of the day.

The only other times you feel this secure is right after you eat any meal or snack (unless you're consciously cheating on a diet and are dealing with guilt issues). This is the high side of the cycle, this is when you feel that everything is OK, "my stomach is full and I don't feel like I need anything except to sit here and relax for a minute. This is how you feel at the end of Thanksgiving Dinner, Christmas Dinner, New Years Day dinner, Easter Dinner, etc, etc, etc. This is also the end of every meal you eat, to some extent. This is the glucose hitting your bloodstream, waiting to give you fuel for energy. This is also the start of glycation and the hunger cycle.

It's the start of glycation because all that glucose you just put into your blood by eating your starchy grains, is now floating all through your blood after being broken down to glucose, starting with the saliva in your mouth. That means that before it hits your stomach, your blood glucose levels are reacting.

This is the start of the hunger cycle to which there is no end until you stop feeding it. When your blood glucose levels fall and your stomach starts to shrink just a little bit after the digestion of your meal, that triggers your stomach to release Ghrelin, your hunger hormone. That's the hormone that nobody on a carbohydrate diet can resist. That's because many of those on a carb diet must satisfy that Ghrelin hormone. Once they get hungry they feel the need to satisfy their hunger usually with some form of carbohydrate more than anything else. This is the low side of the cycle that drives people to abhorrent behavior because of their need.

This hunger and satiety cycle influences almost every other cycle our bodies go through. It's what's behind all the behavior, of those that are on a carbohydrate diet. This is the cycle that drives people into the use and abuse, of social media to slander, attack, and accuse without evidence, others they disagree with. As PBS's late **GWEN IFILL** said, "we have to guard against how we treat each other". We should remember it was cancer that took Gwen from us. If this cure had been publicized 10, 20, or 30 years ago, Gwen would still be here giving us her newscast.

This manner in how we treat each other is one of the reasons why I'm writing this book, about what this food source that Monsanto has given us to eat is doing to everyone who eats it. Up until I watched **FOOD, INC,** (Monsanto only played a small part in my equation. I didn't realize they were behind this to the extent that they actually are. I now see that they are a much larger part of it than I suspected.)

What their grains do with their glycating destruction starts with premature aging. It does that by driving fat production and the glycation factor that influences all modern disorders. That figures into everything glycation plays a factor in. Glycation is another name for inflammation. I know this. I've experienced the release of the addiction. The evidence in my books proves this. I know why we behave like the society that we do. It has to do with what we eat.

Nobody will believe me until they heed my advice and kick their own addiction. Only then, can they see the true light? I can guarantee the light you'll see is a light of freedom, true freedom. Freedom from the cycle of hunger that drives virtually every other cycle. If you can eliminate this cycle, you can eliminate everything this cycle creates and drives, starting with obesity and diabetes and moving on to glycation. That will go far to improve not only health, but mental attitudes, and hence better emotional outcomes and less strife.

That is true freedom, freedom from the cycle of hunger, freedom from the cycle of addiction. Freedom from the wild roller coaster ride of emotional swings. The freedom I experience is true freedom as this cycle does not affect anybody on a purely ketogenic diet. We're not subject to the hunger cycle that the carb diet requires. By the same token, we're not subject to the glycation cycle of destruction either. This cycle is also at the root of all violence and terrorism, as it's subject to the same hormonal changes that control your emotions, as explained above. These emotions are just slightly altered because of their influence on the glucose fluctuations in your blood.

To control the glucose fluctuations, the easiest way is to control what feeds the cycle. That means to control the cycle you need to control the introduction of glucose into your body. Controlling the flow of sugars (carbs and fructose) is the only way you can control the blood glucose fluctuations.

As easy as this may sound, that may be furthest from the truth. Controlling the inflow of carbs into your body is as difficult as fighting any addiction, because that's exactly what you're doing, fighting an addiction. That's also why you must break the addiction, addictions kill prematurely and you can live without this addictive food. This brings me to the conclusion that a ketogenic diet is an optimal diet for a society to be following on, for the best health of that society. The ketogenic diet not only removes the hormonal control out of the equation, it removes hunger and glycation out of the equation. That makes it a truly win, win, win diet for everyone to follow.

The problem here is sticking to a ketogenic diet. We'll cover that here because it's not only important, it's vital to convert to the ketogenic diet to save yourself and our society as a whole. This is also how curing hunger can also cure terrorism by curing abhorrent behavior by removing your emotions from the hunger cycle. This removal of your emotions from the hunger cycle has multiple other benefits for your emotional behavior. It puts those emotions back in your control and not the control of the industry that promotes the masturbation of them. It also returns other emotional control you'd thought you'd lost years ago. The control you lost was a relinquishing of control to the industry that has addicted you. This isn't your fault. You've always eaten carbs and sugar. The fact that they were considered healthy at one time is an indication of their addictive nature. (If the body needs it, it must be healthy!) We now know, that science was skewed.

To be able to stick to a ketogenic diet means that you must break the addiction. Once it's broke, you'll know it and you'll know it firmly, distinctly. It's a feeling I still remember clearly, three years later. It's a feeling of freedom. It's a feeling of freedom from dependence on a substance that is as satisfying as it as dangerous.

That is what makes it so dangerous, the fact that is so satisfying, so satiating, so hormonal fluctuating. That also makes it emotionally fluctuating. That makes you prone to emotional outbursts and fits of terrorism, yourself. (Frightening people with the use of force is terrorism, by strict definition.) That makes any threat, terrorism, to some extent. Those who make the most threats (bullies) tend to be the most terroristic. If you control your emotions and not let what you eat control them, that gives you more control over your emotional reactions and the consequences of those emotional reactions. This is a small synopsis of the control that glucose has on your actions and reactions.

I, being on a ketogenic diet, do not experience this control of my emotions or actions or reactions due to glucose influence. I've learned how to live without that influence. I learned that three years, two weeks ago. It may have been the best day of my life. But I have to admit that sticking to a ketogenic diet is difficult to get into. It took me over two years to transform into the diet I've been on since I started writing my books.

One thing I know is that I could have never accomplished this without being on this diet. I've not only overcome severe chronic pain, but I've also overcome pre-diabetic conditions as well as high blood pressure, chronic constipation from the drugs that were prescribed, near obesity, and brain drain more than anything else. Being on my ketogenic diet has sharpened my brain to a point I wish it could have been when I was in school. Boy, would my life have been different? This is why I want to help you succeed at your attempt to convert, it's that important for our society if we're to end hunger and terrorism.

In order to do that, I recommend stopping buying everything that raises your blood glucose more than 50 pts on the glycemic index. This will help keep your blood glucose levels from reaching glycating or hunger cycling proportions. This is the starting point that I used when I started three years ago. I cut out bread first. That was the hardest because that included everything that flour is used in. To do otherwise is not giving up the bread. After the magic came from giving up the bread, I switched those calories to calories from higher fiber carbs like vegetables and fresh fruit. I was still reluctant to put dairy in my diet then, as I still have some Almond Milk in my fridge, I didn't realize it then because my knowledge hadn't grown to the point to where I decided to go completely ketogenic, so I was still putting more sugar in my body than what I am now, where I'm experiencing the improvements in my mental functions as well as my physical abilities. I'm actually healing my paralysis, little by little. My right side is actually getting more functional every day that I remain on this diet,

That is why I decided to convert to a completely keto diet after two years of simply a low carb diet. That may have got me to my weight goal, but it wasn't getting me my brain back. Quitting bread prompted me to quit all grains and starchy carbohydrates like potatoes and beans. That felt so great, I decided to go completely keto approximately one year ago. That's when I started my website and started writing all the information that I'm packing into three books. If anyone else were doing this I would think it phenomenal. But because it's myself doing this, I'm just driven to get this information out there where the public can see it. Killing my mother has become my driving force to get this known. My ability to accomplish this working in a state of paralysis, to me is what's phenomenal. For that, I have to thank Dr. Perlmutter. Thank you, Dr. Perlmutter, I couldn't have done this without your book or advice.

For those who want something to kill? I've got something for you to kill. Kill your hunger cycle. Kill it before it kills you first. Monsanto may have different ideas, though. Their profits depend on your hunger cycle. Their drug industry depends on your hunger cycle. Your hunger cycle drives you to eat more and more carbs to satisfy that hunger cycle. If you want to kill something worth killing, kill your hunger cycle and do it as quickly as you can. The following report from Wikipedia shows why;

The influence of funding on research and the management of conflicts of interests *as explained from The New England Journal of Medicine (Aug 19, 1993)*

"Conflict of interest" in the field of medical research has been defined as "a set of conditions in which professional judgment concerning a primary interest (such as a patients welfare or the validity of research) tends to be unduly influenced by a secondary interest (such as financial gain)."]

In the early 1900s private companies such as the Carbolic Smoke Ball Company, Mrs. Winlow's Soothing Syrup among other snake medicine remedies were solicited around the world and were the cause of many deaths due to misinformation. Information was not readily available to consumers nor was it required of the pharmaceutical producers to inform their customers of the ingredients that they were consuming. Samuel Hopkins Adams was an investigator to uncover the wide corruption and falsehoods that existed within the American pharmaceutical industry. He is quoted saying: "Gullible America will spend this year some seventy-five millions of dollars in the purchase of patent medicines. In consideration of this sum, it will swallow huge quantities of alcohol, an appalling amount of opiates and narcotics, a wide assortment of varied drugs ranging from powerful and dangerous heart depressants to insidious liver stimulants; and far in excess of all other ingredients, undiluted fraud."

Regulation of industry-funded biomedical research has seen great changes since Samuel Hopkins Adams declaration. In 1906 Congress passed the Pure Food and Drugs Act of 1906. In 1912 Congress passed the Shirley Amendment to prohibit the wide dissemination of false information on pharmaceuticals. The Food and Drug Administration was formally created in 1930 under the McNairy Mapes Amendment to oversee the regulation of Food and Drugs in the United States. In 1962 the Kefauver-Harris Amendments to the Food, Drug, and Cosmetics Act made it so that before a drug was marketed in the United States the FDA must first approve that the drug was safe. The Kefauver-Harris amendments also mandated that more stringent clinical trials must be performed before a drug is brought to the market. The Kefauver-Harris amendments were met with opposition from industry due to the requirement of lengthy clinical trial periods that would lessen the period of time in which the investor is able to see a return on their money. In the pharmaceutical industry, patents are typically granted for a 20-year period of time, and most patent applications are submitted during the early stages of the product development. According to Ariel Katz on average after a patent application is submitted it takes an additional 8 years before the FDA approves a drug for marketing. As such this would leave a company with only 12 years to market the drug to see a return on their investments. After a sharp decline of new drugs entering the US market following the 1962 Kefauver-Harris amendments economist Sam Petlzman concluded that cost of loss of innovation was greater than the savings recognized by consumers no longer purchasing ineffective drugs. In 1984 the Hatch-Waxman Act or the Drug Price Competition and Patent Term Restoration Act of 1984 were passed by Congress. The Hatch-Waxman Act was passed with the idea that giving brand manufacturers the ability to extend their patent by an additional 5 years would create greater incentives for innovation and private sector funding for investment.

The relationship that exists with industry-funded biomedical research is that of which industry is the financier for academic institutions which in turn employ scientific investigators to conduct research. A fear that exists wherein a project is funded by industry is that firms might negate informing the public of negative effects to better promote their product. A list of studies shows that public fear of the conflicts of interest that exist when biomedical research is funded by industry can be considered valid after a 2003 publication of "Scope and Impact of Financial Conflicts of Interest in Biomedical Research" in The Journal of American Association of Medicine. This publication included 37 different studies that met specific criteria to determine whether or not an academic institution or scientific investigator funded by industry had engaged in behavior that could be deduced to be a conflict of interest in the field of biomedical research. Survey results from one study concluded that 43% of scientific investigators employed by a participating academic institution had received research-related gifts and discretionary funds from industry sponsors. Another participating institution surveyed showed that 7.6% of investigators were financially tied to research sponsors, including paid speaking engagements (34%), consulting arrangements (33%), advisory board positions (32%) and equity (14%). A 1994 study concluded that 58% out of 210 life science companies indicated that investigators were required to withhold information pertaining to their research as to extend the life of the interested companies' patents. Rules and regulations regarding conflict of interest disclosures are being studied by experts in the biomedical research field to eliminate conflicts of interest that could possibly affect the outcomes of biomedical research.

This is pretty much the definition of what Monsanto has accomplished in the last 40-50 years and they seem to be doing their level best to increase their power and influence. It's their food that glycates your blood. It's their food that addicts you to eat more and more of their food. It's their food that creates the hunger cycle that drives your behavior. It's this company that is forcing farmers to purchase their seed to grow the crops to put on your table to eat. That means that it's this company that is responsible for over 45,000 deaths every day, across the world from ECC, Excessive Carbohydrate Consumption. ECC is the deadliest addiction mankind has ever been exposed to. Monsanto, who's infiltrated their execs into the offices of the USDA and the FDA and the departments that control all the agencies and offices within them, controls all. From planting to harvesting to processing to treating, Monsanto has their hands in everything. Can you trust a corporation that's dedicated to owning your hunger? If they own your1183 hunger, they own you.

This has given them unprecedented control over what you eat. That has given them full control over the diseases and disorders, all who eat their food will acquire. That is something I can virtually guarantee. Why? It lies in the science of a glucose diet, the deadliest diet man can eat. Thank you, Monsanto, but I disrespectfully decline your offer to buy your drugs and live life as you see fit.

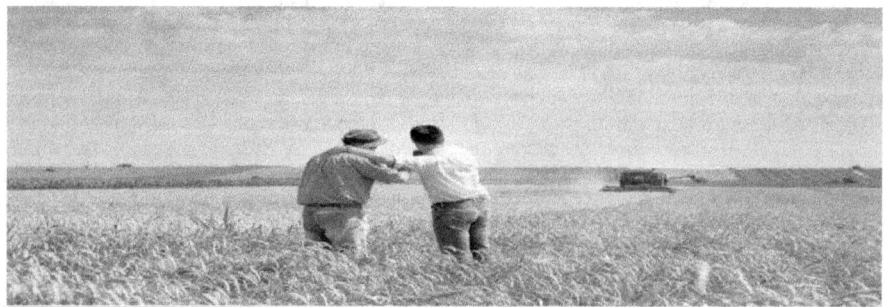

CHAPTER 17

GOD'S ANSWER

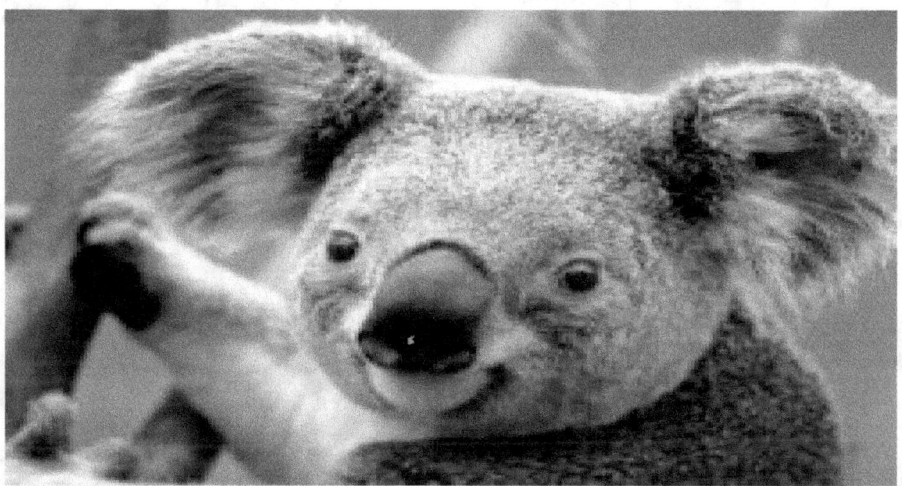

The state of our current food supply industry has forced me to reconsider my beliefs in God. It appears that this industry is pure evil with the rampant destruction this industry is content with allowing.

In their quest for profits, they're pulling off quite possibly the most devious deception ever perpetrated on the American people and the world. This can be only be achieved by pure evil or pure greed. My belief is its greed. I don't believe in evil, except for corporate evil, which is another word for greed.

Since greed is a form of evil, I guess we can consider greed, evil. That makes corporate greed, evil is done on an industrial level, or pure evil or as Christians would put it, the devil incarnate. This has forced me to reassess my beliefs in God. I don't believe in God anymore, at least, not the God I was brought up to believe in. That God is too rigid.

I don't believe in a God that is rigid. God is not rigid. Rigid is the antithesis of God. I don't believe in God as much as I live in God. God is not a He or a She as God is not anyone being. God is All Beings, all life either in harmony or discord. God is forever changing along with life and the changing of man. As a man thinks, so thinks God. This idea that God is rigid and never changing, that God is the same today as it was 10,000 years ago or 2000 years ago, is not the faith that Christ taught me. Because I still believe in the Word, I still believe in what Christ taught. What Christ taught is for us to love one another as we love ourselves. I'd like to share how my God works to shape our lives.

Belief in a rigid God is the root of all religious strife, and subsequently most all wars. Most everyone who believes in God believes their God is rigid and never changes. This is how they base their whole set of beliefs, their *isms* wherever their faith takes them, whether they're Catholic, Protestant, Jewish, or Muslim. Their God is a rigid God, One that never changes and who's views never change. It's this attitude of a rigid, never changing the idea of what's sacrosanct, that makes everybody "right by God/Allah" and unwilling to bend and this is what leads to war and terrorism. That's the God I used to worship. I believed in the Word, the Word of Christ.

I still believe in the Word. I just believe as I believe Jesus wanted us to believe, without reservation, without fear and anger, but with Love and Understanding. That is the God I worship but I don't worship a supreme being. What I never realized is, that Word is also my Word. It's also your Word. It's everybody's Word. That is what represents God at any one moment. It's the thoughts and actions and consequences of every living being that comprise Life on earth. That is what God is. It's the good thoughts along with the bad thoughts. This is how God shapes our future, with either thought of Love, the good thoughts or through the god of fear and anger, with bad thoughts.

That puts more importance on our emotions as those are the emotions of God or god. This value of our emotions is regulated, more than anything else, by what we eat and yes carbs do play a part in it. God is different today. God, in Jesus' time, was a god of fear throughout most of the world. But in some civilized parts, there were pockets of civility. These were the villages and towns, where civilization existed and our beliefs of helping and kindness were born. This is also where religion was born.

The people gathering together with common interests were and are the people who make up how God acts and reacts. Whether it is good or bad behavior, it's Us working through God that influences how God operates and how God works. God works through either Love or hate. Is the voice of your God that you hear a Voice of Love or is it a voice of hate?

That, more than anything else dictates what your God is usually like, as God is different at different times. I hope you're beginning to see, your God or god is your inner voice working to tell you how to act and react to each other through god (God). God is Us, All of Us. We work through our inner voices and how we influence each other. This is how God or god works. This is how We work through God (god), whether it be a God of Love or a god of fear and hate.

Therefore God is always moving. God is always changing because of this movement. That means that God is not rigid. God is forever changing just as life changes, constantly and always. That is the forever in God. God is Us, All of Us, together and always changing to meet Our needs. The only quality about God that remains the same is the way in which We work with each other through our emotions. If we can control our emotions, we control God. If we can't control our emotions, god controls us.

The whole point I'm trying to make here is, what controls your emotions, you or your food? The evidence that I've presented in these books is that your diet can control your emotions more than you realize. Carboholics are controlled by their emotions, with their diets and not common sense, whereas ketogenics control their emotions themselves with their diets. The difference is carboholics are controlled by their diet whereas ketogenics control their diet and hence, control their emotions.

That may be why it's easier for us to add the kindness to make life easier. (This comes from our instinct to go back to save our family members while running for our lives from calamity or predators.) This desire to save the family in our Paleolithic days gradually turned into a benevolent civilization when as learned to cultivate wheat. The wheat itself made it malevolent.

God changed at that time. God became more of a God of love instead of just a god of fear. This God of Love's influence grew with the emergence of the church and organized religion. That's also how religions try to control the masses. Most western religions use fear for that control, whereas eastern religions use the consequences of actions cycle or karma, to control the masses.

As this cycle exists today, it controls little greed for money, nor does it do much to control the greed for power and it only controls those who fear god. It's the fear of punishment that controls this god, thinking that will prevent the wrongdoing in the first place. By leaving in the god of fear and anger, they're hoping the fear part would easier control the masses. Thus the mantra *"Fear God and you fear nothing else"* was born. This is the foundation of western religions that have a supreme being, like Hebrew, Islam, Christianity, and almost all modern religions, like LDS and Jehovah's Witnesses (two religions based on Christianity except they don't believe in the Trinity).

Being based on Christianity also means that they're based on the Hebrew beliefs about there being a supreme being that controls all. The problem is, there isn't. They don't understand that God isn't 1 rigid supreme being that controls all. God is multiple beings acting unified to create and change our own manifestations in each of our own little worlds. This can completely alter our perception of how God controls our lives because all of us are God if we're united in Love. But then all of us are god as well if we're united in fear.

The question one must ask themselves, in this case, is what God or god do you want to be part of? Do you want a rigid god of fear to control your life or do you want an all-inclusive God of Love, assisting you in that control? This points to why it's important to believe in the God of Love. The God of Love has learned to go past the risk/reward phase of humanity to the *"do it because it's better for humanity"* phase. This is a major step in conquering fear, as it's fear that drives evil. It just happens that fear is driven by hunger. The risk/reward cycle is also driven by hunger.

Many times that's why iniquity happens in the first place. It's the *risk/reward* cycle that promotes it. Too often the risk of achieving the reward is a stronger desire than that of their fear of God (especially when that god doesn't appear to discipline or reward anyone for their actions). This belief can be a fallacy when one doesn't fear God. Without the fear, there's no reason for discipline negating the need for the belief, in turn negating the need for religion. This is the inherent problems with western religions that use this risk/reward cycle for its discipline.

This places much more importance on the diet, as that's the only thing that can replace religion. We've always used the fear of religion to control our emotions, but the real control was from our diet of carbohydrates. Since we've lost that risk/reward cycle that religion used to use to control our emotions, our emotions have gotten out of control. The only way we can truly control them is to control what we eat. This, in turn, gives us control over our hormones and emotions, putting us in control of God instead of a god controlling of us. (Currently, that god is Monsanto and its industries.)

Because most Christians are blind to the real motivation behind any iniquity, they believe them to be acts of God, because their God never changes and he uses these acts as rewards or punishment. He just disciplines and rewards. They're caught trying to solve today's problems, with yesterday's solutions, but their solutions are eons old. They're old as civilization, dating to 2000 years ago, for Christians, 1400 Years for Muslims. 10,000 years for Hebrews (their Bible dates to 10 century BCE). That's about how long each of these religions has existed, all out of the seed of Abraham. The God he Worshiped has become the God of these peoples. It's the very same God worshipped differently in every manner, except one, he is a rigid God in their eyes, one whose ideas never change and this is what directs us all to conflict.

They called the hated god the devil 2000 - 8000 years ago. We know now, the hated god isn't the devil, it's us. We are God, so we get to take the responsibility for how our God lives and works within us. This is why we have to protect how we think and work through God. When we create fear, hate, and anger, it drives violence because the only way to fight fear is with anger. Too often it becomes too easy to turn that anger into antagonism and this is where the danger lies. We're experiencing that now. God has all of a sudden turned into an angry god. (I refuse to capitalize the god of hate, as that isn't the God of Love). I believe that God is supposed to be synonymous with Love. That means that God can't hate, as hate has no place in God of Love.

Once all of these religions realize that God is not rigid, but moving, always moving and always changing, that changes Gods perspectives completely. No longer can we ASSUME what God is thinking. What God is thinking about is always changing, and that will never change. That means that God is forever changing to meet our new and different values and needs. That means that God is never the same God to everyone or everything, nor are God's values and needs to everyone. As man's needs and values change, Gods needs and values change also. How we shape that change only history will tell.

I know what you're thinking, needs? Does God have needs? Uh…yeah. God has needs. The Bible says that God needs our love. That's what the first commandment is, "to Love God with all your heart and mind." If God is all of us, doesn't that mean if we're to love God, we're to love everybody? Isn't that what Jesus was trying to teach us, to love one another as if you love yourself? The point I'm trying to make is that God needs love and that means that We need love because We are God. The Bible says that exactly when it tells us what God's name is. It is I AM. That means that I AM God. That also means that You are God along with everybody else.

As life changes, God changes along with it. God's attitudes change because God is Life. Life forever changes so God forever changes. That changes everything. All of a sudden it's OK to be gay or lesbian, bisexual or transsexual. It's OK to be a different race. None of us are exactly alike as we have to accept the differences in others to be part of a God of Love. God accepts all and loves all. *Accepts*, is the key word here. If God accepts the differences in others, we accept it because we are God and we are always right, because God is always right. That points to your choices, it's your choice to work through a God of Love or a god of hate. Which do you think would make life easier?

God is testing us right now with a possible anti-Christ in the oval office running the free world. An antichrist is a god of hate and our President used a god of hate to promote his candidacy. That makes him a being who uses a god of hate to achieve his goals. This is the definition of an antichrist, one who uses fear and hate to achieve goals of greed and power. This representation of what we see as a god, right now, is full of hate and anger, and he uses that fear and hates to drive the masses into frenzies of anger and antagonism. It's the god of hate that could ruin this country…..and subsequently, the world.

There are those who say they believe in God but deep down inside, they really don't. They think they do but they don't display the traits of someone who truly follows God. They display the traits of someone who follows a god, but only for convenience purposes. They want to believe in the idea of going to heaven because they're afraid of death. They believe in a corporate god, a god of greed and acquisition, a god of possessions and power, not in a God of Love. Those who say they believe in God but really don't, believe this fantasy of God as a punisher or rewarder who's going to rescue them from their iniquities at the end of their mortal lives.

This behavior is also indicative of a carbohydrate diet and the risk/reward cycle, which brings me to my point in this book series. Glucose is an addiction that builds dependence as it makes you hungry, to begin with, and the more you eat, the hungrier you get. That makes this food (which has always been a staple) very dangerous to eat now and stay healthy. Because the hunger cycle is part of the risk/reward cycle, Monsanto's done a very good job of making it very addictive. It's far more addictive now than it's ever been in history.

God being "almighty who controls everything" that watches over us all the time is only partially true. This belief is only partly true, in that God does see everything, but not through one being.

God sees everything only because God is everyone. Only all beings can see all things, therefore God cannot be a single being, but multiple beings acting as an entity of its own.

Modern Christians believe their God to be a supreme being to give them a father figure who can scold them for their iniquities. (All of the iniquities involve greed for money or power of some sort.) Without punishment for wrongdoing, there's no reward for not doing wrong. This is the basis of our ethics. Some have it. Too many don't.

Christians feel that they should be punished for their evil-doing, not knowing that the evil-doing in itself is going to end up punishing them by the karma their actions generated. If they knew that in the first place, they'd think twice before they acted. Usually, it's greed for money or greed for power that makes people misuse the guidelines that God has given them through the Hebrew Nation on how to treat each other. Instead of treating each other like God asks us to, too many supposedly Christians treat each other with suspicion, fear, and hate. These are the actions of a god of fear and hate and not the God they profess to believe in. This makes most Christians liars by holding onto their belief in a rigid god of fear.

I mentioned that our guidelines or ethics were given to us by a Hebrew god, which is where they come from. All of our values are based on the Ten Commandments from the old testament to the Bible and Torah. These values also show up in the Quran.

(This risk/reward system grew out of our Paleolithic past when running from predators was more important than helping the young or old to keep up with the rest of the group. This is basically what our two-party system has worked out to be, now. One party wants to keep running from the "predators", whereas the other party wants to help those who can't run as fast.) Who's right?

That depends on where your risk/reward cycle plays. Does it play in the carbohydrate domain or does it play in the ketogenic domain? The carbohydrate domain plays with hunger whereas the ketogenic domain doesn't. Hunger may be one of our biggest influences when it comes to greed as hunger is a threat to security.

If one can control their hunger cycle, they have better control of the security, as their hunger can't pose a threat to the security. Most Christians are too wrapped up in their addiction to realize this. Most don't even know that it's the carbs that create and maintain this hunger cycle. This makes the carbs implicit in the iniquity that goes on throughout the world.

Christians need the risk/reward cycle to end their life cycle because of their fear of the unknown. This fear is a direct result of spreading fear and anger throughout their lifetime. All they experience in their own lives, in dealing with God (dealing with everybody in general), is the manner in which they treat other people. The way they treat others is the way in which they will be treated, with either fear and anger or Love. This is how life ends also, with fear or Love.

Those who fear, treat other people with fear. It's what they know best. Often it's the only manner in which they know how to treat each other. It's this treatment or others that's displays, Gods, works within all of us. Those who treat others with Love, Understanding, and Respect worship the God of Love. Those who treat others with hate, suspicion, and disdain worship the god of fear and hate. That gives Us the power to manifest how God is going to act and react to any situation. That gives Us the power to be God. Hence We are God.

Once you realize that the unknown is the fullness of God and all God wants is Love, you realize that the unknown is Love, it's a loving embrace of all those who have gone on before us, and when you look at death in that manner, in the same manner, that you treat everyone during life, with love and respect, you discover that there really is nothing at all to fear, except for the fear itself.

That's because of what God needs. The only thing that God needs is our love. God needs it because we need it. The reason most fear death is because they fear to go to hell. Here's a new flash; there is no hell except for what you make. That means that you make your own hell or heaven by the way you influence other people and the impact you've had within the workings of God, day in and day out, throughout your life.

Working with a God of Love leads you to an afterlife of Love. Leading a life of fear, hate and anger are going to lead you to an afterlife of that same fear and hate that you professed your whole life long. What you do throughout your life dictates how your death will manifest itself after you die, so it's your choice what you experience after you die. You can experience Love and all of Gods wonders, or you can experience fear and hate when you die. How you live your life, is what you experience in death. You can expect to see that "on the other side" after you die.

Yet too many old faiths hang on to the traditional reward/punishment cycle and they do this with a rigid God, one that never changes, not even from when man's needs were far from what they are now. They do this to control the faith. That is not the way God works. Instead of the faith controlling the people in my world, the people control the faith. Only in this way can God be forever changing and loving.

But today's religions worship a rigid God, one that never changes, not even from when man's needs were far from what they are now. (That's due to their carb diet, which is as old as civilization.) Their rigid beliefs date back to the cradle of civilization as well, as they still believe strictly, every word in the Bible or Quran, or Torah tells them, about how their faith started and continued until today, never changing.

This has led most foundational and Evangelistic faiths to believe in age-old customs and beliefs that were valid in their time, but they are, no longer. Time is the one thing that God can't control. Time changes everything, as time represents life, forever changing. That means that God can't control the change, only time can. That gives Time power over God because time always changes and makes God change.

If time is more powerful than God, should we worship time or should we just use it as wisely as possible? Maybe that's the best way to worship God. That puts us in control of time, which in turn puts us in control of God. Finally, something that makes sense. That means, we can't assume what God wants, as God is us. Saying "what God wants" is code for what that person wants. They just can't take responsibility for saying it themselves, they have to say 'it wants God wants', putting the responsibility on God and not themselves for their choice.

That is one thing we individually have as God, as God has given us that right. It has to do with the right to live. To live you must make choices. Life is nothing but a string of choices, whether good or bad. That is the right to live, the right to make choices. It's those choices we make as God that is written about in the history books of the future. How one's history is written, is dictated by how they live their life. Did they live their lives through a God of Love or a god of fear and hate?

Hence, We are God. You, I, and everyone else in our world, We are All God. We make up what we want to see expressed in God. Whether it's good or bad, it's what we want. And because We are God, We know what God wants, whether good or bad. How we express our will, shows how we want our God to be, whether it's a god of hate or a God of Love. We all live, love-hate and work through God as God is always moving through us making us make our choices to do such. It's always our choices that makeup what God wants, whether we Love it or hate it.

The exciting thing is our world is growing and that means that God is growing. What used to be our whole world 1,000s of years ago was minute compared to today's world. We live in a much bigger world now. (Even though the size of the world hasn't changed, our view of the world and our perspectives have changed. What we see now is much more than what we experience in the past.) Our world is forever growing. That is the definition of life, the right and ability to grow and as growth means life and life are really Love, that means that growth can only happen through Love. If you want to use fear, hate, and anger, don't expect too much growth.

Will We make God Good, filled with Love? Or will we make god evil, filled with fear, hate, and anger? Which God would you prefer? Would you rather have growth? Or would you rather have stagnation and death? God or god can only manifest their kind of world that we live in. I know which one I want. hate is driven by a carb diet. Love doesn't have to be. All that means is that Love is saner than fear, hate, and anger. Fear hate and anger are driven by cycles of hunger. Love is driven by cycles of inclusion, collaboration and the improvement of our society itself.

As life changes, God changes. God's attitudes change because God is Life. Life forever changes so God forever changes. That really does change everything. Can you believe in a changing God? I do. My God accepts and loves everything and everybody, simply because everybody is God, whether filled with hate and fear or filled with Love. The one filled with Love is much better for your health and thus, much healthier for God and that's why I choose a God of Love to live through. What kind of God/god do you live through?

Do you live through the same corporate god that most people live through? It's a god of greed. It's the god that says he who dies with the most toys wins. Does that sound like a very wise god? It's this god of greed that leads to mistrust of your fellow man and the rest of god. This makes having anything to do with this god of greed means dealing with mistrust and deceit. That sounds too much like dealing with a god of mistruth and lies. This is not the god of an ethical people. This is the god of people who operate with fear and anger. It's also a god of people addicted to a hunger cycle. This is not the kind of god I want in my world. I can't believe this kind of god. My God isn't that destructive.

I don't believe in god. I Live through God because I am God, at least a part of God. I believe that was Christ's Word that He was trying to spread 2000 years ago and that's why I follow the Word. I believe in the Word, for I am part of the Word. Thank you, Jesus! (Have you ever wondered why we capitalize the first letter of our names like we do God's?)

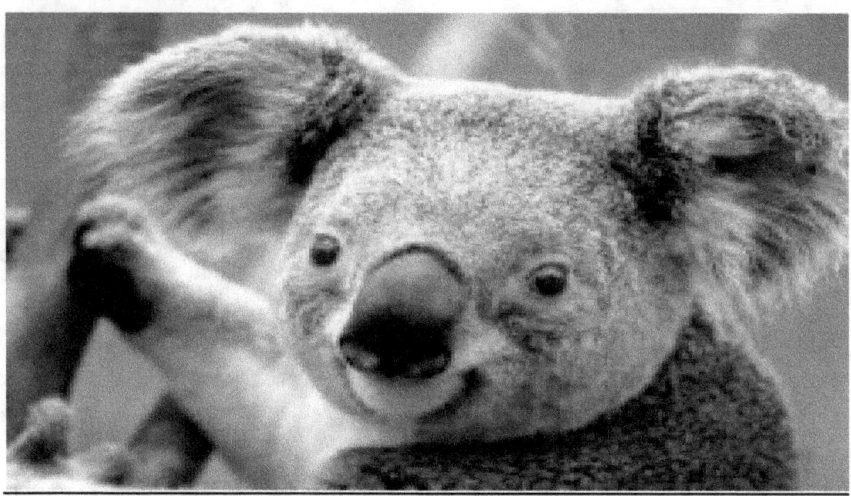

Chapter 18

Evolution of the Human Diet

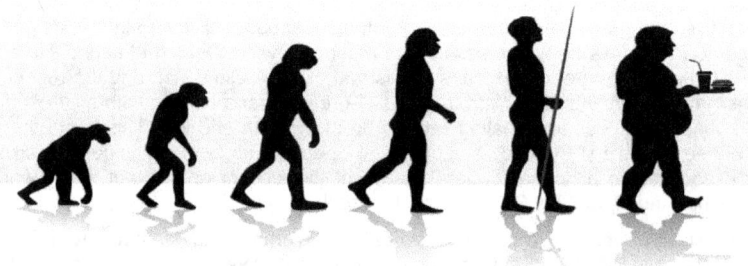

HOW OUR ADDICTION STARTED

There was a time in our evolutionary history when our species ate pretty much nothing but carbs, as we were all herbivores while we were apes and chimpanzees. Although chimps are omnivorous, they prefer fruit over anything else. This is probably due to the sugar content in fruit and probably where our addiction to carbs started. However, as we evolved, our diet evolved along with us due to our need for more protein to feed our hungry brains, so we needed to alter our diet to meet that need. As our ancestors left the trees and moved onto the savannah in Africa, we were growing smarter and to meet that demand, our brains needed to grow. For our brains to grow, we needed more protein and we found it in the animal life that was around us. Although this food may have been harder to find, it was easier to eat, once obtained. But we also found grains on the savannah, they were really easy to pick

Because it was harder to hunt rather than gather, our brains needed to adapt. This was basically our next step to modern man. It's this adaptation that's the hallmark of homo Sapiens. We're able to adapt better than any other species, ever, and it's this ability to adapt that's made us as strong and smart as we are. Homo Sapien is Latin for wise man, so maybe we should be labeled as homo Adaptare or adaptable man as that's the true reason our species has thrived and grown as well as it has. The true reason for our intelligence is that we have the ability to adapt as much as we do. This is why I think that homo Sapiens, who have now interbreed with most other homo species, throughout our evolution and incorporated them into our genome, have earned the right to a new title of homo Adaptare. We truly are a species apart, even from homo Sapiens. It was hybridization along with our change to a higher protein diet, that enabled our brains to grow so much.

Homo Sapiens were hunter-gatherers. We as homo Adaptares are neither hunters nor gatherers anymore. We've adapted into controllers of our environment while becoming destroyers of our physiology. (That's due to our diet, which I'll get into later.) We're the first species with the ability to do this and it's this one trait of our species that sets us apart as much as it does. This one trait has made us the smartest mammals in earth's history. Other species may have lasted longer than homo Sapiens, but their development didn't allow them the latitude that homo Sapiens had the luxury of enjoying, with the expanded Temporal and Parietal lobes in their brains, allowing them the ability of speech and better navigation. This is what makes us adaptable. This is what's also allowed us to advance exponentially more than other homo species in the short time we've been here. 200,000 years is a blink of an eye in evolutionary terms. Especially when you take into account our ancestors started out of the trees 6-7 million years ago and our homo genus started around 3-4 million years ago.

Neanderthals came out of Africa as homo Erectus and thrived for 400,000 years in Europe, Asia and even into the Americas. There's Neanderthal DNA in all of us except for those on the continent of Africa due to the interbreeding of homo Sapiens and Neanderthals. Our species, homo Sapiens came out of Africa roughly 200,000 years later and ultimately absorbed the Neanderthals DNA into our DNA as modern man, through interbreeding. A characteristic that I find interesting in the Neanderthal is that their brains were larger than ours, yet they didn't have the capacity for speech because of the shape of their craniums. Their brains weren't as evolved as much as the homo Sapiens' cranium was and the portion of the brain that regulates speech couldn't form in the homo Erectus cranium as it had in the homo Sapiens'.

This lack of speech, though, didn't prevent the Neanderthals from thriving in their environments in Europe and Asia. How were they able to survive for so long without the ability of speech? It seems to me that their inability to communicate as well as homo Sapiens, prohibited them from evolving as the homo Sapiens did.

It was our transformation to life on the savannah that aided our brains more than our life in the trees, as the grassland foods were a lot more diversified, increasing the protein in our diet. Grains come with more protein than fruits, but they still have the glucose, so we started eating grains as well as meat from the small game we were able to find and this added to the protein in our diet allowing our brains to develop more than that of the homo Erectus, our closest ancestor whose diet was limited to meat and very little grains.

Our transformation from herbivores to omnivores manifested more, somewhere close to when our transformation from ape to human was in the Homo Habilis species when we started eating more meat as a species, whether it was because our brains required more protein, while learning how to live in the savannah or whether our brains grew because of our change in diet, it's easy for me to see that when homo Habilis was alive, it started eating more meat which means that there was more protein in our diet allowing both our brains and bodies to grow larger. This would evolve into our healthiest diet in the Homo Erectus species. This species evolved larger brains, as had the Neanderthals.

Even many the earliest homo Sapiens like Cro-Magnon man[2] had larger cranial capacities than those of modern man, yet they were Homo Sapiens. This is directly due to their diet higher in protein than carbohydrates. It's also due to the fact that they went hungrier more often than what we have since we first cultivated grasses. This absence of food or going hungry is what we call fasting today and it's been found to be the healthiest state in which one can keep their body because of the growth hormones and anti-oxidants that it generates.

I'll bet that you didn't know that your body produces growth hormones when you're hungry. They enable your body to heal itself from virtually anything. This state also ramps up your production of anti-oxidants so high, you couldn't eat enough anti-oxidant foods in a lifetime to match what you can produce, on your own, in one day simply by going without food. This is why fasting has been a part of health care for the last 2500 years. It' just been forgotten about recently when we discovered that we could create a drug to treat anything (That's where our current health crisis is, in the assumption that a drug will cure anything when it will only treat a patient and nothing more. That in itself leads only to more and more treatments and never a valid cure. That's because there's no money in a cure, as cures are final. so the money is in treatment, ongoing treatment. The cure I propose in these books is in your diet. Something that costs you next to nothing to change, Actually, this diet will save you millions of dollars in medical costs.)

The evolution of Homo Sapiens allowed their craniums to evolve in a manner that allowed them to incorporate speech into their society, affording them a much quicker path to modern man. Neanderthals didn't have this luxury, yet they lasted for over 400,000 years. Modern man has only been around for maybe 200,000 years at most. Some archaeologists still believe we've only been about 100,000 yrs, although fossils have been found in NW Africa that is dated at over 330,000 years old. DNA has confirmed the age of this species as having the earliest DNA that is still in modern man today. As homo Sapiens have evolved over our 200k-300k years, our brains have grown smaller, due to the grain diet our species has been on for that time.

Grains have a tendency to shrink the brain and since our civilization has been cultivating, surviving on, and using these grains (many time as a wedge) to control people with, it's no wonder that they've had as much influence that they've had, on our physiology, society, and most importantly, our brains. Our bodies benefited from the added protein, which forced our bodies to grow taller along with our bipedalism, but our brains benefited more due to the easily obtained glucose to fuel it as well as the added protein to enable it to grow as well. It was our migration to the savannah that increased our diet of protein, allowing our brains to grow and evolve faster than that of homo Erectus in Europe. It was the grains of the savannah that promoted the development of our craniums to allow to develop speech and it was this ability to communicate better than advanced homo Sapiens so much quicker than the homo Erectus Neanderthal. We lived right alongside homo Erectus, hunted with them, ate with them and even breed with them, eventually incorporating them into our own genome. Yet, for 400,000 years, they survived without the ability for verbal speech.

This is why homo Sapiens advanced as fast as they did. As homo Sapiens, we are very adaptable, more so than any other species. Glucose is the primary food of the brain and it this glucose that's enabled our species to become so adaptable. Our brains can work on ketones, but glucose is the preferred fuel and I think that the grasses in the savannah allowed our species to develop our brains quicker than that of the homo Erectus Neanderthals in Europe and Asia as the climate was much more severe there and didn't allow the growth of the grasses until the climate warmed closer to that of what it is today. Due to Neanderthals' inability to obtain the mental capacity as that of homo Sapiens, their evolution was stunted until homo Sapiens entered their world and started interbreeding with them and eventually incorporated them into our species. In Africa, homo Erectus evolved into homo Sapiens, yet in Europe, they didn't. This is due to the fact that the grains have the ability to shrink our brains, however, their brains may have still worked better on glucose than on the ketones at that time in our evolution. I can see where the addition of grasses in our diet is ultimately what shrank the brain to make it smaller than that of homo Erectus and even earlier homo Sapiens like the Cro-Magnon.

Without the capacity for speech that homo Sapiens acquired, Neanderthals still had the capacity to survive the harshest environments and thrive for as long as they did, yet just like every other species homo Sapiens have come across, they too eventually succumbed to us when we absorbed them into our species by interbreeding with them [1]. Most species we just killed off to survive. Extinctions took place on every continent after a man showed up. It wasn't until the 20th century AD that we started to recognize our faulty control of the environment and what we were doing to wipe out completely, other species on our planet. Homo Sapiens have had a tendency to kill off many other species to extinction throughout our history. Wherever homo Sapiens have propagated, larger game animals disappeared. After our emergence on every continent, the larger species of mammals disappeared, due to our hunger and superiority. Our hunger has driven us to our current status as supreme ruler of our realm by forcing us to feed that hunger. Only recently have we started to care about our environment and the ecosystems that go with it, yet still we're having problems reconciling our hunger cycle and ecology. It seems, our hunger cycle wins out every time.

Hunger is the driving force of every species and homo Sapiens are least immune to this phenomenon due to our history of a carbohydrate diet. Our diet has transformed from this carbohydrate/herbivore diet when we were apes to an omnivorous diet as we left the trees to forage in the grasslands. It was during this time that we started eating more meat and fat because it provides more protein for the body and brain. It was during this time that our brains started to grow more, and in order to keep our brains growing more than previously, we needed more protein to keep up with the growth. This was also the beginning of our species growing taller so we could hunt for the game on the savannah. This is due to the higher protein content in the grains than that of the fruit that we ate while up in the trees. This higher protein content not only allowed us to grow us taller, it developed our brains faster, much faster. Our migration onto the savannah allowed us the protein needed to grow our brains larger while still providing enough glucose to allow our brains to work more efficiently.

Because grains were so easy to eat, we learned to cultivate them and made them the majority of our diet. This allowed our brains to work better because glucose is the fuel that the brain uses most and grains readily break down into glucose. (It's so important to the brain, that our bodies developed the ability to create our own glucose, through the process of gluconeogenesis.) Ketones are fuel for the body as well as the brain but there is still a portion of the brain that needs glucose. That's why our bodies have the ability to generate its own glucose. This ensures that we don't need to eat it because when we do, we get sick. We don't get sick right away, that takes years to manifest, but the diseases will manifest. It's written in the science of digestion and there's nothing we can do about it if we continue to eat it. This may be how man has learned to survive longer than any other species, as well. For all the good that carbs do for the body, they still damage it.

I attribute our superiority to our hunger cycle because that cycle drives everything. That means that I have to attribute our speedy evolution to carbs. It is carbs after all that create the hunger cycle, and thus they're responsible for our evolution. Our drive to have more to satiate our hunger cycle also drives greed for more territory, money, and power to satisfy that hunger cycle. This is and has been what's driven a modern man to be superior to all other species. This is why I contend that we've evolved again, from homo Sapiens into homo Adapatares, adaptable man. Our next adaptation will be in outer space, as we now have the ability to go one step further by ending our need for carbohydrates. Our bodies have the ability to generate its own glucose, so I contend that we don't need carbs at all. All we really need is protein and fat, which our bodies have evolved to digest easier than carbs. Carbs require that you eat a lot for the same number of calories of what you can get from fat. That in itself makes fat a much easier to eat and higher octane food than what you can get from carbs. Since fat requires much less quantity to supply us with the needed energy, it only makes sense that fat will make a much better food for when we are in space and can't carry that much food with us.

That's what makes a ketogenic diet so important, it doesn't come with sugar or glucose. Both of those are completely foreign to a ketogenic diet and that's what makes the ketogenic diet so important. Due to this lack of glucose, it lacks one other very important factor, the hunger cycle. This is the deadliest factor of a carbohydrate diet. The fact the glucose creates hunger makes it a very deadly substance. It also guarantees that those who continue this cycle will get sick in the future and up addicted to a cycle of medication to combat those illnesses. This is also why a ketogenic diet is too important. It's the next step in our evolution. It's this step that will prepare us for space travel and space is the only environment we haven't mastered fully.

As I've previously stated, man cannot survive in space on a carbohydrate diet because they require so much food to sustain our need for calories. A diet of fat and protein will be necessary to travel to the stars, simply due to the lack of food needed to supply the necessary calories for survival. The other, more important factor in this equation is hunger. No carbs mean no hunger. How much easier do you think space travel will be without a hunger cycle? I'll give you a clue right now, it'll be much, much easier. With hunger cycles driving all abhorrent behavior, doing away with them will transform our species into a species that operates almost solely with our brains. I can actually see smaller humans in the future with larger craniums and brains making us even smarter than we can ever imagine.

I believe that this is happening in our galaxy as I write this. According to astrophysics every galaxy and a black hole in the center of it and every black hole bends time and space because of the intense gravity inside the black hole. Astrophysics claims that time speeds up inside these black holes. I contend that if time speeds up, so does evolution. That means that if there is life near our center, it's had to evolve more rapidly than ours, due to its proximity to the center of our galaxy. That tells me that any civilization is going to be advanced much further than ours also. That also tells me that the closer you get to the center of our galaxy, the more advanced societies you'll find, along with the most advanced species. Could these species be the little men with big heads that we often see as aliens? Could they be traveling from deep inside our galaxy? Have they evolved that far? The only way we may know this is to look closer inside our own galaxy toward that black hole. Can we find more advanced civilizations on other worlds closer to the center of our galaxy? What will these discoveries tell us when we find them? My mind is just starting to fill with questions.

This explains a lot. If time and evolution does speed up nearer the center of the galaxy, there have to be more advanced civilizations than ours and if evolution brings about smaller beings with larger brains, that would explain why aliens who visit our planet are as small they are. We can learn from that. These creatures travel through space, yet they're smaller creatures than what we are, leading me to believe that as our species evolves we will grow smaller with larger brains. I see this as the only manner in which we will be able to leave this planet. We have to make ourselves like them, bigger brained with smaller bodies to sustain us while traveling in space. I believe that this will be our evolution into homo Adaptare, a smaller much more intelligent species. When we do evolve into that, we won't be able to sustain ourselves on carbs at all, and because of that our diet will have to be fats and proteins only.

This all points to the next evolution of our diets, a ketogenic diet. None of our species live in trees anymore, nor do we live on the savannah. As we evolved, so did our diet into one that's most beneficial for the homo Sapien. Now, it's time to evolve our diet once again to one that will be most beneficial for homo Adaptare, which can only be a diet completely void of carbs. That's where the ketogenic diet fits into our world. Only a ketogenic diet will allow our species to evolve to our next evolutionary species. The ketogenic diet feeds our bodies exactly what they need and nothing more. The ketogenic diet allows for fasting without stress, which forces the body to heal itself without the need for medication. Fasting also produces the same hormones that allow for more brain growth. These are the same hormones you get from exercising and points to the fact why exercising and fasting is so healthy for us. It's what our ancestors went through, to allow them to evolve quicker than the other species. As our ancestors stood taller, our gate came easier and we used much fewer calories to move, than we previously used, allowing more protein to be dedicated to our brains allowing them to grow faster than other species. As we lost our hair and started perspiring, we obtained the ability to outrun our game because our bodies could cool themselves when our prey couldn't. This action of running on empty stomachs set our bodies up to produce the growth hormones that our brains needed as well as our bodies, to make us superior. It was the production of these growth hormones combined with the increase of protein in our diets that allowed us to grow our brains and propel our species into the evolutionary step, homo sapiens. Now, it's time to move into our next evolutionary step; Homo Transformare.

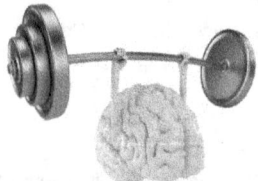
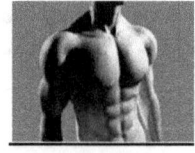

<u>AFTERTHOUGHTS</u>

I may not be a doctor, but I can still add up evidence. I've accomplished little due to the disabilities that I've had to live with for the majority of my adult life. Prior to this book, I've accomplished little, especially in the last 32 years.

I started writing this book for my mother when I published my website, Save Your Dignity, and continued writing post after post after post of what I found to be devastating news that I thought the whole world should know. So I added more and more until my book filled out. My mother was fighting cancer for the third time. Both my sisters are diabetic and I was on my way to being diabetic. My father was borderline diabetic for a number of years. He still takes medication to inhibit his own body's production of glucose. (Unfortunately, this is the only clean glucose in his body and points to the desire of our pharmaceutical industry to keep us addicted to their drugs.) This is all because we've always eaten bread, pasta, cereals, pastries and all other grain foods we could find. We thought we were supposed to. It was recommended. Weren't grains at the bottom of the food pyramid for 50 years?

I figured this out and I don't have a degree more than an A.A. degree and a digital electronics diploma. Yet, because of my disability, I was motivated enough to try to learn how I could retrieve that which I had lost over 30 years ago to a drunk driver running a red light.

I used to have learning disabilities that were completely unrecognized 40-50 years ago when I was young. I was just labeled as a rambunctious typical boy. I walked home from school the first recess of the first day of my second year. I missed the part where the teacher said she was going to review what we learned the previous year. So at first recess, I walked home, only to have my mother march my right back.

My reason, which I thought valid, was that I wasn't learning anything new. It was the same stuff that we learned last year and I thought, I've got better things to do than to sit here and relearn what I already know, so I walked home, where I had better things to do.

I didn't realize this, at the time. Neither did my mother. But it was a sign of my ADD. This ADD that I was inflicted with, I can see now was a direct result of my diet, which happened to be a diet high in carbohydrates. Actually, it was very high in carbs. Mom thought that's what she was supposed to feed us. It's what she fed her siblings when she had to take care of them after her father died, when she was 12 and her mother had to go to work to support the family.

At that time, this food that she unwittingly addicted us to was not nearly as dangerous as it is today. Today it's been completely modified to feed more people out or less acreage of land used to grow the crop, and this modification has made this food dangerous to consume, now. The same parcel of land that used to produce a dozen loaves of bread now produces hundreds of loaves of bread. My question is how can the same land still pack as many nutrients in hundreds of loaves, as it did with just a few dozen?

I contend that it can't. I contend that it's this mass production of this wheat, that's easier for the farmer, seed companies, and agrochemical companies to make a buck from, that's killing America and the rest of the world that consumes it. It may be giving pharmaceutical companies a booming business, but it's killing everyone who can't break the hold of its addiction.

What I've learned in the last 6 months could fill volumes. To me, what's amazing is that I've retained a much greater portion of what I've learned than I ever have in the past. This is solely due to the diet I've been on for the last 2½ years, 6 months in particular.

What makes me qualified to make the statements that I've declared in the book, is the fact that I've lived through it. I've been through the worst that this grain and food can put anyone through. Spending a month in a coma due to a drunk driver is the worst expression that this addiction can do to anyone except kill them. In some cases, the latter of the two is preferential as the former leaves its victim with life-changing injuries that are, most of the time, irreversible. I get to live with hemiplegia and it affects everything I do. Never-the-less, I kicked the addiction and I was addicted in the worst way.

My thinking is if I can kick it anyone should be able to. But then I realize that there are millions if not billions who are addicted worse than I ever was. This is evident in the obesity, diabetic, CVD, cancer and dementia epidemics that are so prevalent today. I also think, that if this diet can do this much to straighten me out, as bad as shape as I was in, to level out my emotions that have already been adjusted by a severe closed head injury, why couldn't it do the same thing for anyone else, whose brain damage may be different than mine, but never-the-less, still exists? Because of the nature of this food, everyone who's consumed it for any length of time has brain damage.

Although their damage is quite different from mine, it's still brain damage and I know firsthand what brain damage does to a person. I know what severe brain damage does. I know what it's like to forget things. I know what it's like having trouble remembering things. I know what it's like to have mood changes that are completely out of character. Sounds a lot like Alzheimer's doesn't it? I can empathize with those losing their memories, as well as those who have to take care of them. I've been there. I've done that, more than once or twice or even three times. I'm well experienced with it.

That in itself gives me the authority to state what I've stated throughout this book. Does one need a degree to see what this food is doing to us physically and well as what it's doing to our society? A little research was all I need to see the damage being inflicted on the American people. The studies aren't that hard to find. You just have to look for them. I just can't help but wonder, were these studies hidden on purpose? Did an industry, more interested in their bottom line, shade the reports of these studies, in an attempt to keep them stifled?

If an industry links itself with another industry that benefits each other, from the harm that one industry does, does that make them accomplices? We know how much the pharmaceutical industry takes from you for the treatment of all the disorders and diseases that this food inflicts upon you. Where would Bayer be without your headaches? Making crop seed? From what you've read here, in article 22 Bayer has already had in hands in both. So has Monsanto, Syngenta, and a few others.

This alarms me and it should you. This is a clear-cut case, that what you don't know, is clearly killing you. To me, it's also the biggest ruse and crime ever committed on the American public. This is a change we must implement immediately if not sooner, but addiction keeps us from doing that.

I thought that was a good reason to write this book....and still, I wonder

WHY ARE THEY STILL PROMOTED LIKE THEY ARE?

WHERE IS THE RECOMMENDATION FROM MORE DOCTORS

TO STOP EATING THEM?

WHERE IS THE RATIONALITY TO IT?
THERE ISN'T ANY EXCEPT FOR ADDICTION AND GREED

WHERE IS THE OUTRAGE?

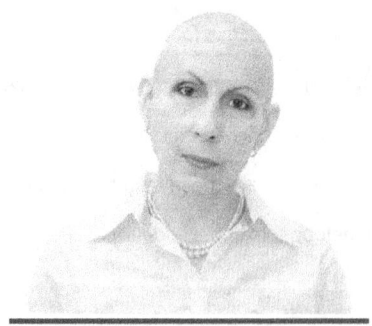

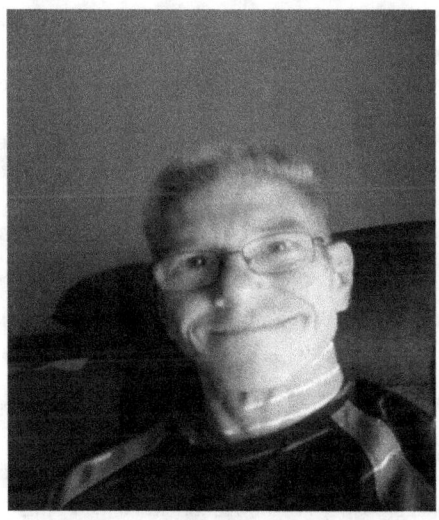

ABOUT THE AUTHOR

<u>No one knows how hard it is for me to appear normal.</u>

Living with hemiplegia.

At one time, I was just as I appeared to be, normal. But that was quite a while ago. Now it's a whole different story. Now, appearing normal is my biggest disability because nothing on the inside of me is as it appears on the outside. It takes more effort and energy than I can ever explain in one document just to appear normal. This statement, for example, I started it 30 minutes ago. I do the best I can and I don't hunt and peck type.

I took typing in the summer of my ninth grade and even though I never had the opportunity to use it, it stuck with me and came back a soon as I started typing again ten years ago. Even though I can type approximately 35 words a minute, I can't do it without errors. But those aren't the only errors that I encounter when I type out a document of this nature. In order for the document for portraying an accurate account of my experiences, feelings, both physical and emotional, and actions, both wanted and unwanted, I constantly need to re-read it as I type it.

Even though my fingers are the most guilty parties, because of the multitude of times I *fat-finger* what I'm trying to type, they're not the main factor in my inability to finish this document in a timely manner. The main factor is my inability to concentrate on what I'm writing about.

For that reason, I'll make a list of the problems that I get to deal with every day and how they impact every aspect of my life that I can think of while I write this, knowing that there will be things that I will miss and need to update at a later time when I remember them.

- **Weakness on right side, all the time**
- **Slowness on right side, all the time**
- **Difficulty with balance, bowel control, vision in right eye, all of the time**
- **Trouble swallowing, hearing, holding on to things, most of the time**

- **The difficulty with memory, (mostly forgetfulness & short-term memory) creating problems with understanding, reasoning, judgment, analyzing, deciding…etc, this happens every time I need to use these skills.**
- **Difficulty maintaining attention, keeping focused and intent to finish projects, and tasks. this happens whenever I need to concentrate on a task or project or focus on getting a job done. I call it neurological ADD.**
- **Think, speak, hear and read dyslexic, and I do it quite often**
- **Easily frustrated because of my inabilities often vocalizing my frustration at the top of my voice without control, hesitation or contemplation, too often**

All of these manifestations evolved after the severe closed head injury I sustained on December 24, 1984, as the result of a drunk driver running a red light and t-boning the car I was riding in. All of these problems are a direct result of the two bruises on my brain and strokes I sustained while comatose for 4 weeks due to that head injury.

For clarification purposes, I've now been working on this document for a little over 3 hours, to get this far and modified it again 5 hrs, later.

I will now try to explain how each of these manifestations affects the different parts of my life;

- **Weakness and slowness on right side**

I suffer from multiple problems all on the right side of my body. These problems include but are definitely not limited to all the troubles and difficulties listed above, such as swallowing, hearing, vision, coordination, the speed of movement, difficulty holding on to things – I'm always dropping things because I can't always feel my grip on them. I live with constant numbness (pins and needles) throughout my whole right side. My wrist always feels like it has a bunch of rubber bands around it that are always pulling and resisting every time I move a muscle. I never feel this on my left side. Every muscle on my right side has this *elastic* feeling.

 My hip replacement is on the right hip probably because of my weakness on that side as well as my hernia, and chronic backache in my lower back on right side. My right-hand flops around every step I take, making it impossible to appear completely normal. Evidence of this can only be seen by an astute observer watching me walk. Whenever I take a step, my right-hand flops around because of the lack of control I have over it. It's like my hand is held on my wrist by a bunch of rubber bands.

Because my right side is slower than my left, my right foot gets caught dragging behind, causing me to stumble. While just casually walking, it takes constant effort to walk without limping, due to the weakness on my right side. This is something that can be easily seen by everybody every time I run. I cannot run without a very noticeable limp. Even walking fast can't be done without a noticeable limp. I don't like walking fast or running because of the problems I've had in the past with balance. A slow and weak right leg won't work properly causing me to stumble or fall almost all of the time. It gets worse the more tired I get. I seldom walk anywhere without stumbling at least once because my right leg gets lazy and won't lift enough to clear the ground.

To avoid any of these problems, it takes an enormous amount of effort and energy. To appear normal, it takes even more effort and energy.

- **Trouble swallowing, hearing, holding on to things**

I often get food caught in my throat when several attempts to swallow it fail. I attribute that to the weakness on my right side no allowing my throat muscles to work as efficiently as the muscles on my left side where I didn't suffer any paralyzes. I have the same problem holding on to things. Because I can't always feel what I'm holding in my right hand, I often drop what I'm holding on to. Things seem to slip through my fingers more than they do with anybody else. Of the hearing problems, I have, only hearing dyslexicly is probably a result of the head injury. The tinnitus I have is probably due to the direct impact of the cars involved in the accidents that caused my injuries and the neck injury I received in another car accident in March of 1993. I say that the dyslexic hearing is a result of my head injury because of the trouble I have with my short-term memory and not being able to recall the meaning of a particular word immediately. I often hear words spoken in reverse order because of this. I often speak my words in reverse order because of the same reason.

- **Difficulty with balance, bowel control, vision in right eye**

My balance is always questionable. Although I don't often lose my balance while on both feet, I can definitely balance on my left leg better than on my right leg. My right leg doesn't have the same amount of strength, endurance or ability to make the slight muscle changes necessary for balance, as my left leg has. That last reason alone is the major reason my balance problems persist.

The most embarrassing problem that I have to deal with because it can sometimes be messy, is my ability to withhold a bowel movement. I attribute this to two factors; 1. That I'm not taking opioid medication anymore and enjoying a diet richer in fruits and vegetables and 2. The weakness of my sphincter muscles to retain the fecal matter in my colon. Knowing that I always have at least two bowels movements each day, usually in the morning, I often have to stay close to a bathroom in the often case that I'll have to go a third or fourth time during the morning hours. I'm constantly making adjustments for this problem alone for there are times when I've had accidents while away from home.

Concerning the vision in my right eye, the clarity of the vision in my right eye grows weaker on its own, sometimes while I'm typing and can visually witness it and sometimes while I'm sleeping and wake up with diminished focus. Sometimes while I'm typing on my computer, I can remember when I realized a diminished focus in my right eye just recently. This wasn't the first time this has happened either. It's happened at least 3 times in the past 15 years. But it's only happened in my right eye.

- **The difficulty with memory, (mostly forgetfulness & short-term memory) creating problems with understanding, reasoning, judgment, analyzing, deciding…etc, this happens every time I need to use these skills.**

This is quite often the most difficult disability to hide as it's always mistaken for stupidity or ignorance when it's almost always a case or either poor judgment and poor decision making due to the inability of my brain to remember and think rationally and in a timely manner. When given time to organize my thoughts, I can prove to be very intelligent. Living without the ability to use this gift has proven to be a downfall for me. This is where my lack of short-term memory has had the most effect on my life. Frustration hits me hard when I try to accomplish something I should be able to do in a specific amount of time and can't. I either mess up the whole project, right at the finish of the project or can't even come close to finishing it in the time I should be able to. This often manifests itself in a very loud and very vulgar output that I have absolutely no control over. Anger issues are a common problem with head injuries of the nature I sustained and I think they're due exactly to this reason.

- **Difficulty maintaining attention, keeping focused and intent to finish projects, and tasks. this happens whenever I need to concentrate on a task or project or focus on getting a job done. I call it neurological ADD.**

This is caused by the same problems as my above problem with judgment and reasoning. When you can't remember what to focus on, how can you focus on anything? Lack of short-term memory impacts a life more than almost anything else. You can never begin to understand what it does to interrupt a life until it happens to you and you have to live with it. These are *"shoes that not everybody gets to walk in"*, meaning only a few can fully understand the impact that no short-term memory has on a life, and half of those that can, are complete invalids. The other half are like me but you can usually see their disabilities. With me, you can't because of the trouble, effort, and energy I put out to look like I'm not disabled. I'm not a complete invalid, just an unseen invalid.

- **Think, speak, hear and read dyslexic often**

I can't remember living with this problem before the head injury so I attribute this disability as well to my neurological damage. Quite often I'll say something dyslexic or hear something dyslexic. Since my thinking is often dyslexic, I often type out my thoughts dyslexic as well. And this doesn't even come close to the number of times I read dyslexic. I see a lot of words and numbers backward or letters within the word out of order. This always causes me to go back and re-read what I just read. I also have to re-read what I just read because I can't remember specific titles or names that I just read. You can only begin to fathom the problems that this can cause while I get to realize the full gamut of problems it actually does cause.

- **Easily frustrated because of my inabilities often vocalizing my frustration at the top of my voice without hesitation or contemplation**

This is the most damaging behavior caused directly by the neurological damage I sustained. Because of my recurring inabilities to complete projects and tasks, and verbalizing my frustrations in a vulgar manner, I'm always left feeling completely shamed from the action that I just presented, completely out of my control. I have no control over this behavior because all of my actions are actually reactions to my inability to complete or complete accurately, any project or task that I work on. It doesn't seem to matter how many times I say the serenity prayer when the frustration of my own inabilities decides to rear its ugly head, I have absolutely no control over how my brain is going to direct me to act. Again, you can only imagine the problems this kind of behavior can cause while I have to realize the full gamut of those problems.

I realize that the problems I experience are problems that a lot of other people experience, but how many people experience all of these problems on a daily basis, on an hourly basis or with the frequency that I do?

These are disabilities connected simply with the neurologic damage I live with, not the other disabilities I live with, in the form disabling pain in my back and groin and sometimes my hip. My back is sore when I get out of bed in the morning until I get back into bed at night, due to the degenerative disc disease and scoliosis I live with. The groin/testicular pain that I live with, comes on every afternoon, as I sit working at my desk. That pain has gotten severe enough to make me nauseous, at times. For twenty years, I've tried every known type of pain relief known to man, including opioid medication, nerve blocks, TENS, SCENAR, acupuncture, massage, topical balms, all without permanent success. The longest relief I've ever gotten was from acupuncture. Most treatments lasted for a couple days, yet sometimes I had limited relief on the third day. This pain is the result of a hernia procedure that left what I was told is my genitofemoral nerve but I'd rather think it's my Ilioinguinal nerve because that's the nerve that branches out to the anterior scrotal nerve, trapped in scar tissue, which is where my pain emanates from.

The hip pain I experience is due to the hip replacement I had two years ago. I experience a stabbing pain when I need to pivot on that hip, that almost takes my leg out from under me. I can walk up to ¼ mile painlessly. Thereafter the pain just keeps getting worse until I can sit or lay down.

My daily pain levels are as follows;

- Back pain – 2 when I wake up, 7 when I get out of bed with jabs to 8 or 9 following certain movements, 4 as I sit at my desk and work, 7 when I get up from my chair, 4-6 as I walk with right leg steps being very painful in the 8-9 range. When I go to bed at night the pain level as around the 4-6 range.

- Testicular/groin pain doesn't present itself until afternoon, depending on how long I need to sit at my desk. When it does it starts out in the 3-5 range increasing steadily in intensity for the rest of the day sometimes to the 8-10 range. (This is the pain that has made me suicidal.)

- Hip pain ranges from 0 when I wake up and get out of bed to 4-6 depending on how much I'm on my feet and walking. Twisting on that leg often provokes a stabbing pain jumping to 8 and often causes me to stumble.

I've now spent 4 hours on day 2 for this document to this point. I've updated it twice today after 3 times yesterday. I ended up spending about 8 hours on it yesterday.

I've had to live with this condition for the last 30 years, some of the pain for 40 years and some for only 20 years. I've searched for cures for my pain to no avail. I've even requested that my right testicle is removed, thinking that if there was nothing there to create the pain, the pain wouldn't exist, but was told time after time that I would have to live with phantom pain. So, I live with pain, sometimes massive pain, the kind that doubles you over.

This last edit took another 3 hours and includes 6-7 updates within the whole document. Even though I've updated this document 5 or 6 times, I'm still not sure I've listed everything necessary. Something keeps nagging at me that I just can't remember. All I can say is that when something affects every aspect of your life, as my neurological problems do mine, it's hard to cover everything in one document.

That was my last edit until I thought of some other things, while at church this morning that I should put in here. Now I just have to remember what they were…oh yes, the testicular pain that usually doesn't start until afternoon; that happens every day except Sundays when it hits me every Sunday in the morning while at church, from having to sit in a pew for hours. Something else came to mind while in church this Morning, sure wish I could remember what it was…Oh yes, OCD, Obsessive Compulsive Disorder. Even though it hasn't been diagnosed, I think I do have a problem with it due to my ADD. Because I have to keep my mind occupied, I have this obsession with the game FreeCell. But then I had my obsessions before the head injury as well. They were just a little more difficult pursuits than what I'm capable of now, like bowling and golf and any other sport I was invited to play. Now, my obsessions are playing card games on the computer when I'm waiting on hold or any other time when I have nothing else to do. Thank God I do that when I'm alone. (FYI- the last edit started over 6 hours ago, but I only spent about 5 hours typing and editing it. That's 6 days so far to complete this.)

Addendum: While not being able to understand any part of a paragraph I read, I re-read it two hours later with complete understanding. Every word that I didn't know before, my mind was able to recall when I read it the second time. My mind had 2 hours to work on the meaning of those words that I couldn't recall earlier without me even thinking about it. Not being able to recall the definitions as I was reading the paragraph, wouldn't allow me to understand it. But, I never would have understood it if I didn't re-read it because I couldn't remember it.

About the author has not been edited due to the fact that I wanted to leave in the errors that were in the original document, so you could see some of the difference in my transformation.

3 years ago after suffering from chronic severe pain for 20 years and taking opioids and anti-depressants for the pain, I had to endure 16 of those years, I decided something had to change. On top of the drugs I was taking for pain, I was taking drugs to counteract the side effects of the opioids and anti-depressants and they weren't killing the pain. The pain was always there, I was overweight from the drugs I was taking and I had had enough, I'd tried every form of pain relief that I could find, from acupuncture 2-3 times a week for years at a time, (that was expensive) to TENS treatments to SCENAR therapy to massage therapy to pain blocks (after I had 5 treatments in 5 months, the doctor refused to inject me again, saying that he'd already injected me with too many steroids), yet the blocks worked for about 30 days, then quit, so I had to go back for another. For 4 years I carried an internal nerve stimulator that I'm sure to cost the insurance plenty of money. That thing worked excellently to mask the pain, but it didn't kill it. The pain was always there under the stimulation however the stimulation masked the pain really well. I used that device so much I wore it out after a couple years and had to have it replaced. The SCENAR is the only device that killed the pain but it didn't last much more than one day. That's why I needed a change, so I changed the last thing I could think of changing, my diet. I quit eating bread. Two weeks later and 10 lbs lighter, magic started to happen. Even though It was the toughest thing I've ever had to accomplish, I quit. I ate no more bread, pasta, crackers, tortillas and potato chips and cut way back on the sodas. Actually, I replaced those with juices, which were better at the time, but I've since quit those also. In the last three years, I've modified my diet to a completely ketogenic diet, concentrating my diet on dairy products (milk mostly). I keep my weight at 10 lbs below my prescribed weight and without eating much of anything all day long, I don't get hungry and I don't get sick. That is the largest blessing of a ketogenic diet. Because I can't afford the treatments and the drugs, I'll keep my ketogenic diet.

The bonus I get from staying on my keto diet is multiple, no inflammation, much, much less pain and believe it or not, no mosquito bites. Mosquitoes like sugar and due to the lack of glucose flowing through my blood, mosquitoes can't smell it on my breath. They smell acetone on my breath, which means that I don't have glucose in my body. I like that benefit. I can remember times when I had over 70 mosquito bites on my body at any one time. Argh, was that itchy. It's so nice to not have to deal with that now. No glucose was all it took. That in itself is as good a reason as any, to give up your addiction and go keto.

Sherri always told me to,

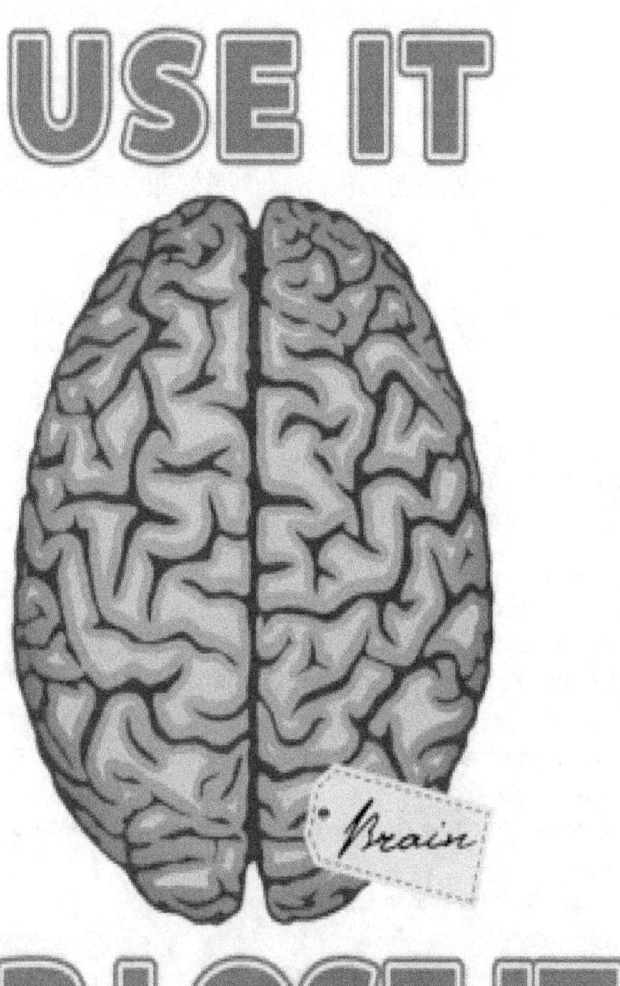

PMC report credits for book II
Garlick RL, Mazer JS, Chylack LT Jr, Tung WH, Bunn HF.

J Clin Invest.

page 327 credits:

(Eker *ET AL.*, **2006**; Bellaloui *ET AL.*, **2009**) (Bellaloui *ET AL.*, **2009**)

Page 328 credits:

(Nielsen *ET AL.*, **1985**; Logan *ET AL.*, **1989**; Pricolo *ET AL.*, **1998**; Cottone *ET AL.*, **1999**; Corrao *ET AL.*, **2001**; Green *ET AL.*, **2003**) (Ames *ET AL.*, **1993**; Coussens & Werb, **2002**) *(Lu ET AL., 2013; María ET AL., 1996) (Hernanz & Polanco, 1991)*

page 338 credits:

Hsia TC[1,2], Yin MC[3,4], Mong MC[5].

PMID: 27517907

PMCID: **PMC5000686** DOI: **10.3390/ijms17081289** [PubMed - in process] **Free PMC Article**

page 339 credits:

Nass N1, Ignatov A2, Andreas L3, Weißenborn C2, Kalinski T3, Sel S4.

page 346 credits:

(Broxmeyer, 2002; Díaz-Corrales *ET AL.*, 2004; MacDonald, 2006; Miklossy *ET AL.*, 2006)

Roundup® Trademark of Monsanto - image from Wikipedia.

Evolution Of The Human Diet page 442

[1] **The phenotypic legacy of admixture between modern humans and Neanderthals**
HHS Author Manuscripts • PMC4849557

[2] **Cro Magnon Man**: Wikipedia

It's Time for a Cure Too -- Roy Knight Jr